# THE ABDOMINAL AORTIC ANEURYSM
## Genetics, Pathophysiology, and
## Molecular Biology

ANNALS OF THE NEW YORK ACADEMY OF SCIENCES
Volume 1085

# THE ABDOMINAL AORTIC ANEURYSM
## Genetics, Pathophysiology, and
## Molecular Biology

Edited by M. David Tilson III, Helena Kuivaniemi, and
Gilbert R. Upchurch, Jr.

Published by Blackwell Publishing on behalf of the New York Academy of Sciences
Boston, Massachusetts
2006

Library of Congress Cataloging-in-Publication Data

The abdominal aortic aneurysm : genetics, pathophysiology, and
molecular biology / edited by M. David Tilson III, Helena
Kuivaniemi, and Gilbert R. Upchurch, Jr. – 2nd ed.
    p. ; cm. – (Annals of the New York Academy of Sciences,
ISSN 0077-8923 ; v. 1085)
    Includes bibliographical references.
    ISBN-13: 978-1-57331-657-6 (paper : alk. paper)
    ISBN-10: 1-57331-657-1 (paper : alk. paper)
    1. Abdominal aneurysm–Pathophysiology. 2. Abdominal
aneurysm–Molecular aspects. 3. Abdominal aneurysm–Genetic
aspects. I. Tilson, M. David. II. Kuivaniemi, Helena. III. Upchurch,
Gilbert R. IV. Series.
    [DNLM: 1. Aortic Aneurysm, Abdominal–genetics–Congresses.
2. Aortic Aneurysm, Abdominal–physiopathology–Congresses.
W1 AN626YL v.1085 2006 / WG 410 A134 2006]

    Q11.N5 vol. 1085
    [RC693]
    500 s–dc22
    [616.1'38]
                                                        2006032975


The *Annals of the New York Academy of Sciences* (ISSN: 0077-8923 [print]; ISSN: 1749-6632 [online]) is published 28 times a year on behalf of the New York Academy of Sciences by Blackwell Publishing, with offices located at 350 Main Street, Malden, Massachusetts 02148 USA, PO Box 1354, Garsington Road, Oxford OX4 2DQ UK, and PO Box 378 Carlton South, 3053 Victoria Australia.

**Information for subscribers:** Subscription prices for 2006 are: Premium Institutional: $3850.00 (US) and £2139.00 (Europe and Rest of World).
Customers in the UK should add VAT at 5%. Customers in the EU should also add VAT at 5% or provide a VAT registration number or evidence of entitlement to exemption. Customers in Canada should add 7% GST or provide evidence of entitlement to exemption. The Premium Institutional price also includes online access to full-text articles from 1997 to present, where available. For other pricing options or more information about online access to Blackwell Publishing journals, including access information and terms and conditions, please visit www.blackwellpublishing.com/nyas.

**Membership information:** Members may order copies of the *Annals* volumes directly from the Academy by visiting www.nyas.org/annals, emailing membership@nyas.org, faxing 212-298-3650, or calling 800-843-6927 (US only), or +1 212-298-8640 (International). For more information on becoming a member of the New York Academy of Sciences, please visit www.nyas.org/membership.

**Journal Customer Services:** For ordering information, claims, and any inquiry concerning your institutional subscription, please contact your nearest office:
**UK:** Email: customerservices@blackwellpublishing.com; Tel: +44 (0) 1865 778315; Fax +44 (0) 1865 471775
**US:** Email: customerservices@blackwellpublishing.com; Tel: +1 781 388 8599 or 1 800 835 6770 (Toll free in the USA); Fax: +1 781 388 8232
**Asia:** Email: customerservices@blackwellpublishing.com; Tel: +65 6511 8000; Fax: +61 3 8359 1120
**Members:** Claims and inquiries on member orders should be directed to the Academy at email: membership@nyas.org or Tel: +1 212 838 0230 (International) or 800-843-6927 (US only).

Printed in the USA.
Printed on acid-free paper.

**Mailing:** The *Annals of the New York Academy of Sciences* are mailed Standard Rate. **Postmaster:** Send all address changes to *Annals of the New York Academy of Sciences*, Blackwell Publishing, Inc., Journals Subscription Department, 350 Main Street, Malden, MA 01248-5020. Mailing to rest of world by DHL Smart and Global Mail.

**Disclaimer:** The Publisher, the New York Academy of Sciences, and the Editors cannot be held responsible for errors or any consequences arising from the use of information contained in this publication; the views and opinions expressed do not necessarily reflect those of the Publisher, the New York Academy of Sciences, or the Editors.

*Annals* are available to subscribers online at the New York Academy of Sciences and also at Blackwell Synergy. Visit www.annalsnyas.org or www.blackwell-synergy.com to search the articles and register for table of contents e-mail alerts. Access to full text and PDF downloads of *Annals* articles are available to nonmembers and subscribers on a pay-per-view basis at www.annalsnyas.org.

The paper used in this publication meets the minimum requirements of the National Standard for Information Sciences Permanence of Paper for Printed Library Materials, ANSI Z39.48_1984.

ISSN: 0077-8923 (print); 1749-6632 (online)
ISBN-10: 1-57331-657-1 (paper); ISBN-13: 978-1-57331-657-6 (paper)

A catalogue record for this title is available from the British Library.

### Digitization of the *Annals of the New York Academy of Sciences*

An agreement has recently been reached between Blackwell Publishing and the New York Academy of Sciences to digitize the entire run of the *Annals of the New York Academy of Sciences* back to volume one.

The back files, which have been defined as all of those issues published before 1997, will be sold to libraries as part of Blackwell Publishing's Legacy Sales Program and hosted on the Blackwell Synergy website.

Copyright of all material will remain with the rights holder. Contributors: Please contact Blackwell Publishing if you do not wish an article or picture from the *Annals of the New York Academy of Sciences* to be included in this digitization project.

ANNALS OF THE NEW YORK ACADEMY OF SCIENCES
*Volume 1085*
*November 2006*

# THE ABDOMINAL AORTIC ANEURYSM
## Genetics, Pathophysiology, and
## Molecular Biology

*Editors*
M. DAVID TILSON III, HELENA KUIVANIEMI, AND
GILBERT R. UPCHURCH, JR.

This volume is the result of a conference entitled **The Abdominal Aortic Aneurysm: Genetics, Pathophysiology, and Molecular Biology,** held on April 3–5, 2006 in New York City, sponsored by the New York Academy of Sciences with the Columbia University College of Physicians and Surgeons.

## CONTENTS

## Part II. Animal Models: Pathophysiology and Biomechanical Aspects

## Part III. Enzymology—Another Approach to Interventional Pharmacology

**Part IV. Biological Aspects of Endovascular Devices to Repair AAA**

**Part V. Genetics and Immunology in AAA**

**Part VI. Short Papers**

§

**Financial assistance was received from:**

- National Heart, Lung, and Blood Institute, National Institutes of Health
- Arkansas Community Foundation
- Macy Foundation
- Yamaguchi University
- Cook Group Inc.
- Endologix Inc.
- Medtronic Inc.
- WL Gore & Associates, Inc.

# Introduction

The co-organizers and I are delighted to welcome this audience to the Tenth Anniversary Symposium sponsored by the New York Academy of Sciences and Columbia University CME, on the subject of the pathobiology of the abdominal aortic aneurysm (AAA). The registrants have come from more than 10 countries. They are a literate audience on the subject of AAA and other aneurysmal conditions. The platform presenters are carefully chosen top authorities from several fields of expertise, and the poster presenters have offered many fine abstracts. We trust that the quality of this assemblage guarantees an informative meeting.

The organizers also express sincere appreciation to the following organizations: the National Heart, Lung, and Blood Institute of the National Institutes of Health (1R13HL083677), the Arkansas Community Foundation, the Macy Foundation, Yamaguchi University, Cook Group Inc., Endologix Inc., Medtronic Inc., W.L. Gore & Associates, Inc., and anonymous private parties. It is doubtful that it is possible to mount a multidisciplinary meeting on receipts from registrants alone, and this meeting would not be happening without the support of these contributors.

Finally, this meeting is the twentieth anniversary of the first multidisciplinary symposium on AAA pathobiology, which I hosted at Yale in 1986. There are a few fossils from that first meeting in attendance today, but I believe that only two of the speakers are dinosaurs from the Dark Ages of AAA research. This is good. Younger scientists have repopulated the field at the same time that knowledge on the subject has grown by orders of magnitude.

My personal thanks go to Drs. Upchurch and Kuivaniemi for their efforts as co-organizers. They recommended many of the speakers and helped me keep abreast of new developments in the field of AAA research. During the planning process, our differences of opinion on some subjects were resolved through many exchanges of e-mail, and decisions were reached by consensus.

Especially for young investigators present at this meeting, the organizers are grateful to have had the opportunity to introduce you to each other. You will meet many people who approach the AAA problem from perspectives that are novel to you, and no doubt you will form friendships and collaborations that will be a source of pleasure for you as your careers progress. We expect that numerous opportunities will arise for you to make important new contributions to the AAA field in multidisciplinary partnerships with your new colleagues and associates.

Ann. N.Y. Acad. Sci. 1085: xiii–xiv (2006). © 2006 New York Academy of Sciences.
doi: 10.1196/annals.1383.050

Welcome to New York, and we hope that the meeting will be as rewarding as your highest expectations.

—M. DAVID TILSON III
*Ailsa Mellon Bruce Professor of Surgery*
*Columbia University in the City of New York*
*St. Luke's/Roosevelt Hospital Center*
*New York, New York, USA*

# Views in Research on Abdominal Aortic Aneurysms

Aortic aneurysms represent increasingly common vascular conditions with life-threatening implications. They affect more men than women and are the 15th leading cause of death in the United States. When prehospital deaths are included, the overall mortality following rupture of an aortic aneurysm exceeds 75%, including emergency surgical intervention.

Abdominal aortic aneurysms (AAAs) are known to be associated with advanced age, male gender, cigarette smoking, atherosclerosis, hypertension, and genetic predisposition. While these epidemiological associations are widely recognized, the specific relationships between various risk factors and the development of aneurysm diseases are not well understood. Current research in the area of AAA encompasses: (a) investigations on the genetic and environmental factors associated with development of aortic aneurysms, (b) mechanistic studies on the fundamental pathophysiology of aortic degeneration and aneurysm formation, (c) elucidation of the role of biomechanical stresses in the biology of the aortic wall, and (d) development of novel treatment strategies to prevent and treat aortic diseases. Many of these studies have been supported through recent initiatives from the National Heart, Lung, and Blood Institute.

Examining the etiology of AAA led to the traditional belief that atherosclerosis was an active component of the process of aortic dilation. In addition to the physical presence of atherosclerosis in aneurysmal tissue, the development of these two diseases appears to be promoted by similar risk factors, including smoking, hypercholesterolemia, and elevated blood pressure. However, as data accumulate, the debate continues as to whether atherosclerosis is an active participant in the development and progression of AAA or is a consequence of aneurysms. Although it will be difficult to prove definitively whether there is a role for atherosclerosis in AAA formation, these research efforts will have important therapeutic implications for the treatment of AAAs.

Genetic studies of AAAs indicate that approximately 15% of the patients have a positive family history for AAA, and segregation studies have favored a major recessive gene as the cause of familial aggregation of the disease. A gene

Address for correspondence: Momtaz Wassef, Ph.D., Atherosclerosis Research Group, Division of Heart and Vascular Diseases, National Heart, Lung, and Blood Institute, Two Rockledge Center, 6701 Rockledge Drive, Suite 10196, Bethesda, MD 20892. Voice: 301-435-0550; fax: 301-480-2858.
   e-mail: wassefm@mail.nih.gov

Ann. N.Y. Acad. Sci. 1085: xv–xvii (2006). © 2006 New York Academy of Sciences.
doi: 10.1196/annals.1383.020

locus for the condition has been mapped to a location distinct from the loci identified for other aortic diseases indicating the presence of genetic heterogeneity in this disease. Thus, identification of families with aortic diseases as well as with mapping and identifying the defective genes causing the condition are critical for understanding the disease process and identifying individuals at risk for this life-threatening condition.

The histopathological features of human AAAs are characterized by chronic transmural inflammation, destructive remodeling of the elastic media, and depletion of medial smooth muscle cells. Defining the cellular and molecular mechanisms underlying the distorted architecture of aneurysms and elucidating the pathophysiology of these processes are important areas of investigative focus. Translation of knowledge regarding the pathophysiology of aneurysms, as obtained from basic studies and animal models, is also an extremely fruitful area for translational and clinical development.

Significant heterogeneity occurs in the distribution of aneurysm disease along the length of the aorta. This may be expected owing to the multiple embryonic cellular origins of the aorta, which contribute to the regional heterogeneity that exists in the biology of the aorta. Therefore, studies are required to test the regional heterogeneity of aneurysm in response to various preventive treatments and to further define the structural heterogeneity of the aorta in health and disease.

It is clear that the risk of aneurysm rupture is directly related to the hemodynamic stresses placed on the degenerative aortic wall as well as the capacity of this tissue to resist tensile stress. Recent studies have helped to define the manner in which hemodynamic stresses are altered in AAAs and have demonstrated that stress distribution is largely a function of aneurysm size and geometry. New methods to measure aortic wall stress are now being used to better define the effect of wall tension and the presence of mural thrombus on the underlying biology of AAAs. The development of imaging techniques to map tensile wall stress is also beginning to provide a new and exciting tool to evaluate risk of rupture in aneurysms of different sizes.

Although basic research studies have led to a better understanding of aneurysm diseases over the past two decades, there has also been growing appreciation that fundamental knowledge regarding the process of aneurysmal degeneration is still quite limited. In addition, there is no proven effective pharmacological intervention for intact aneurysms, and surgical repair is the predominant mode of treatment at substantial financial costs. Thus, the relatively high prevalence of aortic aneurysms in the general population and the limitations of current clinical treatments have clearly indicated an urgent need to investigate the cellular and molecular nature of aneurysm disease and its component mechanisms as well as translational research to develop new therapeutic strategies.

In summary, many aspects of AAA genetics, pathophysiology, and molecular biology will be discussed in this symposium. As a result, it is hoped that highly integrative and synergistic research programs will be initiated to address the pathophysiology and clinical management of aneurysmal diseases employing interdisciplinary scientific approaches and experimental strategies. We will need to investigate potential new mechanism-based pharmacological interventions to treat and suppress the expansion of small aneurysms; identify the genetic basis for an inherited predisposition to aneurysmal degeneration; develop and refine (minimally) noninvasive approaches for the early detection of arterial aneurysms; examine potential novel surgical approaches and design new biomaterials for the management of aneurysm diseases; define cellular and molecular factors and signals involved in the initiation and progression of the aneurysms and determine features of the inflammatory response that might reflect patient-specific susceptibility to the disease; and finally initiate and promote awareness programs for the diagnosis and treatment of aortic aneurysms.

## CONFLICT OF INTEREST STATEMENT

Momtaz Wassef participated in an uncompensated capacity on his own time. Although he is employed by the National Heart, Lung and Blood Institute (NHLBI) of the National Institutes of Health within the United States Department of Health and Human Services, no support was received and no endorsement should be inferred.

—MOMTAZ WASSEF
*National Heart, Lung, and Blood Institute*
*National Institutes of Health, Bethesda, MD, USA*

# Epidemiology of Aortic Aneurysm Repair in the United States from 1993 to 2003

JOHN A. COWAN, JR., JUSTIN B. DIMICK, PETER K. HENKE,
JOHN RECTENWALD, JAMES C. STANLEY,
AND GILBERT R. UPCHURCH, Jr.

*University of Michigan Cardiovascular Center, Ann Arbor, Michigan, USA*

ABSTRACT: The epidemiology of abdominal aortic aneurysm (AAA) disease has been well described over the preceding 50 years. This disease primarily affects elderly males with smoking, hypertension, and a positive family history contributing to an increased risk of aneurysm formation. The aging population as well as increased screening in high-risk populations has led some to suggest that the incidence of AAAs is increasing. The National Inpatient Sample (1993–2003), a national representative database, was used in this study to determine trends in mortality following AAA repair in the United States. In addition, the impact of the introduction of less invasive endovascular AAA repair was assessed. Overall rates of treated unruptured and ruptured AAAs remained stable (unruptured 12 to 15/100,000; ruptured 1 to 3/100,000). In 2003, 42.7% of unruptured and 8.8% of ruptured AAAs were repaired through an endovascular approach. Inhospital mortality following unruptured AAA repair continues to decline for open repair (5.3% to 4.7%, $P = 0.007$). Mortality after elective endovascular AAA repair also has statistically decreased (2.1% to 1.0%, $P = 0.024$) and remains lower than open repair. Mortality rates for ruptured AAAs following repair remain high (open: 46.5% to 40.7%, $P = 0.01$; endovascular: 40.0% to 35.3%, $P = 0.823$). These data suggest that the numbers of patients undergoing elective AAA repair have remained relatively stable despite the introduction of less invasive technology. A shift in the treatment paradigm is occurring with a higher percentage of patients subjected to elective endovascular AAA repair compared to open repair. This shift, at least in the short term, appears justified as the mortality in patients undergoing elective endovascular AAA repair is significantly reduced compared to patients undergoing open AAA repair.

KEYWORDS: abdominal aortic aneurysm; repair; endovascular

Address for correspondence: Gilbert R. Upchurch, Jr., M.D., Section of Vascular Surgery, 1500 E. Medical Center Dr., Taubman Health Center, Ann Arbor, MI 48109-0329. Voice: 734-936-5790; fax: 734-647-9867.
e-mail: riversu@umich.edu

Ann. N.Y. Acad. Sci. 1085: 1–10 (2006). © 2006 New York Academy of Sciences.
doi: 10.1196/annals.1383.030

## INTRODUCTION

Dramatic improvements have been made during the past 50 years in the overall diagnosis, management, and treatment of abdominal aortic aneurysms (AAAs). Early detection programs, improvements in risk factor control, and a better understanding of the progression to rupture have allowed physicians and surgeons to make better treatment decisions.[1-4] Furthermore, recognizing the potential benefits of regionalizing these complex procedures to high volume centers and specialized surgeons may further improve treatment outcomes.[5-7] The advent and dissemination of endovascular approaches to AAAs will likely expand the number of patients in the population undergoing AAA repair. These facts will be crucial in managing the increasing elderly population at risk for AAAs in the United States.

Unfortunately, the mortality for ruptured AAAs has improved little in recent decades.[2,5] While some evidence suggests the rate of ruptured AAAs in the general population is decreasing, certain populations, including those of lower socioeconomic status and the uninsured, have significantly higher rates of rupture.[5,8] Measures to provide minimum preventative services or screening to manage AAAs before rupture may be needed if outcomes are to continue to improve. The objective of this investigation was to provide a population-level analysis of AAAs treated in the United States from 1993 to 2003.

## METHODS

All clinical data were obtained from the Nationwide Inpatient Sample (NIS) for the years 1993 to 2003. The NIS is a 20% random, stratified sample of discharges from nonfederal hospitals in the United States.[9] The database is maintained by the Agency for Healthcare Research and Quality (AHRQ) as part of the Healthcare Costs and Utilization Project (HCUP). The clinical sample was derived in a two-step process using International Classification of Diseases, Ninth Revision, (ICD-9) procedure and diagnostic codes. First, all patients underwent repair of an AAA either *open* (ICD-9, 38.34 aorta resection and anastomosis; 38.44 replacement of abdominal aorta; 38.64 excision of aorta; 39.52 other repair of aneurysm) or *endovascular* (ICD-9, 39.71 endovascular abdominal aorta repair). The endovascular code did not come into use until the year 2000. Second, diagnostic codes for both *unruptured* AAAs (ICD-9, 441.4 abdominal aneurysm without mention of rupture; 441.9 aortic aneurysm of unspecified site without mention of rupture) and *ruptured* AAAs (ICD-9, 441.3 abdominal aneurysm, ruptured; 441.5 aortic aneurysm of unspecified site, ruptured; 441.6 thoracoabdominal aneurysm, rupture) were used to ensure the sample included only treatment for AAAs rather than other conditions. Population estimates of AAA repair utilization were made using discharge sampling weights provided by the NIS and information provided by the United States Census Bureau.[10] Basic demographics were reported and tested for changes over time. Mortality, length of stay (LOS), and total charges were also calculated. Total charges were adjusted to the year 2003 dollar values using the consumer price index (CPI) for inpatient hospital services.[11]

Statistical analyses were carried out using analysis of variance (ANOVA) for patient age, chi-square for gender, race, and mortality, and Mann–Whitney U test for LOS and charges. All analyses were performed using SPSS software package (SPSS version 12.0, SPSS Inc., Chicago, IL, USA). $P < 0.05$ was considered significant for all analyses.

# RESULTS

The overall sample yielded 94,825 cases of treated AAAs (80,183 unruptured, 14,642 ruptured) over the 11 years of study. The mean age of the population was 72.0 years and was higher for patients with ruptured AAAs (TABLE 1). Females comprised 20.8% of patients. Overall mortality, LOS, and total charges were significantly higher for patients presenting with rupture.

Marked differences in the demographics and overall outcomes between open and endovascular repair were observed (TABLES 2 and 3). Years 2000 to 2003 were used in the comparisons since endovascular repair was not separately coded prior to that time. Patients who underwent endovascular repair for unruptured AAAs were more likely to be male and older. Mortality and LOS were less for endovascular repair, while total hospital charges were more for

**TABLE 1. Demographics and outcomes for patients who underwent AAA repair in the NIS from 1993 to 2003**

| | | Aneurysm type | | |
| | Total | Unruptured | Ruptured | $P^*$ |
|---|---|---|---|---|
| Number | 94,825 | 80,183 | 14,642 | — |
| Patient age in years $\pm$ *SD* | 72.0 (8.1) | 71.8 (8.0) | 73.1 (8.7) | <0.001 |
| Female (%) | 20.8% | 20.7% | 21.4% | 0.063 |
| Caucasian race (%) | 92.2% | 92.5% | 90.8% | <0.001 |
| Comorbid conditions | | | | |
| COPD† | 23.7% | 23.9% | 22.8% | 0.003 |
| Diabetes mellitus | 8.2% | 8.6% | 6.1% | <0.001 |
| History of myocardial infarction | 9.5% | 10.4% | 4.8% | <0.001 |
| Inhospital mortality | 10.4% | 4.2% | 44.8% | <0.001 |
| Median LOS in days‡ | 7 (5 to 11) | 7 (5 to 10) | 9 (2 to 17) | <0.001 |
| Median hospital charges‡ | $44,977 | $43,085 | $65,004 | <0.001 |
| | ($31,463 to | ($30,754 to | ($38,596 | |
| | $68,736) | $63,062) | $121,658) | |

*ANOVA for patient age; chi-square for gender, race, and mortality; Mann–Whitney U test for LOS and charges.

† COPD = Chronic obstructive pulmonary disease; ‡ = interquartile range.

**TABLE 2. Demographics of patients who underwent open versus endovascular repair for an unruptured AAA in the NIS from 2000 to 2003**

| | Aneurysm repair type | | |
| --- | --- | --- | --- |
| | Open | Endovascular | $P*$ |
| Number | 22,672 | 9,392 | – |
| Patient age in years ± $SD$ | 71.7 (8.2) | 73.4 (8.1) | <0.001 |
| Female (%) | 22.7% | 15.9% | <0.001 |
| Caucasian race (%) | 90.8% | 90.9% | 0.878 |
| Comorbid conditions | | | |
| COPD† | 25.6% | 22.2% | <0.001 |
| Diabetes mellitus | 9.8% | 12.6% | <0.001 |
| History of myocardial infarction | 10.8% | 15.3% | <0.001 |
| Inhospital mortality | 4.4% | 1.3% | <0.001 |
| Median LOS in days‡ | 7 (5 to 10) | 2 (1 to 4) | <0.001 |
| Median hospital charges‡ | $43,462 | $51,877 | <0.001 |
| | ($30,913 to $66,185) | ($38,369 to $72,146) | |

*ANOVA for patient age; chi-square for gender, race, and mortality; Mann–Whitney U test for LOS and charges.
† COPD = Chronic obstructive pulmonary disease; ‡ = interquartile range.

endovascular repair. Patients treated for ruptured AAAs were of similar age, gender, and race comparing open and endovascular approaches. Mortality was less in the endovascular cohort, although did not reach statistical significance.

**TABLE 3. Demographics of patients who underwent open versus endovascular repair for a ruptured AAA in the NIS from 2000 to 2003**

| | Aneurysm repair type | | |
| --- | --- | --- | --- |
| | Open | Endovascular | $P*$ |
| Number | 4,439 | 271 | – |
| Patient age in years ± $SD$ | 73.1 (9.0) | 73.6 (9.0) | 0.334 |
| Female (%) | 22.8% | 23.3% | 0.851 |
| Caucasian race (%) | 88.8% | 86.0% | 0.218 |
| Comorbid conditions | | | |
| COPD† | 24.6% | 26.6% | 0.471 |
| Diabetes mellitus | 7.6% | 9.6% | 0.230 |
| History of myocardial infarction | 5.0% | 7.4% | 0.078 |
| Inhospital mortality | 42.7% | 36.7% | 0.052 |
| Median LOS in days ‡ | 9 (2 to 18) | 8 (2 to 15) | 0.205 |
| Median hospital charges ‡ | $69,611 | $71,926 | 0.555 |
| | ($41,535 to $129,935) | ($45,266 to $132,925) | |

*ANOVA for patient age; chi-square for gender, race, and mortality; Mann–Whitney U test for LOS and charges.
† COPD = Chronic obstructive pulmonary disease; ‡ = interquartile range.

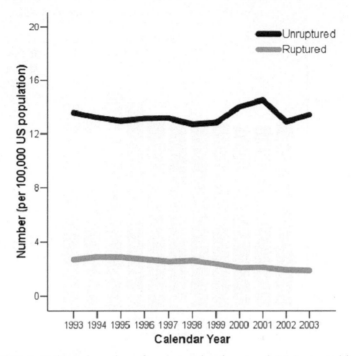

**FIGURE 1.** Estimated number of unruptured and ruptured AAAs treated in United States hospitals from 1993 to 2003.

Overall rates of treated unruptured and ruptured AAAs remained relatively constant during the period of study (unruptured 12 to 15/100,000; ruptured 1 to 3/100,000) (FIG. 1). In 2003, 42.7% of unruptured and 8.8% of ruptured AAAs were repaired using an endovascular approach (FIG. 2). Mortality for unruptured AAAs repaired by open means decreased from 5.3% to 4.7% ($P = 0.007$). Endovascular AAA repair mortality rates from 2000 to 2003 were statistically decreased (2.1% to 1.0%, $P = 0.024$). Mortality rates for ruptured AAA treated by open repair decreased significantly, while the mortality for endovascular repair did not significantly change (open: 46.5% to 40.7%, $P = 0.01$; endovascular: 40.0% to 35.3%, $P = 0.823$) (FIG. 3).

## DISCUSSION

AAA disease in the United States is still a disease primarily of the elderly male patient with more than 15,000 deaths in the year 2000 secondary to aortic disease.[12] Other well-documented risk factors for the development of an AAA include tobacco use, the presence of hypertension, atherosclerosis in other vascular beds, and hypercholesterolemia.[3]

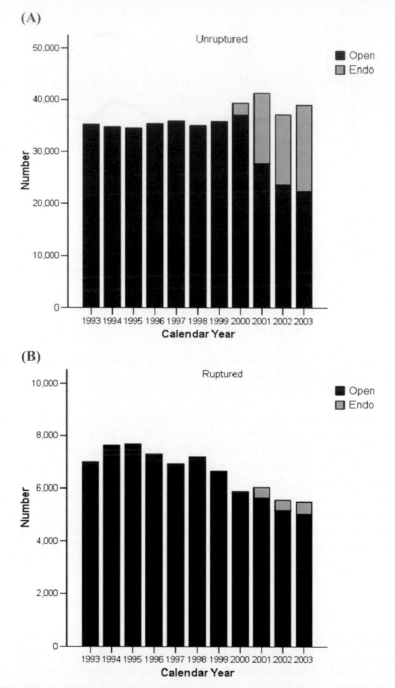

**FIGURE 2.** Estimated number of AAA repairs, by type, performed in the United States from 1993 to 2003. (**A**) Unruptured. (**B**) Ruptured.

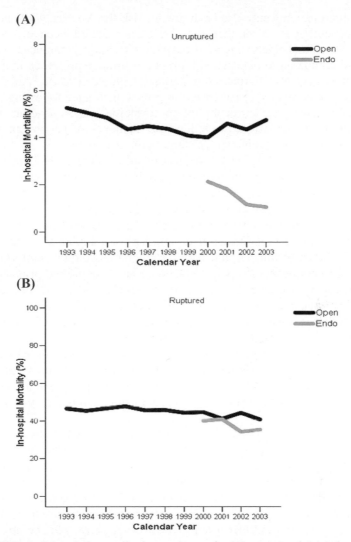

**FIGURE 3.** Inhospital mortality by repair type for (**A**) unruptured AAA (open: 5.3% to 4.7%, $P = 0.007$; endovascular: 2.1% to 1.0%, $P = 0.024$). (**B**) ruptured AAA (open: 46.5% to 40.7%, $P = 0.01$; endovascular: 40.0% to 35.3%, $P = 0.823$).

Certain recent studies have suggested specific subsets of patients who may be at increased risk for AAA development and rupture. Englesbe reported on 1, 557 patients who underwent heart, kidney, or liver transplantation and were screened for AAAs.[13] Cardiac transplant patients in particular, when screened for AAAs at a high rate (87% were screened), had a 5.8% prevalence of AAAs. In addition, among those transplant patients with AAAs, the rate of aneurysm rupture was 22.5% per year with a mean diameter of only 6.1 cm.

Uninsured patients may also be at greater risk for AAA rupture and dying more frequently even when their intact AAA is repaired electively. A recent study by Boxer and others suggested that patients without insurance or who had Medicaid compared to patients with private insurance presented more often with ruptured AAAs.[8] Furthermore, patients without insurance had a higher mortality rate compared to patients with private insurance following elective AAA repair, even after correcting for comorbidities. These findings suggest screening programs designed to reduce the incidence of patients presenting with ruptured AAAs should perhaps target noninsured patients.

The incidence of AAAs in the general population of the United States should predictably be increasing with the aging population. However, the present data suggest that the numbers of patients undergoing elective AAA repair have remained relatively constant. This has been the case despite the introduction of less invasive diagnostic and therapeutic technology, which often serves to lower the threshold for intervention. Clearly, there are many examples in the vascular surgery literature in which a "less invasive" therapy, even if it is inferior in the long term to conventional operative therapy, has become the primary mode of treatment of a disease. Examples of the accelerated use of less invasive technology have been documented in the endovascular treatment of patients with aortoiliac occlusive disease[14] as well as in the treatment of patients with renovascular hypertension secondary to renal artery stenosis.[15] It is possible that the total number of patients undergoing AAA repair in the United States has recently remained stable despite the introduction of less invasive technology, secondary to a number of large randomized trials suggesting that the threshold diameter for AAA repair should be increased from 5 cm to 5.5 cm, especially in males.[4,16,17]

A shift in the treatment paradigm of patients with AAAs is occurring over time with a higher percentage of patients undergoing elective endovascular AAA repair compared to open AAA repair. In the short term, this is clearly justified as mortality following elective endovascular AAA repair is significantly less than open AAA repair. This difference in outcome has occurred despite increased comorbidities such as prior myocardial infarction and more diabetics in the endovascular group. However, endovascular therapy entails greater costs reflected by increased hospital charges as documented in this study.

Clearly, the paradigm for elective AAA repair has changed.[18–20] Nowygrod and colleagues examined national data from the NIS and statewide data from four states and also documented a significant shift in the treatment paradigm in patients undergoing elective AAA repair.[18] While also using the NIS, but examining AAA repair only as the primary procedure code, the authors noted that endovascular AAA repair was used for 43% of total AAA repairs. Data from the Center for the Evaluative Clinical Sciences revealed that the rates of AAA repair per 1,000 Medicare enrollees, despite the introduction of endovascular AAA repair, were similar to levels observed in the mid 1990s.[19] This report documented that inpatient reimbursements for AAA repair had fallen modestly since 1991. Dillavou and colleagues, also using the Medicare database, noted that endovascular AAA repair was more often undertaken in the elderly with lower mortality especially in older patients compared to open AAA repair.[20] They also reported average elective AAA repair hospital charges that were not different for patients undergoing open or endovascular repair. However, endovascular repair was reimbursed more poorly by Medicare. This occurred even with more patients in the endovascular AAA group classified as DRG 111 (major cardiovascular procedure without complications), supporting a higher reimbursement level.

Importantly, two reasons may exist to explain why fewer patients are presenting with ruptured AAAs. First, strategies aimed at reducing modifiable risk factors such as quitting smoking and treating hypertension may have had a positive effect on aneurysm development and subsequent rupture. Second, screening programs may be having their intended affect, namely allowing early elective AAA repair and lessening the number of late ruptured AAAs. In the setting of relatively constant numbers of patients undergoing elective AAA repair, it appears that endovascular technology has not accelerated the rate of total AAA repair.

While not specifically addressed with the data from the current studies, individual centers of excellence have demonstrated remarkably low mortality rates following ruptured endovascular AAA repair.[21,22] Although greater numbers of patients having ruptured AAAs will need to be treated endovascularly before significant decreases in mortality can be realized with the endovascular approach, this technology has the potential to significantly lower the staggering mortality accompanying open ruptured AAA repair.

## REFERENCES

1. BREWSTER, D.C., J.L. CRONENWETT, J.W. HALLETT, JR., *et al.* 2003. Guidelines for the treatment of abdominal aortic aneurysms. Report of a subcommittee of the Joint Council of the American Association for Vascular Surgery and Society for Vascular Surgery. J. Vasc. Surg. **37:** 1106–1117.
2. HELLER, J.A., A. WEINBERG, R. ARONS, *et al.* 2000. Two decades of abdominal aortic aneurysm repair: have we made any progress? J. Vasc. Surg. **32:** 1091–1100.
3. LEDERLE, F.A., G.R. JOHNSON, S.E. WILSON, *et al.* 2000. The aneurysm detection and management study screening program: validation cohort and final results. Arch. Intern. Med. **160:** 1425–1430.
4. LEDERLE, F.A., S.E. WILSON, G.R. JOHNSON, *et al.* 2002. Immediate repair compared with surveillance of small abdominal aortic aneurysms. N. Engl. J. Med. **346:** 1437–1444.
5. WAINESS, R.M., J.B. DIMICK, J.A. COWAN JR., *et al.* 2004. Epidemiology of surgically treated abdominal aortic aneurysms in the United States, 1988 to 2000. Vascular **12:** 218–224.

6. DIMICK, J.B., J.A. COWAN, JR., J.C. STANLEY, *et al.* 2003. Surgeon specialty and provider volumes are related to outcome of intact abdominal aortic aneurysm repair in the United States. J. Vasc. Surg. **38:** 739–744.

7. BIRKMEYER, J.D. & J.B. DIMICK. Potential benefits of the new Leapfrog standards: effect of process and outcomes measures. Surgery **135:** 569–575.

8. BOXER, L.K., J.B. DIMICK, R.M. WAINESS, *et al.* 2003. Payer status is related to differences in access and outcomes of abdominal aortic aneurysm repair in the United States. Surgery **134:** 142–145.

9. HEALTHCARE COST, AND UTILIZATION PROJECT (HCUP). Nationwide Inpatient Sample, 1993-2003. Rockville, MD: Agency for Health Care Research and Quality.

10. U.S. CENSUS BUREAU. Population estimates. Available at: http://eire.census.gov/popest/estimates.php (accessed July 1, 2004).

11. U.S. Department of Labor. Bureau of Labor Statistics: http://www.bls.gov (accessed February 2004).

12. NATIONAL CENTER FOR HEALTH STATISTICS. Deaths, percent of total deaths, and death rates for the 10 leading causes of death in selected age groups, by race and sex: United States. 2000. National Vital Statistics Report, 2002. Accessed at www.cdc.gov/nchs/fastats/pdf/nvsr50´16t1.pdf on 15 November 2004.

13. ENGLESBE, M.J., A.H. WU, A.W. CLOWES & R.E. ZIERLER. 2003. The prevalence and natural history of aortic aneurysms in heart and abdominal organ transplant patients. J. Vasc. Surg. **37:** 27–31.

14. UPCHURCH, G.R., JR., J.B. DIMICK, R.M. WAINESS, *et al.* 2004. Diffusion of new technology in health care: the case of aorto-iliac occlusive disease. Surgery **136:** 812–818.

15. KNIPP, B.S., J.B. DIMICK, J.L. ELIASON, *et al.* 2004. Diffusion of new technology for the treatment of renovascular hypertension in the United States: surgical revascularization versus catheter-based therapy, 1988–2001. J. Vasc. Surg. **40:** 717–723.

16. ASHTON, H.A. , M.J. BUXTON, N.E. DAY, *et al.* 2002. The Multicentre Aneurysm Screening Study (MASS) into the effect of abdominal aortic aneurysm screening on mortality in men: a randomised controlled trial. Lancet **360:** 1531–1539.

17. UNITED KINGDOM SMALL ANEURYSM TRIAL PARTICIPANTS. 2002. Long-term outcomes of immediate repair compared with surveillance of small abdominal aortic aneurysms. N. Engl. J. Med. **346:** 1445–1452.

18. NOWYGROD, R., N. EGOROVA, G. GRECO, *et al.* 2006. Trends, complications, and mortality in peripheral vascular surgery. J. Vasc. Surg. **43:** 205–216.

19. CENTER FOR THE EVALUATIVE CLINICAL SCIENCES. DARTMOUTH- CMS- FDA COLLABORATIVE. 2005. Trends and Regional Variations in Abdominal Aortic Aneurysm Repair. Dartmouth Atlas of Health Care: Studies of Surgical Variation. 1–24.

20. DILLAVOU, E.D., S.C. MULUK & M.S. MAKAROUN. 2006. Improving aneurysm-related outcomes: nationwide benefits of endovascular repair. J. Vasc. Surg. **43:** 446–452.

21. OHKI, T., F.J. VEITH, L.A. SANCHEZ, *et al.* 1999. Endovascular graft repair of ruptured aortoiliac aneurysms. J. Am. Coll. Surg. **189:** 102–113.

22. HECHELHAMMER, L., M.L. LACHAT, S. WILDERMUTH, *et al.* 2005. Midterm outcome of endovascular repair of ruptured abdominal aortic aneurysms. J. Vasc. Surg. **41:** 752–757.

# A Biomechanics-Based Rupture Potential Index for Abdominal Aortic Aneurysm Risk Assessment

## Demonstrative Application

JONATHAN P. VANDE GEEST,[a] ELENA S. DI MARTINO,[b] AJAY BOHRA,[c] MICHEL S. MAKAROUN,[c] AND DAVID A. VORP[a,c]

[a]*Department of Bioengineering, University of Pittsburgh, Pittsburgh, Pennsylvania 15219, USA[1]*

[b]*Institute for Complex Engineering Systems, Carnegie Mellon University, Pittsburgh, Pennsylvania 15213, USA*

[c]*Division of Vascular Surgery, Department of Surgery, University of Pittsburgh, Pittsburgh, Pennsylvania 15219, USA*

ABSTRACT: Abdominal aortic aneurysms (AAAs) can typically remain stable until the strength of the aortic wall is unable to withstand the forces acting on it as a result of the luminal blood pressure, resulting in AAA rupture. The clinical treatment of AAA patients presents a dilemma for the surgeon: surgery should only be recommended when the risk of rupture of the AAA outweighs the risks associated with the interventional procedure. Since AAA rupture occurs when the stress acting on the wall exceeds its strength, the assessment of AAA rupture should include estimates of both wall stress and wall strength distributions. The present work details a method for noninvasively assessing the rupture potential of AAAs using patient-specific estimations the rupture potential index (RPI) of the AAA, calculated as the ratio of locally acting wall stress to strength. The RPI was calculated for thirteen AAAs, which were broken up into ruptured ($n = 8$ and nonruptured ($n = 5$) groups. Differences in peak wall stress, minimum strength and maximum RPI were compared across groups. There were no statistical differences in the maximum transverse diameters (6.8 $\pm$ 0.3 cm vs. 6.1 $\pm$ 0.5 cm, $p = 0.26$) or peak wall stress (46.0 $\pm$ 4.3 vs. 49.9 $\pm$ 4.0 N/cm$^2$, $p = 0.62$) between groups. There was a significant decrease in minimum wall strength for ruptured AAA (81.2 $\pm$ 3.9 and 108.3 $\pm$ 10.2 N/cm$^2$, $p = 0.045$). While

[1]Currently at the Department of Aerospace and Mechanical Engineering, University of Arizona, Tucson, Arizona, USA.

Address for correspondence: David A. Vorp, Ph.D., Department of Bioengineering, University of Pittsburgh, Technology Drive, Suite 200, Pittsburgh, PA, 15219, USA. Voice: 412-235-5142; fax: 412-235-5110.

e-mail: vorpda@upmc.edu

Ann. N.Y. Acad. Sci. 1085: 11–21 (2006). © 2006 New York Academy of Sciences.
doi: 10.1196/annals.1383.046

the differences in RPI values (ruptured $= 0.48 \pm 0.05$ vs. nonruptured $= 0.36 \pm 0.03$, respectively; $p = 0.10$) did not reach statistical significance, the $p$-value for the peak RPI comparison was lower than that for both the maximum diameter ($p = 0.26$) and peak wall stress ($p = 0.62$) comparisons. This result suggests that the peak RPI may be better able to identify those AAAs at high risk of rupture than maximum diameter or peak wall stress alone. The clinical relevance of this method for rupture assessment has yet to be validated, however, its success could aid clinicians in decision making and AAA patient management.

KEYWORDS: abdominal aortic aneurysm; stress; strength; rupture

## INTRODUCTION

Abdominal aortic aneurysms (AAA) are characterized by structural remodeling resulting in the gradual weakening and expansion of the aortic wall. AAA can typically remain stable until the strength of the aortic wall is unable to withstand the forces acting on it as a result of the luminal blood pressure, resulting in AAA rupture. Since AAAs are often asymptomatic, impending AAA rupture can occur without warning. The clinical treatment of AAA patients presents a dilemma for the surgeon: surgery should only be recommended when the risk of rupture of the AAA outweighs the risks associated with the interventional procedure.

This clinical dilemma has led researchers to investigate several different predictors of AAA rupture. The most common clinical quantitative measure of aneurysm rupture risk has been the maximum transverse diameter.[1] Some of the other predictors proposed in the literature include cyclic strain via ultrasound,[2] intraluminal thrombus (ILT) volume,[3] enlargement rate,[4,5] and stress.[6] Since AAA rupture occurs when the acting wall stresses exceed the tensile strength of the degenerated AAA wall, we and others have advocated the use of biomechanical principles to assess AAA rupture severity.[6–17] For example, we reported methods to noninvasively estimate the wall stress distribution in patient-specific computer models of AAA using the finite element method (FEM).[11] Using FEM, two recent studies evaluated ruptured and electively repaired AAA, and suggested that peak wall stress as opposed to maximum diameter may better identify those AAAs at high risk.[6,17]

Our FEM-based AAA wall stress analysis technique has undergone several stages of improvement since our original report. These have included the inclusion of the commonly found ILT[15] and the anisotropic AAA tissue behavior[14] into the computer models of AAA. Though these changes have led to improvements of estimations of AAA wall stress over previous techniques,[6–10,12,13,16] this quantity alone is theoretically insufficient to predict AAA rupture potential. That is, since AAA rupture occurs when the stress acting on the wall exceeds its strength, the prediction of AAA rupture should include both the wall stress distribution as well as the wall strength distribution. To facilitate this, we have developed techniques for noninvasively estimating AAA wall strength distribution. We may then define a rupture potential index (RPI) as the ratio of the acting wall stress to the wall strength. Therefore, the maximum RPI value for a particular AAA would represent its rupture potential. When the RPI approaches a value of 1, rupture of that AAA would be imminent. We believe the RPI to be a more reliable criterion than those previously proposed for assessing patient-specific rupture potential including the widely accepted maximum transverse diameter criterion.

## METHODS

There were 13 AAAs simulated in this work that were broken up into two groups: nonruptured repairs ($n = 5$, N1–N5) and ruptured repairs ($n = 8$, R1–R8). Nonruptured AAAs were those that had CT scans at least 1 year apart with the latter scan providing evidence that the AAA remained quiescent. For these simulations, the images from the earlier CT scan were used to reconstruct the AAAs. Ruptured AAAs were defined as those with CT scans taking place no more than 1 year prior to AAA rupture. The RPI was calculated for each AAA using patient-specific estimations of wall stress and wall strength as described below. The diameters of the AAAs in both groups combined ranged between 5.0 cm and 8.1 cm in maximum diameter.

### *Stress Estimation*

The wall stress simulations use our well-established three-dimensional reconstruction and FEM-based techniques.[11,14,16] Specifically, the locally acting wall stress was estimated using FEMs with the following assumptions. The intraluminal thrombus was included in the FEM stress simulations and was modeled as hyperelastic incompressible isotropic material. Following recent investigations within the authors' laboratory,[19,20] the AAA wall was modeled as an anisotropic material with a preferred stiffening in the circumferential direction. Each of the patient-specific AAA stress simulations resulted in spatially varying estimations of local wall stress.

### *Strength Estimation*

The wall strength was estimated using a mathematical model developed using linear regression techniques, which accounts for the spatially varying influences of local ILT thickness and aneurysm wall dilation as well as the

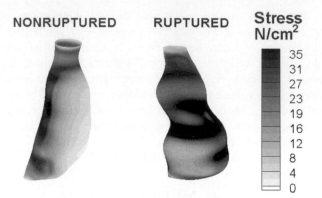

**FIGURE 1.** Representative comparison of the stress between an electively repaired (nonruptured) AAA (maximum diameter = 6.7 cm) and a ruptured AAA (diameter = 7 cm).

global influences of sex and familial history.[14,15] Using multiple linear regression and mixed-effects modeling techniques, the final statistical model for local wall strength was given by

$$\text{STRENGTH} = 72.9 - 33.5^*(\text{ILT}^{1/2} - 0.79) - 12.3^*(\text{NORD} - 2.31) \\ -24^*\text{HIST} + 15^*\text{SEX} \tag{1}$$

where strength has units of N/cm$^2$, ILT$^{1/2}$ is the square root of ILT thickness whose units are in cm, NORD is a dimensionless parameter for local normalized diameter, HIS is a dimensionless binary variable (1/2 for positive family history, -1/2 for no family history), and SEX is a dimensionless binary variable for gender (1/2 for males, -1/2 for females). Inspection of equation 1 provides several insights as to its physical meaning:

- For two patients with the same gender and identical AAAs, the one with family history has a AAA that is globally weaker by 12 N/cm$^2$ compared to the one without family history.
- For two patients with the same family history and identical AAAs, a female will have a AAA that is globally weaker by 7.5 N/cm$^2$ compared to a male.
- For any two points within any given AAA with the same NORD, an increase in ILT$^{1/2}$ of 1.0 results in a corresponding decrease in strength of 33.5 N/cm$^2$.
- For any two points within any given AAA with the same ILT$^{1/2}$, an increase in NORD of 1.0 results in a corresponding decrease in strength of 12.3 N/cm$^2$.

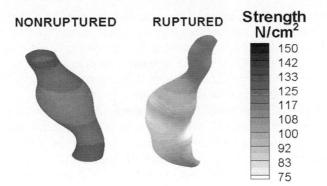

**FIGURE 2.** Representative comparison of the strength between a nonruptured AAA (maximum diameter = 5.8 cm) and a ruptured AAA (diameter = 6.1 cm).

## *RPI*

The RPI is defined as the ratio of local wall stress to local wall strength:

$$RPI_i = \frac{Stress_i}{Strength_i} \qquad (2)$$

The subscript i in equation (2) corresponds to a given (X,Y, Z) location on the AAA wall. Once the stress for a given node in the finite element simulation was determined, the locally acting wall strength was calculated for this node using equation (1). The 3D distribution of RPI is then calculated by dividing each node's stress and strength values. The calculation of the locally acting RPI for a given AAA was done in a Matlab script specifically designed for this purpose.

Maximum transverse diameters, mean and peak wall stresses, mean and minimum wall strengths, and mean and peak RPI values were compared between the ruptured and nonruptured groups using a Students *t*-test, with $P = 0.05$ indicating significance.

## RESULTS

There were no statistical differences in the maximum transverse diameters between ruptured and nonruptured AAAs ($6.8 \pm 0.3$ vs. $6.1 \pm 0.5$, $P = 0.26$). A representative comparison of the stress distributions for a ruptured (maximum diameter = 7.0 cm) and nonruptured AAA (maximum diameter = 6.7 cm) is shown in FIGURE 1. We found no significant differences in peak stresses between the nonruptured and ruptured AAA groups ($46.0 \pm 4.3$ vs. $49.9 \pm 4.0$ N/cm$^2$, respectively; $P = 0.62$). There was also no significant difference between the mean stresses for the nonruptured and ruptured AAA ($20.4 \pm 1.7$ vs. $20.7 \pm 2.6$, $P = 0.95$).

A representative comparison of strength distributions for a ruptured (maximum diameter = 6.1 cm) and nonruptured (maximum diameter = 5.8 cm) AAA is shown in FIGURE 2. The minimum wall strength values were $81.2 \pm 3.9$ and $108.3 \pm 10.2$ N/cm$^2$ for the ruptured and nonruptured AAA models, respectively ($P = 0.045$). The average wall strength values were $102.8 \pm 3.4$ and $124.5 \pm 5.8$ N/cm$^2$ for these two groups ($P = 0.005$).

FIGURE 3 shows a representative comparison of RPI distribution for a ruptured (maximum diameter = 5.20 cm) and nonruptured (maximum diameter = 5.23 cm) AAA of nearly equivalent maximum diameter. While the differences between ruptured and nonruptured peak RPI values ($0.48 \pm 0.05$ vs. $0.36 \pm 0.03$, respectively; $P = 0.10$) did not reach statistical significance for the numbers of AAA studied here, the $P$-value for the peak RPI comparison was lower than that for both the maximum diameter ($P = 0.26$) and peak wall stress ($P = 0.62$) comparisons. This result suggests that the peak RPI may be better able to identify those AAAs at high risk of rupture than maximum diameter or peak wall stress alone.

Representative stress, strength, and RPI distributions for one AAA are shown in FIGURE 4. The peak RPI for this AAA was 0.34, which can be interpreted the corresponding location on this AAA as being at 34% of its capacity to withstand mechanical wall stress. The results for maximum transverse diameter, peak wall stress, minimum wall strength, and RPI between the ruptured and nonruptured groups are summarized in TABLE 1 and FIGURE 5.

## DISCUSSION

The formation of an aneurysm within the abdominal aorta presents a dilemma requiring clinicians to predict when the risk of rupture outweighs that associated with intervention. The most commonly used criterion for AAA

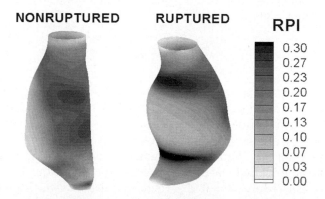

**FIGURE 3.** Representative comparison of the RPI between an electively repaired AAA (nonruptured, maximum diameter = 5.23 cm) and a ruptured AAA (diameter = 5.20).

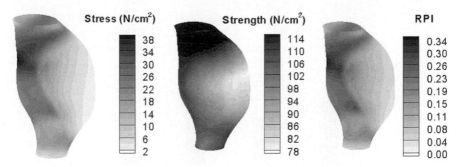

**FIGURE 4.** Three-dimensional distributions of AAA wall stress, strength, and RPI for a representative AAA.

rupture prediction is the maximum diameter criterion, which is typically based on a cut-off value of 5.5 cm.[1] Other parameters that have been proposed as potential predictors of AAA rupture include the AAA expansion rate,[20–22] wall stiffness,[2] increase in ILT thickness,[23] volume of ILT,[3] wall tension,[24] and peak AAA wall stress.[6,17] All of these approaches are empirical in nature and, as such, fail to take into account the physical aspects that control AAA development and rupture.

Because AAA rupture occurs with mechanical failure of the aneurysm wall, we have developed a purely biomechanics-based RPI for the purposes of assessing AAA severity. This index includes patient-specific noninvasive estimations of both AAA wall stress and strength. Comparisons of peak RPI values for ruptured and nonruptured AAAs suggest an improvement in rupture prediction using the current methodology as opposed to the maximum diameter criterion or with peak wall stress alone. In fact, for the limited numbers in this investigation ($n = 5$ nonruptured vs. $n = 8$ ruptured), the noninvasively estimated

**TABLE 1. Maximum diameter, minimum strength, and maximum RPI for all AAAs in this study (NRUP–nonruptured, RUP–ruptured)**

|  | Max diameter (cm) | | Max stress (N/cm$^2$) | | Min strength (N/cm$^2$) | | RPI | |
|---|---|---|---|---|---|---|---|---|
|  | NRUP | RUP | NRUP | RUP | NRUP | RUP | NRUP | RUP |
|  | 7.9 | 7.1 | 53.0 | 33.5 | 90.6 | 89.5 | 0.41 | 0.31 |
|  | 5.8 | 6.6 | 41.4 | 54.5 | 130.7 | 85.1 | 0.31 | 0.64 |
|  | 5.0 | 7.7 | 58.9 | 64.0 | 132.8 | 95.7 | 0.44 | 0.51 |
|  | 5.2 | 8.1 | 36.5 | 55.1 | 104.6 | 68.8 | 0.27 | 0.55 |
|  | 6.7 | 6.7 | 40.1 | 44.4 | 82.9 | 68.5 | 0.38 | 0.57 |
|  |  | 7.0 |  | 67.3 |  | 70.5 |  | 0.60 |
|  |  | 5.2 |  | 42.3 |  | 92.4 |  | 0.38 |
|  |  | 6.1 |  | 34.3 |  | 78.8 |  | 0.28 |
| Mean | 6.1 | 6.8 | 46.0 | 49.9 | 108.3 | 81.2 | 0.36 | 0.48 |
| Sem | 0.5 | 0.3 | 4.3 | 4.0 | 10.2 | 3.9 | 0.03 | 0.05 |

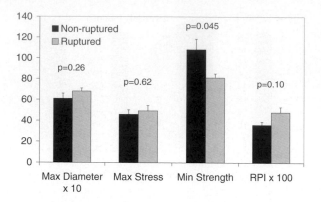

**FIGURE 5.** Comparison of group mean peak diameter, peak wall stress, and RPI between ruptured ($N = 8$) and nonruptured AAAs ($N = 5$).

values of wall strength better identified those AAAs that eventually ruptured compared to using maximum diameter and stress alone.

There are several limitations to this work including a variety of assumptions used in the FEM-based estimation of AAA wall stress. One of these assumptions is that the material properties for all AAA patients can be modeled using one constitutive (stress–strain) relation. This assumption stems from the inability to noninvasively derive a constitutive relation on a patient-specific basis. While such a relation would be ideal, the error arising from using a population-wide anisotropic constitutive model can be assessed by analyzing the stresses on AAA simulations in which the upper and lower 95% confidence interval constitutive models are used. Using a representative AAA, the error in peak wall stress was found to be 2.4% for the upper and 1.8% for the lower 95% confidence interval simulations, respectively. These results are similar to those reported previously in which the upper and lower 95% confidence interval variations in isotropic AAA wall constitutive parameters resulted in less than 4% change in peak wall stress.[25] The same type of analysis was performed by Di Martino and Vorp on the ILT, which resulted in a maximum variation of 10% on the AAA wall stress due to large yet physically reasonable variations in mean ILT model parameters.[26] These results suggest that the peak wall stress acting on an individual AAA is relatively insensitive to the errors introduced using a set of mean or population-wide model parameters.

The limitations associated with the noninvasive estimation of AAA wall strength have been discussed in detail elsewhere and are briefly described here. As with any modeling technique, there are certain limitations that should be kept in mind regarding the statistical model for wall strength estimation used here. Due to restrictions associated with open surgical procedures, the current model was derived from AAA wall samples from the anterior region of the AAA only. Ideally, samples should be obtained from the anterior, posterior, and both lateral regions of AAA. Recent reports on the variability in AAA wall strength as a function of location[27] suggest this may be an important factor to consider whenever using the proposed statistical model.

It is also important to note that in this work it is assumed that the tensile strength of the AAA wall can be adequately measured and modeled using uniaxial techniques. The fact that the aorta itself is a complex composite of collagen and elastin fibers suggests that assuming this material fails in a manner similar to a typical engineering material (e.g., steel, etc.) may not be appropriate. In fact, a recent report by Ohashi *et al.* has shown that the biaxial inflation of human thoracic aneurysms results in a preferential tearing of the aortic wall in the longitudinal direction.[28] The actual failure mechanisms responsible for AAA rupture remain unknown. An alternative mathematical description of the gradual dilation and failure of AAAs has recently been derived by Watton *et al.*[29] In this work the AAA is modeled as a two-layered cylindrical membrane using nonlinear elasticity and physiologically realistic constitutive relations to mathematically model the growth of a AAA *in vivo*. While it is clear that the gradual expansion of an AAA corresponds with a reorganization of the extracellular matrix, it remains unclear which of the structural components (e.g., collagen) may be primarily responsible for the eventual failure of the AAA wall.

Finally, the small numbers used in this demonstrative study ($n = 5$ nonruptured vs. $n = 8$ ruptured) are not large enough to warrant any rigorous conclusions. Ongoing work in our laboratory will serve to validate the use of RPI as a reliable means to assess AAA rupture potential on a patient-specific basis. Nonetheless, the results reported here emphasize the importance of including a noninvasive estimation of wall strength in the assessment of AAA rupture (FIG. 5).

In conclusion, this work describes and demonstrates a biomechanics-based RPI, which involves the noninvasive estimation of those factors that influence the mechanical failure of the AAA wall. The clinical relevance of this method for rupture assessment has yet to be validated, however, its success could aid clinicians in decision making and AAA patient management.

## ACKNOWLEDGMENTS

The authors would like to thank the surgical team at the University of Pittsburgh Medical Center, Division of Vascular Surgery, for their participation and insights. This work was funded in part by grants from the National Institutes of Health (# R01 HL60670 and # R01 HL 079313) awarded to D.A.V.

## REFERENCES

1. United Kingdom Small Aneurysm Trial Participants. 2002. Long-term outcomes of immediate repair compared with surveillance of small abdominal aortic aneurysms. N. Engl. J. Med. **346:** 1445–1452.

2. SONESSON, B., T. SANDGREN & T. LANNE. 1999. Abdominal aortic aneurysm wall mechanics and their relation to risk of rupture. Eur. J. Vasc. Endovasc. Surg. **18:** 487–493.
3. HANS, S.S., *et al.* 2005. Size and location of thrombus in intact and ruptured abdominal aortic aneurysms. J. Vasc. Surg. **41:** 584–588.
4. LOBATO, A.C. & P. PUECH-LEAO. 1998. Predictive factors for rupture of thoracoabdominal aortic aneurysm. J. Vasc. Surg. 1998. **27:** 446–453.
5. VARDULAKI, K.A., *et al.* 1998. Growth rates and risk of rupture of abdominal aortic aneurysms. Br. J. Surg. **85:** 1674–1680.
6. FILLINGER, M.F., *et al.* 2003. Prediction of rupture risk in abdominal aortic aneurysm during observation: wall stress versus diameter. J. Vasc. Surg. **37:** 724–732.
7. ELGER, D.F. *et al.* 1996. The influence of shape on the stresses in model abdominal aortic aneurysms. J. Biomech. Eng. **118:** 326–332.
8. HUA, J. & W.R. MOWER. 2001. Simple geometric characteristics fail to reliably predict abdominal aortic aneurysm wall stress. J. Vasc. Surg. **34:** 308–315.
9. INZOLI, F., *et al.* 1993. Biomechanical factors in abdominal aortic aneurysm rupture. Eur. J. Vasc. Surg. **7:** 667–674.
10. MOWER, W.R., W.J. QUINONES & S.S. GAMBHIR. 1997. Effect of intraluminal thrombus on abdominal aortic aneurysm wall stress. J. Vasc. Surg. Official Publication, the Society For Vascular Surgery [and] International Society For Cardiovascular Surgery, North American Chapter **26:** 602–608.
11. RAGHAVAN, M.L., *et al.* 2000. Wall stress distribution on three-dimensionally reconstructed models of human abdominal aortic aneurysm. J. Vasc. Surg. **31:** 760–769.
12. STRINGFELLOW, M.M., P.F. LAWRENCE & R.G. STRINGFELLOW. 1987. The influence of aorta-aneurysm geometry upon stress in the aneurysm wall. J. Surg. Res. **42:** 425–433.
13. THUBRIKAR, M.J., J. J. AL-SOUDI & F. ROBICSEK. 2001. Wall stress studies of abdominal aortic aneurysm in a clinical model. Ann. Vasc. Surg. **15:** 355–366.
14. VANDE GEEST, J.P. 2005. Towards an improved rupture potential index for abdominal aortic aneurysms: anisotropic constitutive modeling and noninvasive wall strength estimation. *In* Department of Bioengineering. University of Pittsburgh: Pittsburgh, PA.1–314.
15. VANDE GEEST, J.P. *et al.* 2006. Towards a noninvasive method for determination of patient-specific wall strength distribution in abdominal aortic aneurysms. Ann. Biomed. Eng. **34(7):** 1098–106.
16. WANG, D.H.J. *et al.* 2002. Effect of intraluminal thrombus on wall stress in patient specific models of abdominal aortic aneurysm. J. Vasc. Surg. **I36:** 598–604.
17. THUBRIKAR, M.J. *et al.* 2003. Effect of thrombus on abdominal aortic aneurysm wall dilation and stress. J. Cardiovasc. Surg. (Torino) **44:** 67–77.
18. VENKATASUBRAMANIAM, A.K. *et al.* 2004. A comparative study of aortic wall stress using finite element analysis for ruptured and non-ruptured abdominal aortic aneurysms. Eur. J. Vasc. Endovasc. Surg. **28:** 168–176.
19. VANDE GEEST, J.P. *et al.* 2004. Development and 3D finite element implementation of a multiaxial constitutive relation for abdominal aortic aneurysms. *In* 2004 ASME International Mechanical Engineering Conference. Anaheim, CA.
20. VANDE GEEST, J.P., M.S. SACKS & D.A. VORP. 2004. Age dependency the biaxial biomechanical behavior of human abdominal aorta. J. Biomech. Eng., In press. **126:** 815–822.

21. BROWN, P.M., D.T. ZELT & B. SOBOLEV. 2003. The risk of rupture in untreated aneurysms: the impact of size, gender, and expansion rate. J. Vasc. Surg. **37:** 280–284.
22. HATAKEYAMA, T., S. HIROSHI & M. TETSUICHIRO. 2001. Risk factors for rupture of abdominal aortic aneurysm based on three-dimensional study. J. Vasc. Surg. **33:** 453–461.
23. LEDERLE, F.A. *et al.* 2002. Rupture rate of large abdominal aortic aneurysms in patients refusing or unfit for elective repair. J. Am. Med. Assoc. **287:** 2968–2972.
24. STENBAEK, J., B. KALIN & J. SWEDENBORG. 2000. Growth of thrombus may be a better predictor of rupture than diameter in patients with abdominal aortic aneurysms. Eur. J. Vasc. Endovasc. Surg. **20:** 466–469.
25. HALL, A.J. *et al.* 2000. Aortic wall tension as a predictive factor for abdominal aortic aneurysm rupture: improving the selection of patients for abdominal aortic aneurysm repair. Ann. Vasc. Surg. **14:** 152–157.
26. RAGHAVAN, M.L. & D.A. VORP. 2000. Toward a biomechanical tool to evaluate rupture potential of abdominal aortic aneurysm: identification of a finite strain constitutive model and evaluation of its applicability. J. Biomech. **33:** 475–482.
27. DI MARTINO, E.S. & D.A. VORP. 2003. Effect of variation in intraluminal thrombus constitutive properties on abdominal aortic aneurysm wall stress. Ann. Biomed. Eng. **31:** 804–809.
28. THUBRIKAR, M.J. *et al.* 2001. Mechanical properties of abdominal aortic aneurysm wall. J. Med. Eng. Technol. **25:** 133–142.
29. OHASHI, T., S. SUGITA, T. MATSUMOTO, *et al.* 2002. Measurement of rupture properties of thoracic aortic aneurysms using pressure-imposed test. *In* Proceedings of Int. Cong. Biol. Med. Eng. Singapore.
30. WATTON, P.N., N.A. HILL & M. HEIL. 2004. A mathematical model for the growth of the abdominal aortic aneurysm. Biomech. Model Mechanobiol. **3:** 98–113.

# The Long-Term Relationship of Wall Stress to the Natural History of Abdominal Aortic Aneurysms (Finite Element Analysis and Other Methods)

MARK FILLINGER

*Section of Vascular Surgery, Dartmouth-Hitchcock Medical Center, Lebanon, NH*

ABSTRACT: For the past four decades, abdominal aortic aneurysm (AAA) rupture risk has been estimated using maximum aneurysm diameter. Although this works relatively well in general, clinicians know that some aneurysms rupture at an unusually small size, while others grow to exceptionally large sizes without rupture. We have demonstrated that finite element analysis (FEA) of AAA wall stress using three-dimensional computed tomography (CT) reconstructions is better than diameter for differentiating AAAs near the time of rupture, and that wall stress is superior to AAA diameter for predicting rupture risk in patients under observation. This article summarizes our current work, future areas of investigation, and issues related to "translational" research for FEA of aortic aneurysms.

KEYWORDS: aneurysm; rupture; wall stress; finite element

For the past four decades, abdominal aortic aneurysm (AAA) rupture risk has been estimated using maximum aneurysm diameter. Although this works relatively well in general, all clinicians know that some aneurysms rupture at an unusually small size, while others grow to exceptionally large sizes without rupture. We have demonstrated that finite element analysis (FEA) of AAA wall stress using three-dimensional computed tomography (CT) reconstructions is better than diameter for differentiating AAAs near the time of rupture,[1] and that wall stress is superior to AAA diameter for predicting rupture risk in patients under observation.[2]

In 2002 in the first report using FEA on a large cohort of AAA patients with and without rupture, our group reported that FEA of AAA wall stress using

Address for correspondence: Mark F. Fillinger, M.D., Dartmouth-Hitchcock Medical Center, Section of Vascular Surgery, One Medical Center Drive, Lebanon, NH 03756. Voice: 603-650-8677; fax: 603-650-4973.
e-mail: mark.fillinger@hitchcock.org

Ann. N.Y. Acad. Sci. 1085: 22–28 (2006). © 2006 New York Academy of Sciences.
doi: 10.1196/annals.1383.037

three-dimensional CT reconstructions is better than diameter for differentiating AAAs near the time of rupture. Moreover, we found that calculated indices previously suggested to better predict rupture risk (e.g., ratio of maximum AAA diameter to normal infrarenal diameter) were not helpful at all.[1]

In 2003 our group reported on the first large series of patients with AAAs under observation, looking at the natural history of aneurysms that had elective repair deferred or were felt to be at low risk of rupture. In that study, we found that wall stress is superior to AAA diameter for predicting rupture risk in patients under observation. It was clear that aneurysm wall stress is elevated well in advance of the time of rupture allowing sufficient time to repair the aneurysm prior to a catastrophic outcome in almost all patients.[2] This study demonstrated for the first time that wall stress can be a useful clinical tool with the potential to replace the method we have used for the past four decades. At this point, the strength of the data and the size of the patient cohort already rival or exceed that of the data for the clinical use of aneurysm diameter to estimate rupture risk.

## REFINEMENTS OF THREE-DIMENSIONAL AND EVEN TWO-DIMENSIONAL ANALYSIS OF AAA

While three-dimensional "stress analysis" is already superior to diameter, it can be improved further. Work continues in three broad categories: refining AAA stress analysis techniques to create a more realistic model for wall stress (and strength); developing techniques to allow widespread use in a simple manner; and investigating markers identifiable on two-dimensional imaging (conventional CT or MR) that may improve prediction of rupture risk over maximum AAA diameter alone.

## REFINING AAA STRESS ANALYSIS TECHNIQUES TO CREATE A MORE REALISTIC MODEL

### *Aortic Bifurcation*

Early in our work, we found that if the aneurysm model is "cut off" at the aortic bifurcation, stress artifacts are located at that site. In trying to extend the method to make it applicable for broad use in a large patient series, we found that we needed to include the aortic bifurcation in the model to make the method clinically useful.[1] Inclusion of the aortic bifurcation is not without its own problems, however, as stress artifacts can arise at this point as well. These artifacts tend to be focal, limited, and mathematically definable, but a perfect method without any requirement for human evaluation has yet to be developed.

## Calcium

Surgeons are well aware that calcified plaque is quite different from the surrounding tissue, and calcific plaque or calcified vascular wall is common in aortic aneurysms. We have investigated the effects of including calcified deposits in the finite element modeling of abdominal aortic aneurysms and early results suggest that the impact may be significant. Calcified plaque tends to elevate the stress locally due to the focal stiffness induced by the plaque itself, causing significant elevations in predicted wall stress for most aneurysms. The degree of elevation in stress is not proportional to the degree or surface area of calcification, however.[3] There may also be effects related to wall strength beyond the effects on wall stress.

## Thrombus

Results show that the presence of intraluminal thrombus may reduce and redistribute the stresses in the aortic wall.[4] Although thrombus is clinically heterogeneous within an individual aneurysm and between patients, adopting a nonhomogeneous thrombus model may not alter the stress distribution substantially.[5] Work from the University of Pittsburgh indicates that population mean parameters for thrombus material characteristics might be used to reasonably estimate the wall stresses in patient-specific aneurysm models.[5] Again, the relationship between thrombus and aneurysm wall strength may be as important or more important than its effect on wall stress, but this relationship remains to be tested on a large scale.

## Realistic Pressurization

To date, aneurysm wall stress models have taken the three-dimensional geometry of a pressurized aneurysm and then applied a pressure load. Although this method is not ideal, it has been used because it is impossible to perform a CT or MR scan on an unpressurized aneurysm sac in a living patient. We have developed a method of estimating the appropriate "zero pressure configuration" of an aneurysm as a means of developing a more realistic model. Results to date suggest that incorporation of the zero-pressure geometry into the model improves aneurysm wall motion predictions (as confirmed by dynamic MR), but does not have a major influence on predicted wall stress.[6]

# DEVELOPING TECHNIQUES TO ALLOW WIDESPREAD USE OF FEA IN A SIMPLE MANNER

A great deal of work is ongoing with regard to creating more realistic mathematical models of aneurysm wall stress and strength. While all of this is extremely important, it is unclear just how much refinement will be necessary to create a clinically useful technique. For example, diameter is far from an ideal method, but has served as a useful clinical tool for decades. As in our early work with more than 100 patients (and now well over 200), aneurysm wall stress alone is clearly superior to maximum aneurysm diameter for predicting wall stress.[2]

Standardizing this method so that it is applicable to a large human population in a relatively automated fashion is not trivial, however.[7] As we model an increasingly large number of aneurysms, we have encountered significant issues that have to be addressed before moving on to a more complex model. One example is the aortic bifurcation artifact mentioned earlier. The bifurcation clearly must be retained, yet can cause artifact of its own. Seemingly simple issues such as the mesh size and method of generation can have substantial effects on predicted wall stress and estimations of rupture risk. Each new refinement to the model (wall calcifications, thrombus, wall strength, zero-pressure configuration, etc.) potentially adds new issues that are not obvious when analyzing a small number of patients, but quickly become problematic when expanding the analysis to more than 100 patients. These issues clearly will have to be addressed before this research can be "translational" and applicable to the 200,000 patients diagnosed with aortic aneurysms each year. Many apparent improvements along the way have done nothing to improve the clinical estimation of rupture risk in our clinical cohort. Despite the need to overcome these hurdles, it is clear that aneurysm wall stress is already superior to diameter in an analysis on the scale of hundreds of patients. We believe that we are nearing a solution that will help decrease artifacts and exceptions requiring human analysis even further.

On the road to a clinically applicable solution, there are other hurdles in addition to the mathematical aspects of estimating rupture risk. More realistic FEAs are a worthwhile goal, but will not be helpful if the clinician has to be able to perform this task. A multicenter study is now underway that allows any interested center to obtain automated aneurysm wall stress analysis without cost over and above the three-dimensional reconstruction, and without requiring any knowledge of finite element method. The process creates a "rupture risk report," which reports on modifiable risk factors for rupture such as smoking and blood pressure as well as how blood pressure affects aneurysm wall stress and rupture risk. The hope is that the more technical aspects of stress analysis can be translated into a simple number that is easily grasped. One proposal for this is an "equivalent diameter"—meaning that if a 5 cm aneurysm has a wall stress typical of a 6 cm aneurysm, it has an "equivalent diameter" of 6 cm, thus giving the clinician a number that they have already incorporated into clinical practice over a number of years. The study group has now expanded to be international in scope, but adequate capacity is available to add new centers.[8] As the method continues to be refined, participating centers will have access to the best methods available without having to resend data.

## METHODS TO EVALUATE RUPTURE RISK BASED ON
## CONVENTIONAL TWO-DIMENSIONAL IMAGING

While work continues to make stress analysis more readily available for clinical practice, we are often asked about information that can be garnered from conventional CT that might help improve the evaluation of rupture risk. Even with a large database of anatomic data, lack of adequate controls is a frequent problem. For example, women have at least a 3-fold higher risk of AAA rupture than men, independent of AAA diameter.[2,9] Other factors such as blood pressure, smoking, and COPD affect rupture risk, and aortic dimensions vary with age.[9,10] Thus, when evaluating morphology of ruptured AAAs, it is appropriate to control for diameter, gender, age, and other demographic variables to the extent that this is possible.

In a recent series, we evaluated the conventional CT morphology of ruptured aneurysms in the context of electively imaged AAAs, matching patients for AAA size, patient gender, and age in an effort to isolate key anatomic variables that might be identifiable without finite element techniques.[10] Records were reviewed to identify all CT scans at Dartmouth-Hitchcock Medical Center or the referring hospital prior to emergency AAA repair for rupture or acute severe pain (RUP). CT scans prior to elective AAA repair (ELEC) were reviewed for age and gender matches to RUP patients. More than 40 variables were measured on each CT. Diameter matching was achieved by consecutively deleting the largest RUP and the smallest ELEC to avoid bias. CT scans were analyzed for 259 patients with AAAs: 122 RUP and 137 ELEC. Patients were well matched for age, gender, and other demographic variables or risk factors.

Maximum AAA diameter was significantly different in the comparison of all patients (RUP $6.5 \pm 2$ vs. ELEC $5.6 \pm 1$ cm, $P < 0.0001$), and the mean diameter for rupture was 5 mm lower in females ($6.1 \pm 2$ vs. $6.6 \pm 2$ cm, $P = 0.007$). Matching for diameter, gender, and age was possible for 200 patients (100 from each group, max AAA diameter $6.0 \pm 1$ vs. $6.0 \pm 1$ cm). Analysis of diameter-matched AAAs indicated that most variables were statistically similar for the two groups including infrarenal neck length ($17 \pm 1$ vs. $19 \pm 1$ mm, $P = 0.3$), maximum thrombus thickness ($25 \pm 1$ vs. $23 \pm 1$ mm, $P = 0.4$), and indices of body habitus such as ([max AAA diameter]/[normal suprarenal aorta diameter]) or ([max AAA diameter]/[lumbar vertebrae L3 transverse diameter]). Multivariate analysis controlling for gender indicated the most significant variables were aortic tortuosity (Odds Ratio [OR] 3.3, indicating no/mild tortuosity has greater rupture risk); diameter asymmetry (OR 3.2 for a 1 cm difference in major-minor axis); and current smoking (OR 2.7, greater risk for current smokers).

In this study, we found that when matched for age, gender, and diameter, ruptured AAAs tend to be less tortuous and yet have greater cross-sectional diameter asymmetry.[10] On conventional two-dimensional CT axial slices, when diameter asymmetry is associated with low aortic tortuosity, the *larger* diameter on axial slices more accurately reflects rupture risk. When diameter asymmetry is associated with moderate or severe aortic tortuosity, the *smaller* diameter on axial slices more accurately reflects rupture risk. Current smoking is significantly associated with rupture, even when controlling for gender and AAA morphology. This type of information can be used without relying on "high-tech" methodology or participation in a multicenter study. Although two-dimensional methods do not currently appear to be as useful as finite element methods, they may be quite useful until the more complex FEA methods are more widely available and less costly to produce.

## CONCLUSION

Progress continues in developing better tools for estimating aneurysm rupture risk using noninvasive methods. Some of these tools are not yet ready for regular clinical use, but others can be utilized in a practical manner now. Multicenter trials may ultimately allow further development of techniques that can be incorporated into daily clinical practice. Notably, a large amount of wonderful work has been performed in this field as will be evidenced by other presentations and papers from this symposium.

## REFERENCES

1. FILLINGER, M.F., M.L. RAGHAVAN, S.P. MARRA, *et al.* 2002. In vivo analysis of mechanical wall stress and abdominal aortic aneurysm rupture risk. J. Vasc. Surg. **36:** 589–597.
2. FILLINGER, M.F., S.P. MARRA, M.L. RAGHAVAN & F.E. KENNEDY. 2003. Prediction of rupture risk in abdominal aortic aneurysm during observation: wall stress versus diameter. J. Vasc. Surg. **37:** 724–732.
3. MARRA, S., D. CHEN, J. DWYER, *et al.* 2005. Effects of including calcified deposits in the finite element modeling of abdominal aortic aneurysms. ASME Bioengineering Conference. June 25 2005, Vail, CO.
4. WANG, D.H., M.S. MAKAROUN, M.W. WEBSTER & D.A. VORP. 2002. Effect of intraluminal thrombus on wall stress in patient-specific models of abdominal aortic aneurysm. J. Vasc. Surg. **36:** 598–604.
5. DI MARTINO, E.S. & D.A. VORP. 2003. Effect of variation in intraluminal thrombus constitutive properties on abdominal aortic aneurysm wall stress. Ann. Biomed. Eng. **31:** 804–809.
6. MARRA, S., M. RAGHAVAN, D. WHITTAKER, *et al.* 2005. Estimation of the zero-pressure geometry of abdominal aortic aneurysms from dynamic magnetic resonance imaging. ASME Bioengineering Conference. June 25 2005, Vail, CO.
7. RAGHAVAN, M.L., M.F. FILLINGER, S.P. MARRA, *et al.* 2005. Automated methodology for determination of stress distribution in human abdominal aortic aneurysm. J. Biomech. Eng. **127:** 868–871.

8. FILLINGER, M. 2004. Aortic aneurysm wall stress analysis: a description and invitation for participation in a multicenter evaluation. Endovasc. Today. July/August 2003. Available at www.evtoday.com.

9. BROWN, L.C. & J.T. POWELL. 1999. Risk factors for aneurysm rupture in patients kept under ultrasound surveillance. UK Small Aneurysm Trial Participants. Ann. Surg. **230:** 289–296; Discussion 296–287.

10. FILLINGER, M.F., J. RACUSIN, R.K. BAKER, *et al*. 2004. Anatomic characteristics of ruptured abdominal aortic aneurysm on conventional CT scans: implications for rupture risk. J. Vasc. Surg. **39:** 1243–1252.

# A Summary of the Contributions of the VA Cooperative Studies on Abdominal Aortic Aneurysms

FRANK A. LEDERLE

*University of Minnesota, Center for Epidemiological and Clinical Research, VA Medical Center, Minneapolis, MN, USA*

ABSTRACT: The Department of Veterans Affairs Cooperative Studies Program has completed two studies on abdominal aortic aneurysm (AAA) and is currently conducting a third. The first, the Aneurysm Detection and Management (ADAM) Study, consisted of both a screening program, which provided information on the prevalence and associations of AAA, and a randomized trial, which found that survival is not improved by repair of small AAA. The second was a prospective observational study to determine the incidence of rupture in patients with large AAA for whom elective repair was not planned due to medical contraindications or patient refusal. AAA in this population had a high risk of rupture, about 10% per year for AAA > 5.5 cm, and 25% within 6 months for AAA larger than 8.0 cm. The third, the Open Versus Endovascular Repair (OVER) Trial, is a multicenter randomized trial comparing long-term survival following two methods of elective AAA repair.

KEYWORDS: abdominal aortic aneurysm; veterans; multicenter studies; mortality; surgical treatment

## INTRODUCTION

One in 20 U.S. veterans over age 50 have abdominal aortic aneurysms (AAA). A total of 35,000 operations to repair AAA are performed each year in the United States, 1,200 of these in the Department of Veterans Affairs (VA). In recognition of the importance of this disease to veterans, the VA Cooperative Studies Program has completed two cooperative studies on AAA and is currently conducting a third. This chapter summarizes these studies.

Address for correspondence: Frank A. Lederle, M.D., University of Minnesota, Center for Epidemiological and Clinical Research, VA Medical Center, Minneapolis, MN 55417. Voice: 612-467-1979; fax: 612-725-2237.

e-mail: frank.lederle@med.va.gov

Ann. N.Y. Acad. Sci. 1085: 29–38 (2006). © 2006 New York Academy of Sciences.
doi: 10.1196/annals.1383.039

# THE ANEURYSM DETECTION AND
# MANAGEMENT (ADAM) STUDY

The first study, the ADAM Study, consisted of both a screening program and a randomized trial conducted over 8 years in 16 VA medical centers. The ADAM Study addressed five questions, which are discussed below.

(1) *Should Small AAA Be Repaired?*

The ADAM randomized trial was designed to determine whether immediate open surgical repair resulted in better survival for patients with small AAA than imaging surveillance with repair reserved for aneurysms that enlarged to 5.5 cm or became symptomatic.[1,2]

Eligible patients were 50 to 79 years of age, had AAA 4.0 to 5.4 cm in diameter by computed tomography (CT) within 12 weeks prior to randomization, and had none of the following: previous aortic surgery, evidence of aneurysm rupture, aneurysm expansion $\geq 1.0$ cm in the past year or $\geq 0.7$ cm in the past 6 months, supra- or juxtarenal aortic aneurysm (defined as anticipated need for reimplantation of a main renal artery), known thoracic aortic aneurysm $\geq 4.0$ cm in diameter, probable need for aortic surgery other than abdominal aneurysm repair within 6 months, severe heart, lung, or liver disease, serum creatinine $\geq$ 2.5 mg/dL, major surgical procedure or angioplasty within the previous 3 months, expected survival less than 5 years, severe debilitation, inability to give informed consent, or high likelihood of noncompliance with the protocol. The vascular surgery team at each participating center agreed to offer randomization to all eligible patients.

A total of 1,136 veterans aged 50 to 79 years with AAA 4.0–5.4 cm in diameter were randomized to immediate open surgical or imaging surveillance every 6 months with repair reserved for aneurysms that enlarged to 5.5 cm or became symptomatic. Follow-up was 3.5 to 8.0 years (mean 4.9 years). The crossover rate was less than 10%; 7.4% of immediate repair patients failed to have aneurysm repair and 9.0% of surveillance patients had repair without reaching 5.5 cm or becoming symptomatic. Mortality, the primary outcome, was more common in the immediate repair group, but the difference was not significant (relative risk 1.21, 95% confidence intervals, 0.95 to 1.54). Survival trends did not favor immediate repair in any of the prespecified subgroups of age or aneurysm diameter at entry. These findings were obtained despite a low total (30 days plus extended inpatient) operative mortality of 2.7% in the immediate repair group. There was also no significant difference in AAA-related deaths with 19 occurring in each group. Twelve surveillance patients had AAA rupture (0.7% per year of follow-up), resulting in eight deaths.

Hospitalizations related to AAA were reduced by 39% in the surveillance group. For most quality-of-life measures and times, there was no difference between the two randomized groups.[3] Immediate repair resulted in an increased prevalence of impotence more than 1 year after randomization, but was also associated with improved scores on the general health scale of the SF-36 in the first 2 years.

Under the surveillance strategy, about one-fifth of elective AAA repair operations are avoided because patients die of other causes before meeting criteria for repair. We concluded that survival is not improved by repair of AAAs smaller than 5.5 cm, even when operative mortality is low, and that these findings support a policy of reserving elective repair for AAAs ≥ 5.5 cm in diameter.

(2) *Who Gets AAA?*

The ADAM study ultrasound screening program was intended not only to identify patients for enrollment into the trial but also to provide information regarding the prevalence and associations of AAA in a cohort large enough to support extensive multivariable analysis.[4,5] Ultrasound screening clinics were established at the 15 participating VA medical centers. All active patients in the database at these centers (those treated in the current or previous fiscal year or having future appointments) who met the study age criteria were sent invitation letters to attend the clinic. The results of the screening program were reported in two cohorts. The first cohort[4] consisted of subjects screened before April 1995 who were essentially all respondents to the initial invitation letter. The second cohort,[5] those screened from April 1995 onward, consisted of active VA patients who responded to repeated mailings and to various advertising and outreach strategies used by the screening clinics. Those aged 50–79 years were included in the analysis. Inadvertent repeat screenings were identified by social security numbers and the later screening was excluded. Subjects who reported having been told previously that they had AAA were also excluded. Before undergoing the ultrasound examination, subjects completed a brief questionnaire addressing demographic information and possible risk factors for AAA. Because aortic diameters of 3.0 to 3.9 cm are more numerous than those 4.0 cm or larger and may not all represent true disease, including them in the regression models could obscure or dilute the effect of the true AAAs. Therefore, we reported separate regression models for AAA 3.0–3.9 cm and AAA 4.0 cm or larger, each compared with "normals" having infrarenal aortic diameters (IAD) less than 3.0 cm.

There were 73,451 veterans aged 50–79 years screened in the first cohort and 52,745 in the second, a total of 126,196. The two cohorts were very similar in their characteristics and results, so they are described here combined. The screened population had a mean age of 66 years and was 97% male (though with more than 2,000 women, it remains one of the largest screened cohorts of women). A total of 75% of those screened had ever smoked and 5% reported a family history of AAA. We detected 5,283 previously undiagnosed AAA $\geq$ 3.0 cm, representing a prevalence of 4.2%. Of these, 1,644 were $\geq$4.0 cm, for a prevalence of 1.3%.

The principal positive associations with AAA included age, smoking, family history of AAA, and atherosclerotic diseases, whereas female sex, diabetes, and black race were the principal negative associations. The excess prevalence associated with smoking accounted for 75% of all AAAs 4.0 cm or larger. The association of smoking with AAA increased significantly with the number of years smoked and decreased significantly with number of years after quitting smoking when these variables were added to the models. After adjustment for number of years smoked (and all other variables), current smokers were more likely than ex-smokers to have AAA. The ADAM study was the first to conclude that diabetes (or its treatment) reduced the likelihood of AAA, further evidence against the traditional view of AAA as a form of atherosclerosis.[6] Despite the much lower prevalence of AAA in women, most important associations with AAA are similar to those seen in men.[7]

(3) *Would Interval Screening be Better Than One Time Screening for AAA?*

To assess the yield of repeat screening, a sample of ADAM screenees were selected for follow-up and ultrasound 4 years after the original ultrasound.[8] Thirteen VA medical centers participated in the repeat screening study, and these centers had screened 15,098 subjects before June 30, 1993 who had both infrarenal and suprarenal aortic diameter $\leq$ 3.0 cm on the initial ultrasound and no history of AAA prior to the initial screening. Of these, 5,151 without AAA on the initial ultrasound (defined as IAD of 3.0 cm or larger) were randomly selected for follow-up and invited for repeat ultrasound screening after an interval of 4 years. Local records and national databases were searched to identify deaths and AAA diagnoses made during the study interval in subjects who did not attend the re-screening.

Of the 5,151 selected, 598 (11.6%) had died (none attributed to AAA), and 20 (0.4%) had an interim diagnosis of AAA. Repeat screening was done on 2,622 (50.9%), of whom 58 (2.2%) had new AAA. The AAA detected at repeat screening were small: 95% were < 4.0 cm and none were $\geq$ 5.0 cm.

Independent predictors of new AAA at repeat screening (based on the questionnaires administered at the original screening) included current smoker (at the time of the original screening) and either coronary artery disease or the composite variable "any atherosclerosis" (whichever was used in the model). Adding the interim and re-screening diagnosis rates suggests a 4-year true incidence rate of 2.6%. Re-screening only subjects with IAD of 2.5 cm or greater on the initial ultrasound would have missed more than two-thirds of the new AAAs. We concluded that repeat screening was of little practical value after 4 years, but repeat screening after longer intervals warranted further study.

(4) *How Should We Define AAA?*

In 1991, the Society for Vascular Surgery recommended that AAA be defined as a 50% or greater increase in IAD compared with the expected IAD based on age, sex, and other factors such as body size.[9] However, values for expected IAD had not been well defined. To assess the effects of age, gender, race, and body size on IAD and to determine expected values for IAD based on these factors, we analyzed data from the first cohort of the ADAM ultrasound screening program.[10] There were 69,905 subjects who had no previous history of AAA and no ultrasound evidence of AAA (defined as an IAD ≥ 3.0 cm). Three methods of modeling body size were considered. The first model was constructed using the independent variables from the questionnaire (height, weight, and waist circumference). In the second model, body mass index (BMI), a measure of obesity, was substituted for weight. In the third model, body surface area (BSA), a measure of body size, was substituted for height and weight. We found that while age, gender, race, and body size (in whatever parameters considered) had statistically significant effects on IAD, these effects were small. Female sex was associated with a 0.14 cm reduction in IAD and black race with a 0.01 cm increase in IAD. A 0.1 cm change in IAD was associated with large changes in the independent variables: 29 years in age, 40 cm in height, 35 kg in weight, 11 kg/m2 in BMI, 0.35 m2 in BSA. Nearly all height–weight groups were within 0.1 cm of the gender means and the unadjusted gender means differed by only 0.23 cm.

The three models performed similarly with each model explaining 34% of the variability in IAD. The majority of this variability was explained by the indicator variables for medical center. Models constructed without these medical center variables explained less than 6% of the variability in IAD. Thus, variation among medical centers had far more influence on IAD than did the combination of age, gender, race, and body size.

We concluded that use of age, gender, race, and body size to define AAA may not offer sufficient advantage over a one-size-fits-all definition to be worth the extra effort.

(5) *How Accurate Is AAA Measurement?*

Data collected during recruitment into the ADAM trial allowed us to report inter- and intraobserver variability of CT measurements of AAA diameter and agreement between CT and ultrasound.11 CT measurement of AAA diameter was used to determine eligibility for randomization into the trial. To ensure consistent measurement throughout the participating centers, all CT scans were read at a central CT laboratory. Most CT scans submitted for central reading had also been read by a radiologist at the participating center, called the "local reading," and many also had recent ultrasound measurements. For quality control purposes, a proportion of the CT scans read by the central laboratory were randomly selected for blinded central re-reading.

We examined interobserver variation in CT measurement of AAA diameter using all CT scans submitted for central reading (regardless of whether the patient was enrolled in the ADAM trial) for which a local reading was also available. We also studied agreement between CT and ultrasound measurement using all ultrasound examinations done within 30 days preceding these CT scans. In addition, all central re-readings done on these CT scans were used to examine intraobserver variation in CT measurement. The central reader used calipers and a magnifying glass to measure the diameter of the aneurysm against the scale provided on the film. AAA diameter by central CT measurement was defined as the maximum external diameter in any direction.

There were 806 interobserver pairs of local and central CT measurements, 70 intraobserver pairs of central CT re-measurements, and 258 CT and ultrasound pairs. AAA diameters were concentrated in a relatively narrow range reflecting the 4.0–5.4 cm eligible range for the ADAM trial. A marked preference for recording by half centimeter was seen in the local CT and ultrasound measurements, a phenomenon known as "terminal digit preference."

Intraobserver variability for the central readings was low, 0.2 cm or less in 90% of the pairs and 70% were within 0.1 cm. This difference between local and central CT measurements was 0.2 cm or less in 65% of pairs, but 17% differed by at least 0.5 cm. The local measurements tended to be smaller than the central measurements, perhaps reflecting a more rigorous search for the maximum diameter by the central reader. The difference between the ultrasound and central CT measurements was 0.2 cm or less in 44% of pairs, and was at least 0.5 cm in 33%. AAA diameter was generally smaller by ultrasound than by CT in this study, though in more than a fourth of cases the ultrasound measurement was larger.

Because the intra- and interobserver variability in CT readings reported in our study were obtained using the same scan for both measurements, a comparison of different CT scans, generating different images from different slices, would be expected to increase variability. In clinical practice, comparison is usually with another test obtained some months earlier. Our comparison of CT with ultrasound done within 30 days more closely reflects clinical practice in this regard.

In conclusion, we found that a high degree of precision was possible in CT measurement of AAA diameter, but this precision was not obtained in practice because of differences in measurement techniques and rounding errors, and differences between imaging modalities further increased variability. Variations in AAA measurement of 0.5 cm or more were common, and this should be taken into account in management decisions.

## NATURAL HISTORY OF LARGE ABDOMINAL AORTIC ANEURYSMS STUDY

Surgery is usually deferred in high operative risk patients until the AAA attains a diameter at which the risk of rupture is believed to outweigh the operative risk. However, few data are available on the rupture risk of large AAA, resulting in substantial disagreement among experts.[12] We therefore undertook a second VA Cooperative Study, the Natural History of Large Abdominal Aortic Aneurysms Study.[13] This was a 5-year prospective observational study conducted at 47 VA medical centers to determine the incidence of rupture in patients with AAA $\geq$ 5.5 cm for whom elective AAA repair was not planned due to medical contraindications or patient refusal.

Patients were excluded if they had evidence of rupture, previous aortic surgery, dissecting thoracic aortic aneurysm, secondary AAA (e.g., Marfan disease), or death expected in the next 30 days. Enrolled patients provided both informed consent and a signed form indicating willingness to have autopsy. The vascular surgery team at each center agreed to offer entry to all eligible patients.

Medical records (including hospital records, nursing home notes, and imaging and autopsy reports) were requested for deaths or AAA repair procedures. Eyewitness accounts were obtained by phone for deaths that occurred outside of health-care facilities. Death certificates were not used to assign cause of death.

A total of 26% of eligible patients refused enrollment. A total of 198 patients were enrolled at 47 Veterans Affairs medical centers between April 1995 and April 2000 and followed through July 2000. All patients but one were male and nearly all had a history of smoking. As expected, study patients were elderly and had high rates of comorbidities, especially coronary artery disease and chronic obstructive pulmonary disease.

Data were analyzed both by initial and attained AAA diameter. Assessment of attained AAA diameter was by follow-up imaging measurements (primarily ultrasound) every 6 months. A total of 72% of follow-up imaging visits were completed.

The study duration was 5 years and mean follow-up was 1.5 years, outcome ascertainment was complete for all patients, and autopsy was performed on 52 of 112 deaths (46%). A total of 45 patients had probable AAA rupture. The 1-year incidence of probable rupture by initial AAA diameter was 9.4% for AAA 5.5–5.9 cm, 10.3% for AAA 6.0–6.9 cm (20% for the subgroup of

6.5–6.9 cm), and 29.5% for AAA $\geq$ 7.0 cm. Much of the increased risk associated with initial diameters of 6.5–7.9 cm was related to an increased likelihood that the AAA would reach 8.0 cm during follow-up, after which more than one-fourth ruptured within 6 months. AAA diameter was the strongest predictor of rupture in terms of variance explained. Prior rate of AAA enlargement was a significant predictor of rupture but not after adjustment for the current AAA diameter.

These findings should help physicians decide when to offer repair of large AAA to patients at high operative risk.

## THE OVER TRIAL FOR AAA

The third VA Cooperative Study, the Open Versus Endovascular Repair (OVER) Trial for AAA, is a 33-center, 9-year study that began in 2002. Its purpose is to compare two methods of elective AAA repair, endovascular grafting, and standard open surgery, in a multicenter randomized trial. The primary outcome is long-term survival; secondary outcomes include morbidity, procedure failures and need for secondary procedures, and cost. The protocol was revised in November 2005 and now calls for 900 patients to be randomized by October 2007 and followed until October 2011. As of the end of April 2006, 600 patients had been randomized.

OVER is the only trial comparing open with endovascular repair in the Western Hemisphere. Two European trials, EVAR-1 and DREAM, reported that the reduction in all-cause mortality seen with endovascular repair at 30 days had disappeared after 2 years.[14,15] It is not clear whether endovascular repair simply delayed deaths, or if late mortality will continue to be increased with endovascular repair due to complications or failure to prevent rupture.[16] Both EVAR-1 and DREAM reported some advantage for endovascular repair in aneurysm-related deaths, but this may be because all early postoperative deaths are classified as aneurysm related whereas late aneurysm-related deaths are easily misclassified as something else (which is why aneurysm-related mortality was not selected as the primary outcome in any of the trials). Determining which procedure leads to lower late total mortality will require longer and more detailed follow-up, and OVER will contribute to this effort. EVAR-1 and DREAM report on procedures performed from 1999 to 2003, whereas OVER will compare procedures done from 2002 to 2007, which may be an important difference for a rapidly developing technology like endovascular repair. Only in the OVER trial is the specific device the patient would receive if randomized to endovascular repair recorded before randomization, allowing for subgroup analysis by endovascular graft compared with true randomized controls for that graft. OVER also includes a cost-effectiveness analysis that uses U.S. utilization and costs.

## REFERENCES

1. LEDERLE, F.A., S.E. WILSON, G.R. JOHNSON, *et al*. FOR THE ANEURYSM DETECTION AND MANAGEMENT (ADAM) VETERANS AFFAIRS COOPERATIVE STUDY GROUP. 2002. Immediate repair compared with surveillance of small abdominal aortic aneurysms. N. Engl. J. Med. **346:** 1437–1444.

2. LEDERLE, F.A. 2002. Small abdominal aortic aneurysms—reply. N. Engl. J. Med. **347:** 1114, 1902 (corr).

3. LEDERLE, F.A., G.R. JOHNSON, S.E. WILSON, *et al*. FOR THE ANEURYSM DETECTION AND MANAGEMENT VETERANS AFFAIRS COOPERATIVE STUDY. 2003. Quality of life, impotence, and activity level in a randomized trial of immediate repair vs. surveillance of small abdominal aortic aneurysms. J. Vasc. Surg. **38:** 745–752.

4. LEDERLE, F.A., G.R. JOHNSON, S.E. WILSON, *et al*. FOR THE ANEURYSM DETECTION AND MANAGEMENT (ADAM) VETERANS AFFAIRS COOPERATIVE STUDY GROUP. 1997. Prevalence and associations of abdominal aortic aneurysm detected through screening. Ann. Intern. Med. **126:** 441–449.

5. LEDERLE, F.A., G.R. JOHNSON, S.E. WILSON, *et al*. AND THE ADAM VA COOPERATIVE STUDY INVESTIGATORS. 2000. The Aneurysm Detection and Management Study screening program: validation cohort and final results. Arch. Intern. Med. **160:** 1425–1430.

6. LEDERLE, F.A., D.B. NELSON, A.M. JOSEPH. 2003. Smokers' relative risks for aortic aneurysm compared with other smoking-related diseases: a systematic review. J. Vasc. Surg. **38:** 329–334

7. LEDERLE, F.A., G.R. JOHNSON, S.E. WILSON, *et al*. FOR THE ANEURYSM DETECTION AND MANAGEMENT VETERANS AFFAIRS COOPERATIVE STUDY. 2001. Abdominal aortic aneurysm in women. J. Vasc. Surg. **34:** 122–126.

8. LEDERLE, F.A., G.R. JOHNSON, S.E. WILSON, *et al*. AND THE ADAM VA COOPERATIVE STUDY INVESTIGATORS. 2000. Yield of repeated screening for abdominal aortic aneurysm after a four-year interval. Arch. Intern. Med. **160:** 1117–1121.

9. JOHNSTON, K.W., R.B. RUTHERFORD, M.D. TILSON, *et al*. 1991. Suggested standards for reporting arterial aneurysms. J. Vasc. Surg. **13:** 444–450.

10. LEDERLE, F.A., G.R. JOHNSON, S.E. WILSON, *et al*. AND THE ADAM VA COOPERATIVE STUDY INVESTIGATORS. 1997. Relationship of age, gender, race, and body size to infrarenal aortic diameter. J. Vasc. Surg. **26:** 595–601.

11. LEDERLE, F.A., S.E. WILSON, G.R. JOHNSON, *et al*. FOR THE ABDOMINAL AORTIC ANEURYSM DETECTION AND MANAGEMENT VETERANS ADMINISTRATION COOPERATIVE STUDY GROUP. 1995. Variability in measurement of abdominal aortic aneurysms. J. Vasc. Surg. **21:** 945–952.

12. LEDERLE, F.A. 1996. Risk of rupture of large abdominal aortic aneurysms: disagreement among vascular surgeons. Arch. Intern. Med. **156:** 1007–1009.

13. LEDERLE, F.A., G.R. JOHNSON, S.E. WILSON, *et al*. FOR THE VETERANS AFFAIRS COOPERATIVE STUDY #417 INVESTIGATORS. 2002. Rupture rate of large abdominal aortic aneurysms in patients refusing or unfit for elective repair. JAMA **287:** 2968–2972.

14. BLANKENSTEIJN, J.D., S.E.C.A. DE JONG, M. PRINSSEN, *et al*. 2005. Two-year results of a randomized trial comparing conventional and endovascular repair of abdominal aortic aneurysms. N. Engl. J. Med. **352:** 2398–2405.

15. EVAR Trial Participants. 2005. Endovascular aneurysm repair versus open repair in patients with abdominal aortic aneurysm (EVAR trial 1): randomised controlled trial. Lancet. **365:** 2179–2186.
16. Lederle, F.A. 2005. Endovascular repair of abdominal aortic aneurysm—round two. N. Engl. J. Med. **352:** 2443–2445.

# Pharmacological Approaches to Prevent Abdominal Aortic Aneurysm Enlargement and Rupture

MARK RENTSCHLER AND B. TIMOTHY BAXTER

*The Methodist Hospital and The University of Nebraska Medical Center, Omaha, Nebraska*

ABSTRACT: Current efforts to limit the mortality from abdominal aortic aneurysm (AAA) are dependent on detection and elective repair. Even by conservative estimates, there are more than 300,000 undetected AAAs in the United States, most of which are small and would not require immediate intervention. Current practice following detection of a small AAA includes education, risk factor management, and serial observation. This approach, based on the statistical probability of death from rupture compared to the morbidity and mortality of repair, can be unsettling to patients and lead to a decline in perceived quality of life. While the pathophysiology of AAA is not completely understood, observations from human tissues and animal studies have identified a number of potential targets for inhibiting aneurysm expansion. It is clear that the prominent inflammatory response identified in aneurysm tissue has a role in promoting aortic expansion. This inflammatory response is thought to account for increased expression of proteolytic enzymes. Recent work has suggested a unifying hypothesis centered on the MAP kinase family affecting both the regulation of matrix synthesis and the expression of proteolytic enzymes. The tetracycline antibiotics and antihypertensive medications that affect the angiotensin-converting enzyme system can inhibit proteolysis. There are adequate preliminary data to support a large prospective randomized trial of doxycycline to prevent aneurysm expansion.

KEYWORDS: aneurysm; tetracycline

## INTRODUCTION

Abdominal aortic aneurysm (AAA) represents a formidable health-related problem in industrialized nations.[1] It has been estimated that 1–2% of the

Address for correspondence: B. Timothy Baxter, M.D., Suite 220, 8111 Dodge St., Omaha, Nebraska, 68132. Voice: 402-393-6624; fax: 402-393-6635.
e-mail: btbaxter@unmc.edu

Ann. N.Y. Acad. Sci. 1085: 39–46 (2006). © 2006 New York Academy of Sciences.
doi: 10.1196/annals.1383.003

general population is affected by this problem. This number increases to 6% if the population screened is predominantly elderly males who have smoked.[2] We are aware of approximately 50 to 60,000 patients who come to medical attention for elective repair, treatment of ruptured aortic aneurysm, or death from ruptured aneurysms each year. However, extrapolating to the population of the United States, it is clear that there is a much larger proportion of aneurysms undetected in comparison to those recognized. One estimate is that there are 360,000 undetected small AAAs in the United States.[3] The current demographics indicate that 29% of the entire population of the United States is now between the ages of 40 and 60 years. During the next 20 years, this group will move into the "at risk" population for aortic aneurysm disease. Recognizing this epidemic, the centers for Medicare and Medicaid services (CMS) have made reimbursement available for one-time aneurysm screening for men over the age of 65 years who have ever smoked. The bill authorizing this (screening AAA very efficiently or SAAAVE) was passed in February 2006. The detection of unrecognized aortic aneurysms will become increasingly common. Since the vast majority of these aneurysms will be below the threshold requiring immediate intervention, it will become imperative that we explore and develop medical treatments for this common problem.

A number of population-based screening studies have now been performed for the problem of AAA. The studies are surprisingly consistent in demonstrating that only a small percentage of aneurysms detected at screening reach or exceed the threshold of 5.5 cm that would warrant immediate intervention.[3] Thus, 90% or more of these aneurysms are small and will require serial observations. Our current practice is to follow these aneurysms at 6- to 12-month intervals with ultrasound or CT imaging. Specific recommendations regarding the interval between follow-up imaging studies based on aneurysm size have been published.[4] While we can reassure these patients that the risk of rupture is extremely low during this period of observation, many find this approach unsettling. A number of studies have, in fact, demonstrated that there is a significant decrease in an individual's perception of his/her health when made aware of the presence of an aneurysm, which will be observed.[5] This may manifest in a number of ways such as anxiety or depression resulting in a decrease in quality of life. Interestingly, this decrement appears to be reversible with definitive repair. Because of our understanding of the anatomy, physiology, and natural history of AAA, we, as physicians and surgeons, have a perspective that may be quite different from the patient. Having seen the rare but memorable bad outcomes of aneurysm repair, we accept serial observation as a safe and cost-effective approach to the problem. We should recognize, however, that the negative effects identified on these quality of life surveys are a measure of our inability to appreciate the full implications of diagnosis and observational treatment of small AAA.

During the past decade, the interventional treatment of AAA has been revolutionized by treatment from within the lumen of the artery. The endovascular approach has decreased acute morbidity at a cost of increased postoperative surveillance with the possible need for additional endograft revision of the AAA. If repair can alleviate the negative quality of life effects of observation of AAA, perhaps offering endograft repair for small AAA (3.5–5.5 cm) makes sense. This approach is, in fact, now being investigated in clinical trials.[6] This strategy overlooks one inescapable fact: the cost. The average cost for endovascular aneurysm repair is approximately $23,000 per patient.[7] With the approved screening strategy for Medicare patients, we will presumably begin to identify a larger proportion of those 360,000 undiagnosed small AAAs. Thus, broadening the indications for endovascular repair to include small AAA will be cost prohibitive unless expenses were drastically reduced or there were an accepted means of stratification that allowed for repair of selected small AAAs. An alternative and more attractive approach would be medical treatment to prevent progression of aortic aneurysms.

The German microbiologist, Robert Koch, established the tenets that define the conduct of quality research. The postulates were developed to study the most important medical problem of the time, bacterial infection. These postulates, with slight modification, can be applied to most scientific endeavors today. How might they be applied to the problem of aortic aneurysm? (See TABLE 1.) Throughout the 1990s aneurysm research focused on the histological, biochemical, and molecular aspects of human aneurysm tissue. Using this information as a background, a number of animal models of aortic aneurysm were developed. The models were evaluated for their abilities to recapitulate the aspects of human aneurysm tissue. While none of these models could precisely mimic the chronic aspects of the human condition, they were found to be valuable because they could reproduce many of the important features of the disease. The next step using the modification of Koch's postulate was to use these models to identify promising therapies that could inhibit the development or progression of aneurysms. The final step will be to translate this work back to the clinical setting and test promising therapies against the disease.

Our current understanding of the development of aneurysmal disease involves a series of steps beginning with an inflammatory response in the infrarenal aortic wall. Since the infrarenal aorta is one of the favored sites for early development of atherosclerosis, it seems likely that this might be the

**TABLE 1. Approach for development of medical treatment for AAA**

1. The histopathologic features of the disease in patients are carefully investigated and described.
2. Animal models that recapitulate the features of the disease in humans are developed.
3. Pharmacologic agents that inhibit aneurysm development in these animal models are identified.
4. Feasibility and safety trials must be done to demonstrate the safety of the pharmacologic agent in patients with aortic aneurysms.
5. The pharmacologic agent is tested in clinical trials in patients with aortic aneurysms.

initial inciting event for aneurysm formation in individuals with a genetic pre-disposition to this problem.[8] In any case, the inflammation is associated with changes in the structural matrix of the aorta. Since the aorta is a large conduct-ing vessel, the main role of the smooth muscle cells (SMC) is the production and maintenance of the structural matrix proteins. Collagen and elastin are the predominant proteins. Since we know that the aorta is capable of maintaining this critical function for 100 years or more in some individuals, one would anticipate that these important proteins would be resistant to damage by en-zymes. The half-life of elastin is measured in decades.[9] Since these proteins do undergo structural changes during growth and development, proteases capable of degrading them are essential. These enzymes are produced at low levels and maintained in an inactive state in the normal aorta. Following the development of inflammation, a complex remodeling process is induced. This results in dis-ruption of the orderly lamellar architecture. In the initial stages of this process, a reparative effort occurs resulting in the accumulation of collagen with no significant attenuation of the aortic wall. Eventually, typically at a point when the aorta reaches twice its normal size, this mechanism fails and the aortic wall becomes susceptible to failure.

That proteases play a role in the aneurysm development and expansion has been well documented by their presence in human aneurysm tissue and by their requirements in animal models of aortic aneurysm. Experimental studies have identified two specific members of the matrix metalloproteinase (MMP) family of the required for aneurysm formation, MMP-2 and MMP-9.[10,11] Both proteases are present in abundance in human aneurysm tissue. Invading inflam-matory cells are believed to be directly responsible for MMP-9 and indirectly for MMP-2 stimulating its production by the resident SMC and fibroblasts. Inhibiting this inflammatory cascade is one potential strategy to attack this problem. Aspirin and statins are two types of anti-inflammatory medications in common use by patients with AAA. Recent experimental work has identified proximal molecular events that alter the milieu of the aortic wall in favoring a proteolytic environment. One member of a family of mitogen-activated kinases, c-jun N-terminal kinase (JNK), appears to work as a switch, simultaneously decreasing matrix production and increasing protease expression.[12] By target-ing JNK overexpression, not only were aneurysms prevented but, remarkably, existing aneurysms were found to regress.

Blocking MMP production is one of the most obvious approaches to the medical treatment of AAA. One potent family of MMP inhibitors is the hy-droxamic acid derivatives. Recognizing the role of MMPs in angiogenesis and tumor metastasis, there was great enthusiasm for the development of these agents during the 1990s. Early clinical trial results were disappointing and fibrosis was an alarming side effect that appeared early in the clinical tri-als. Considering this potential problem and the probable need for long-term treatment of AAA, the risk to benefit ratio is unfavorable, especially in condi-tions that may be treatable by other means. In 1985 the tetracycline antibiotics were found to be active against MMPs.[13] In comparison to the hydroxamate inhibitors, the tetracyclines are much less potent. Subsequent work since the initial discovery has shown that this effect is not related to the antibiotic moiety of the protein. In fact, nonantibiotic-modified tetracyclines have been developed and are effective MMP inhibitors. Doxycycline was shown to inhibit aneurysm formation in a rodent model of aneurysms in 1996.[14] Subsequent work has shown it to be effective in essentially every model of aortic aneurysm in which it has been tested. The plasma levels required to achieve inhibition are similar to those that can be expected in patients taking standard doses of doxycycline.[15] Furthermore, a short course of preoperative doxycycline has been shown to inhibit the MMP content of the aneurysmal aorta.[16] There has been a single small randomized trial assessing the ability of doxycycline to inhibit the growth of aortic aneurysms. At 6 and 12 months, there was no growth noted in doxycycline-treated patients.[17] Taken together, these data suggest that doxycycline could be an effective therapy for treating aneurysms.

In developing a medical treatment for AAA, there are a number of issues to consider. An ideal pharmacologic agent would be curative after a short treatment course. This paradigm occurs in acute infection or uncomplicated peptic ulcer disease. A more likely option for AAA would be long-term treatment that prevents disease progression akin to the approach now taken for atherosclerosis. Growth arrest would be ideal, but decreasing the rate of growth could also have a major impact on the management of AAA. The impact of growth inhibition on the progression of aneurysm expansion is shown in FIGURE 1 considering three scenarios: 30%, 40%, or 50% inhibition of growth rate. Since most patients with AAA are in their seventh or eighth decades, a significant reduction in the aneurysm growth rate may alleviate the need for repair. This is especially true for the high-risk population where all cause mortality is as high as 8% per year.[18] That AAA might be cured by medical treatment is something that many of us had never considered in the past. Yoshimura et al. reported in December 2005 that regression of an existing aneurysm could be achieved in animal models of aortic aneurysm.[12] Some complex and potentially irreversible aspects of chronic disease cannot, however, be recapitulated in these acute models. While regression should be the ultimate goal, inhibiting progression of small aneurysms may be a more achievable goal in the short term. We have learned an important message from two clinical trials assessing the effects of propranolol on AAA growth.[19,20] The therapy failed in both studies in large part because of poor compliance.

Because of their advanced age and the strong association between smoking and AAA, many of the patients have multiple medical problems. Hypertension and elevated cholesterol are common in AAA patients. This raises a number of practical considerations in developing a clinical trial to inhibit AAA expansion. The American Heart Association has developed recommendations and parameters for treatment of hypertension and hypercholesterolemia. Since these Adult Treatment Protocols, which are in their third iteration (hence,

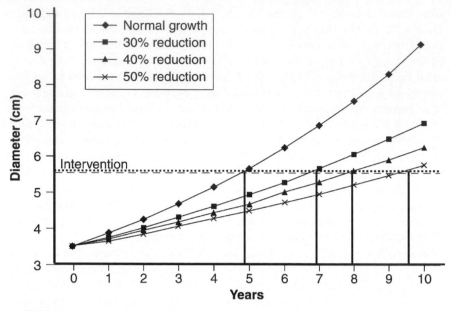

**FIGURE 1.** Aneurysm growth.

ATP III), are accepted as the standard of care, they must generally be adhered to in clinical trials. Thus, while substitution of medications that achieve prescribed goals for hypertension and lipid levels is common in clinical trials, it is much more difficult to develop and recruit patients to a randomized protocol that calls for withholding standard therapy. This is one reason that assessing the role of anti-inflammatory medication such as aspirin or the statins would be difficult to test in a randomized trial. If the therapies to be tested involved newly developed drugs, the arduous task of safety and feasibility testing is required by the FDA. In this regard, setting up clinical studies using existing medications is far more expeditious. The tetracycline antibiotics and antihypertensive working through the angiotensin axis are two potential candidates since they have been shown to inhibit the proteolytic enzymes implicated in AAA.[21]

In summary, AAA is a chronic condition that occurs in the elderly. Based on the average expansion rate for small aneurysms, there is a period of at least 5 years from the point when the aorta is first considered aneurysmal (3.0–3.5 cm) until it reaches a size where intervention would be considered (5–5.0 cm). This period of time represents an opportunity for medical treatment designed to stop or slow aneurysm progression. This approach would be most beneficial to those patients at high risk for repair. There is strong preliminary information to support a clinical trial of doxycycline to inhibit aneurysm expansion.

## REFERENCES

1. NATIONAL CENTER FOR HEALTH STATISTICS. 2002. Deaths, percent of total deaths, and death rates for the 10 leading causes of death in selected age groups, by race and sex: United States, 2000. National Vital Statistics Report. Accessed at www.cdc.gov/nchs/fastats/pdf/nvsr50_16t1.pdf on 15 November 2004.
2. LEDERLE, F.A., J.T. POWELL & R.M. GREENHALGH. 2006. Repair of small abdominal aortic aneurysms. N. Engl. J. Med. **354:** 1537–1538.
3. FLEMING, C., E.P. WHITLOCK, T.L. BEIL & F.A. LEDERLE. 2005. Screening for abdominal aortic aneurysm: a best-evidence systematic review for the U.S. Preventive Services Task Force. Ann. Intern. Med. **142:** 203–211.
4. BRADY, A.R., S.G. THOMPSON, F.G. FOWKES, et al. 2004. UK Small Aneurysm Trial Participants. Abdominal aortic aneurysm expansion: risk factors and time intervals for surveillance. Circulation. **110:** 16–21.
5. LINDHOLT, J.S., S. VAMMEN, H. FASTING & E.W. HENNEBERG. 2000. Psychological consequences of screening for abdominal aortic aneurysm and conservative treatment of small abdominal aortic aneurysms. Eur. J. Vasc. Endovasc. Surg. **20:** 79–83.
6. CAO, P., CAESAR TRIAL COLLABORATORS. 2005. Comparison of Surveillance vs. Aortic Endografting for Small Aneurysm Repair (CAESAR) trial: study design and progress. Eur. J. Vasc. Endovasc. Surg. **30:** 245–251.
7. BERTGES, D.J., R.M. ZWOLAK, D.H. DEATON, et al. 2003. Current hospital costs and medicare reimbursement for endovascular abdominal aortic aneurysm repair. J. Vasc. Surg. **37:** 272–279.
8. MILLONIG, G., G.T. MALCOM & G. WICK. 2002. Early inflammatory-immunological lesions in juvenile atherosclerosis from the Pathobiological Determinants of Atherosclerosis in Youth (PDAY)-study. Atherosclerosis. **160:** 441–448.
9. SHAPIRO, S.D., S.K. ENDICOTT, M.A. PROVINCE, et al. 1991. Marked longevity of human lung parenchymal elastic fibers deduced from prevalence of D-aspartate and nuclear weapons-related radiocarbon. J. Clin. Invest. **87:** 1828–1834.
10. LONGO, G.M., W. XIONG, T.C. GREINER, et al. 2002. Matrix metalloproteinases 2 and 9 work in concert to produce aortic aneurysms. J. Clin. Invest. **110:** 625–632.
11. PYO, R., J.K. LEE, J.M. SHIPLEY, et al. 2000. Targeted gene disruption of matrix metalloproteinase-9 (gelatinase B) suppresses development of experimental abdominal aortic aneurysms. J. Clin. Invest. **105:** 1641–1649.
12. YOSHIMURA, K., H. AOKI, Y. IKEDA, et al. 2005. Regression of abdominal aortic aneurysm by inhibition of c-Jun N-terminal kinase. Nat. Med. **11:** 1330–1338.
13. GOLUB, L.M., M. WOLFF, H.M. LEE, et al. 1985. Further evidence that tetracyclines inhibit collagenase activity in human crevicular fluid and from other mammalian sources. J. Periodontal Res. **20:** 12–23.
14. PETRINEC, D., S. LIAO, D.R. HOLMES, et al. 1996. Doxycycline inhibition of aneurysmal degeneration in an elastase-induced rat model of abdominal aortic aneurysm: preservation of aortic elastin associated with suppressed production of 92 kD gelatinase. J Vasc Surg. **23:** 336–346.
15. PRALL, A.K., G.M. LONGO, W.G. MAYHAN, et al. 2002. Doxycycline in patients with abdominal aortic aneurysms and in mice: comparison of serum levels and effect on aneurysm growth in mice. J. Vasc. Surg. **35:** 923–929.

16. CURCI, J.A., D. MAO, D.G. BOHNER, *et al.* 2000. Preoperative treatment with doxycycline reduces aortic wall expression and activation of matrix metalloproteinases in patients with abdominal aortic aneurysms. J. Vasc. Surg. **31:** 325–342.
17. MOSORIN, M., J. JUVONEN, F. BIANCARI, *et al.* 2001. Use of doxycycline to decrease the growth rate of abdominal aortic aneurysms: a randomized, double-blind, placebo-controlled pilot study. J. Vasc. Surg. **34:** 606–610.
18. EVAR TRIAL PARTICIPANTS. 2005. Endovascular aneurysm repair and outcome in patients unfit for open repair of abdominal aortic aneurysm (EVAR trial 2): randomised controlled trial. Lancet. **365:** 2187–2192.
19. PROPANOLOL ANEURYSM TRIAL INVESTIGATORS. 2002. Propranolol for small abdominal aortic aneurysms: results of a randomized trial. J. Vasc. Surg. **35:** 72–79.
20. LINDHOLT, J.S., E.W. HENNEBERG, S. JUUL & H. FASTING. 1999. Impaired results of a randomised double blinded clinical trial of propranolol versus placebo on the expansion rate of small abdominal aortic aneurysms. Int. Angiol. **18:** 52–57.
21. HABASHI, J.P., D.P. JUDGE, T.M. HOLM, *et al.* 2006. Losartan, an AT1 antagonist, prevents aortic aneurysm in a mouse model of Marfan syndrome. Science. **312:** 117–121.

# Should Usual Criteria for Intervention in Abdominal Aortic Aneurysms Be "Downsized," Considering Reported Risk Reduction with Endovascular Repair?

MARC SCHERMERHORN

*Beth Israel Deaconess Medical Center, Boston, MA, USA*

ABSTRACT: Two randomized trials have demonstrated the safety of waiting until abdominal aortic aneurysm (AAA) diameter reaches 5.5 cm for repair in most patients. Other recent randomized trials have demonstrated lower perioperative mortality and morbidity with endovascular aneurysm repair (EVAR) compared to open surgery. Therefore, it is logical to assume that endovascular repair may change the appropriate threshold for intervention. However, endovascular repair is not as durable as open surgery and is associated with ongoing risks of rupture and reintervention. Decision analysis based on data available in 1998 showed that endovascular repair should not change the threshold for intervention. Since that time retrospective data have emerged to suggest that outcomes with endovascular repair are improved in smaller AAAs, although this may simply represent selection bias and the natural history of small AAAs. Randomized trials are appropriate to determine whether improved endovascular outcomes in small AAAs reduce late rupture and reintervention enough to justify early intervention in patients with appropriate anatomy. In the absence of data from these trials, the threshold for intervention should not be changed.

KEYWORDS: endovascular; aneurysm; threshold; aorta

## USUAL CRITERIA FOR INTERVENTION

The United Kingdom Small Aneurysm Trial (UKSAT) and the Aneurysm Detection and Management (ADAM) trial both demonstrated no benefit to early surgery for small abdominal aortic aneurysms (AAAs) (4.0–5.5 cm).[1,2] An annual rupture risk under surveillance of 1.0% (UKSAT) and 0.6% (ADAM) were offset by the operative mortality in the early surgery groups

Address for correspondence: Marc Schermerhorn, M.D., Beth Israel Deaconess Medical Center, 110 Francis St. 5B, Boston, MA 02215, USA. Voice: 617-632-9971; fax: 617-632-7977.
e-mail: mscherm@bidmc.harvard.edu

Ann. N.Y. Acad. Sci. 1085: 47–58 (2006). © 2006 New York Academy of Sciences.
doi: 10.1196/annals.1383.043

of 5.6% (UKSAT) and 2.2% (ADAM). The inclusion criteria in ADAM were more restrictive of those with severe cardiopulmonary disease, which likely explains the lower operative mortality. Approximately 70% of patients randomized to surveillance eventually underwent repair with an operative mortality of 7.2% (UKSAT) and 2.1% (ADAM).[3] In the U.K. trial, fatal rupture occurred in 5% of men and 14% of women undergoing surveillance. Women were four times as likely to rupture during surveillance as men. Therefore, a lower threshold seems appropriate for women. Compliance with surveillance in general practice may not be as good as in randomized trials. Valentine and associates reported that 32 of 101 patients undergoing AAA surveillance were not compliant despite several appointment reminders and 3 or 4 of these 32 patients experienced rupture.[4] Together, these randomized trials demonstrate that it is safe to wait for AAA diameter to reach 5.5 cm before repair in selected men who would be compliant with surveillance, even if their operative mortality was predicted to be low.

Because all AAAs do not rupture at the same diameter, it would seem prudent to consider other factors that increase rupture risk when deciding whether to repair an AAA in an individual patient. Rupture risk is increased by female gender, smoking status (current > former > never), hypertension, and chronic lung disease.[5–7] Other possible risk factors for rupture include family history, rapid expansion, and eccentric shape (increased wall stress).[8–13]

The operative risk and life expectancy of the patient should also be considered when determining the appropriateness of AAA repair in a given patient.[14,15] In a young and reasonably healthy patient with an estimated operative risk of 1–2%, a long life expectancy, and who is a hypertensive smoker with a 4.8 cm AAA, there is a very high likelihood that the AAA will eventually reach 5.5 cm and there is a finite risk of rupture in the interim. For this patient, it is not unreasonable to recommend surgery at a time when it is convenient for the patient. For the elderly patient in poor health with very high operative risk and limited life expectancy it is reasonable to recommend no surgery even at 5.5 cm or greater. Patient preferences regarding the upfront risk of surgery versus the ongoing risk of rupture must also be considered.

## RISK REDUCTION WITH ENDOVASCULAR REPAIR

### Perioperative Outcomes

Two recent randomized trials have demonstrated lower perioperative mortality and morbidity with endovascular aneurysm repair (EVAR) than open repair in patients with AAA diameter >5.5 cm. The Dutch Randomized Endovascular Aneurysm Management (DREAM) trial showed a 4-fold risk reduction in operative mortality with endovascular repair (4.6% vs. 1.2%) and a 2-fold risk reduction in death or severe complications (9.8% vs. 4.7%).[16] The larger EVAR-1 trial demonstrated a significantly lower 30-day mortality with endovascular repair (1.7% vs. 4.7%).[17] Lower mortality with endovascular repair has also been shown in the general population using administrative data (1.3% vs. 3.8%) despite the fact that the endovascular population tended to be older.[18] Low operative mortality has also been demonstrated in large registries of endovascular repair including EUROSTAR (2.8%) and the Lifeline registry (1.7%)[19,20] These trials also demonstrated shorter procedure time, shorter ICU and hospital length of stay, and decreased blood loss with endovascular repair.

## Mid-Term and Late Outcomes

The EVAR-1 and DREAM trials recently published 4-year and 2-year results (respectively) of open versus endovascular repair.[21,22] The smaller DREAM trial was not designed or powered to examine long-term outcomes. However, the results of the EVAR-1 trial were similar to those of DREAM in that the initial 3% mortality reduction seen with endovascular repair persisted as a 3% reduction in AAA-related mortality at 4 years, but there was no difference in overall mortality at 4 years. Potential reasons for a lack of overall mortality benefit despite a reduction in AAA-related mortality include:

(1) chance;
(2) open repair may have caused the death of frail patients who would have died in the near future anyway; and
(3) complications of endovascular repair that are missed such as death due to rupture that is labeled as cardiac arrest.

Late complications and reintervention were more likely after endovascular repair. Kaplan-Meier estimates of freedom from complications were 59% for endovascular repair and 91% for open repair at 4 years. However, nearly half of the complications with endovascular repair were type II endoleak, which in the absence of AAA sac expansion is typically considered benign. Four year freedom from reintervention was 80% for endovascular repair and 94% for open repair. Endovascular repair was also more costly than open repair. Long-term results of EVAR-1 will be forthcoming. Other randomized trials are underway in the U.S. veteran population as well as in France.

In the EUROSTAR registry, the long-term data are predominantly from stent grafts that have been withdrawn from the market. As of March 2002, 34 ruptures were noted in 4,291 patients entered in EUROSTAR.[23] A total of 74% of these ruptures occurred in patients treated with grafts that are no longer available. The annual rupture risk was 1%.[24] Risk factors for rupture included type I endoleak, type III endoleak, graft migration, and postoperative kinking of the endograft. Conversion to open repair occurred in 2% per year. Of those with at least 1-year follow-up ($n = 1,023$), reintervention of any kind was performed in 18%.[25] Kaplan-Meier estimates of freedom from reintervention were 89% at 1 year, 67% at 3 years, and 62% at 4 years. Again, the majority of reinterventions was performed in those with endografts that were subsequently withdrawn from the market. In a single center study, Verhoeven and colleagues demonstrated a significantly higher rate of reintervention for the Vanguard device compared to the Talent, Excluder, or Zenith devices using Kaplan-Meier analysis.[26]

The Lifeline registry includes data from the IDE clinical trials of four FDA approved devices (Ancure, AneuRx, Excluder, and Powerlink).[20] These trials were conducted at sites with the greatest experience with endovascular repair and typically required strict adherence to appropriate anatomy for stent grafting. In this setting excellent results were obtained. Freedom from AAA-related death was 98% at 6 years. Freedom from rupture was 99% at 6 years. Freedom from conversion to open repair was 95% at 6 years and freedom from reintervention was 78% at 5 years. This demonstrates that with experience, careful patient selection, careful surveillance, and reintervention when needed, excellent long-term results may be obtained with endovascular repair, albeit with a substantial need for reintervention.

After open AAA repair, late complications may also occur. Hallett and colleagues published data with a 6-year mean follow-up on 307 patients undergoing open AAA repair at the Mayo Clinic looking at graft-related complications.[27] Complications included anastomotic pseudoaneurysm 3.0%, graft thrombosis 2.0%, graft-enteric erosion/fistula 1.6%, graft infection 1.3%, anastomotic hemorrhage 1.3%, colon ischemia 0.7%, and atheroembolism 0.3%. Mortality due to graft-related complications was 2.6%. Kaplan-Meier 5-year freedom estimates were 98% for pseudoaneurysm, 98% for graft-enteric erosion/infection, and 98% for graft thrombosis. Biancari and colleagues recently published similar data from 208 open AAA repairs in Finland with a median follow-up of 8 years.[28] Late graft-related complications occurred in 15%. These included proximal pseudoaneurysm 2.9%, distal pseudoaneurysm 8.7%, graft occlusion 5.3%. Overall, 13% of patients required surgical or other invasive intervention. Kaplan-Meier 5-year freedom estimates were 92% for reintervention, and 94% for vascular reintervention. Little data exist regarding the incidence of non-graft-related complications of open AAA repair such as bowel obstruction or incisional hernia, which may require laparotomy.

## MARKOV MODELING OF APPROPRIATE THRESHOLD FOR ENDOVASCULAR REPAIR

If operative mortality for AAA repair were zero and late rupture or reintervention were also zero, we would repair essentially all AAAs regardless of diameter. Because these risks are not zero, one must balance them against the risk of rupture to determine the appropriate threshold for repair. Finlayson and colleagues performed an elegant decision analysis using Markov modeling to determine whether endovascular repair should lower the threshold for intervention.[29] Their analysis was based on data available in 1998. Their base case analysis was for average 70-year-old men. The major assumptions for

TABLE 1. Assumptions from decision analysis by Finlayson and colleagues[29]

| Parameter | Baseline value | Range tested in sensitivity analysis |
|---|---|---|
| Operative mortality | | |
|   Open | 4% | 2–8% |
|   Endovascular | 1% | 0.5–5% |
| Early conversion to open | 5% | 1–15% |
| Late conversion (annual rate) | 1% | 0–10% |
| Operative mortality with early conversion | 11% | 5.5–22% |
| Operative mortality with late conversion | 7% | 3.5–14% |

their analysis (TABLE 1) are remarkably similar to those from subsequent randomized trials and large registries summarized above. They assumed a rupture risk under surveillance of 1% per year for AAA 4.0–4.9 cm, which also was also corroborated by the United Kingdom Small Aneurysm Trial. They did not consider late rupture as this had not been reported widely at the time. They also did not consider late endovascular reintervention separate from conversion to open repair. They did consider that anatomic suitability for endovascular repair may decrease as AAA diameter increases but only to a small extent until the AAA reached 7 cm (2% per cm expansion when <7 cm and 20% per cm expansion for those >7 cm) based on available data at the time.[30] To simulate poor health, operative mortality and morbidity were doubled and age specific life expectancy was shortened to reflect that of a person 8 years older.

They found that endovascular repair did not change the appropriate threshold for repair relative to open repair except in elderly patients in poor health. However, the net benefit of repair (compared with no repair at all) in these elderly patients in poor health was relatively small. In their analysis, they found that endovascular repair consistently resulted in greater quality-adjusted life expectancy compared to open repair but the benefit was very small. In sensitivity analysis the benefit of endovascular repair disappeared when endovascular operative mortality exceeded 3.5% or annual rate of conversion to open repair exceeded 6%. These results were similar to those in a subsequent decision analysis comparing life expectancy after open repair or endovascular repair based on data from EUROSTAR for endovascular repair and Medicare data for open repair.[31] In this report, there was little difference in life expectancy between the two methods, although for younger patients with low operative risk open repair may be preferred while for older patients with higher operative risk endovascular repair may be preferred.

## ENDOVASCULAR REPAIR IN THOSE "UNFIT" FOR OPEN REPAIR

The contention that the threshold for intervention may be reduced in those older patients in poor health is not supported by the recent EVAR-2 trial.[32] In this trial patients with AAAs > 5.5 cm who were not considered suitable for open repair were randomized to endovascular repair or observation. There was no benefit to endovascular repair compared to observation seen in this trial. However, the operative mortality in the "repair" group was high (9.0%). Nine patients (5.4%) randomized to endovascular repair died due to rupture prior to the planned repair. Eight (4.8%) patients died of other causes prior to surgery. Those randomized to repair that in fact underwent repair did so at a median of 57 days. Only 87% had successful implantation of the stent graft. A total of 47 patients (27%) randomized to observation underwent repair against protocol with an operative mortality of only 2%. From these data, it seems that further selection of patients unfit for endovascular repair may be possible and that once such a determination is made repair should be undertaken expeditiously in those deemed fit. However, if life expectancy is short, the benefit of repair is likely to be small, even with low operative mortality as predicted by Finlayson and colleagues.[29]

## OUTCOMES OF SMALL VS. LARGE AAA REPAIR

Several reports have noted that outcomes after endovascular repair are worse for larger AAAs compared with smaller AAAs. Rockman and colleagues noted that larger AAAs treated with endovascular repair were more likely to have endoleaks in general and type I endoleak in particular.[33] Larger AAA diameter was associated with shorter proximal necks and greater neck angulation. Ouriel and colleagues noted that larger aneurysm diameter was associated with more type I endoleaks, device migration, conversion to open repair, and had higher AAA-related mortality and overall mortality.[34] Peppelenbosch and colleagues reported EUROSTAR data demonstrating that larger AAA diameter was associated with increased type I endoleak, systemic complications, perioperative mortality, late rupture, AAA-related mortality, and overall mortality.[35] In the Lifeline registry, larger AAA diameter was also associated with increased late rupture risk, late conversion to open repair, AAA-related mortality, and overall mortality.[20]

It is unknown if such a relationship exists for open surgery. Given these observations, several have suggested that endovascular repair may be more beneficial in smaller AAAs.[34,35] These observations were not available for consideration in the Markov modeling of Finlayson and colleagues.[29] If short necks and greater angulation are associated with larger AAA diameter in retrospective analysis of patients treated with endovascular repair, it begs the question as to whether these characteristics and subsequent outcomes are truly associated with AAA diameter, or if we are simply more likely to "push the envelope" in terms of anatomic suitability in patients with larger AAAs who we do not deem to be good candidates for open repair. The difference in rupture risk and AAA-related mortality may be simply due to the natural history of small AAAs and would be expected to be observed without repair and perhaps with open surgery as well.

## CANDIDACY FOR ENDOVASCULAR REPAIR: SMALL VS. LARGE

If larger AAA diameter is associated with shorter, wider, and more angulated necks, it suggests that candidacy for endovascular repair would decrease with increasing diameter. Armon and colleagues found that AAAs 4–5.5 cm were no more likely to be candidates for endovascular repair than those 5.5–7 cm but that diameter >7 cm was associated with shorter and wider proximal necks.[30] However, Welborn and colleagues found AAAs <5.5 cm had longer necks, less angulation, less tortuosity, and longer iliac landing zones than those >5.5 cm.[36] With each increase in diameter of 1 cm, anatomic suitability for endovascular repair decreased 5-fold. Others have also found a correlation with AAA diameter and suitability for endovascular repair.[37] Arko and colleagues found AAA diameter to be related to neck diameter and length but did not find AAA diameter to be associated with overall suitability for endovascular repair.[38] Resch and colleagues found no correlation between AAA diameter and neck measurements.[39] Lee and colleagues noted that ruptured AAAs had a larger diameter than asymptomatic AAAs and were less likely to be candidates for endovascular repair (46% vs. 74%) due primarily to unfavorable neck anatomy.[40] This was confirmed by others.[41,42] It is unclear if the relationship between rupture and candidacy for endovascular repair is simply confounded by larger diameter of ruptured AAAs, or if there is a true association between anatomic suitability for endovascular repair and rupture at a given diameter.

In the EVAR-1 trial, 54% of patients with AAAs ≥5.5 cm were anatomically suitable for endovascular repair.[17] This number is likely to be dependent on referral patterns, technologic advances, and adherence to the manufacturers' instructions for use. Overall the relationship between AAA diameter and candidacy for endovascular repair remains unclear.

## THE OTHER ENDOLEAK: OPERATING OUTSIDE THE IFU

Several reports have demonstrated inferior results with endovascular repair in those whose anatomy does not meet the criteria outlined in the instructions for use (IFU). Sternbergh and colleagues noted that with excess oversizing (>30%) of the Zenith graft there was a 14% migration rate compared to 1% with ≤30% oversizing.[43] They also noted decreased sac shrinkage (48% vs. 77%) and increased sac enlargement (9.5% vs. 0.6%) with excess oversizing. Connors and colleagues found >20% oversizing to be associated with neck dilation and migration with the AneuRx device.[44] Mohan and colleagues found increased type I endoleak with oversizing <10%.[45] Most device manufacturers recommend oversizing 10–20%. Albertini and colleagues found neck angulation to correspond to type I endoleak and migration.[46] Zarins and colleagues noted that migration and rupture are associated with shorter proximal fixation length and longer distance from the renal artery to the stent graft (graft deployed too low).[47,48] Azizzadeh and colleagues relate that the migration rate was 5% in patients in whom the IFU were followed and 40% in non-IFU patients.[49] Clearly, if endovascular intervention is going to be utilized in small aneurysms, it is imperative that patients be selected with anatomy that is favorable and within the IFU for the specific device to be implanted.

## RANDOMIZED TRIALS

It appears that outcomes after endovascular AAA repair are better in smaller diameter AAAs. Several questions remain.

(1) Are outcomes better because the anatomy is more favorable at smaller diameters or do we choose better candidates for repair at smaller diameters?

(2) Are those with 4–5 cm diameters more likely to be candidates for endovascular repair than those with a diameter of 5–5.5 cm?

(3) If stentgraft failure increases over time and technological advances have already and will theoretically continue to improve outcomes, are we not better off waiting until the diameter (rupture risk) increases?

The UKSAT and the ADAM trial already demonstrated that the majority of patients with small AAAs will ultimately undergo repair due to growth or development of symptoms. By operating on small AAAs (4–5 cm), the operative mortality will cause the death of some patients who would have died at a later date due to other causes without rupture of their AAA. Endovascular repair has lower operative mortality than open repair (used in the UKSAT and ADAM). If by operating on AAAs at a smaller diameter the long-term results are improved compared to those of larger AAAs and future ruptures are prevented, the overall survival may be improved compared to a strategy of waiting until diameter reaches 5–5.5 cm or greater. It is also possible that some patients who would be candidates for endovascular repair at 4–5 cm are no longer candidates at 5.5 cm and therefore would be subjected to the increased perioperative mortality of open surgery. If early intervention does improve outcomes, to what proportion of AAA patients does this data apply (how many patients with small AAAs are suitable candidates)?

Two randomized trials are currently underway to address these issues: the PIVOTAL study (Positive Impact of endoVascular Options for Treating Aneruysms earLy) and the CAESAR Trial (Comparison of surveillance vs.

Aortic Endografting for Small Aneurysms Repair).[50] These trials will compare a strategy of early endovascular AAA repair versus waiting until the diameter reaches 5.0 cm (PIVOTAL) or 5.5 cm (CAESAR). They will assess the proportion of patients with small AAAs who are candidates for endovascular repair, and determine what proportion remain candidates after waiting for AAA growth to the specified diameter. They will compare all-cause mortality, AAA-related mortality, rupture, AAA growth or shrinkage, perioperative and late complications, reintervention, conversion to open repair, quality of life, and costs.

## CONCLUSIONS

Endovascular repair has lower perioperative mortality, morbidity, and lower midterm AAA-related mortality but increased costs, late reintervention, and late rupture risk. Technological advances and appropriate patient selection may decrease late ruptures and the need for reintervention. Based on currently available data, there does not appear to be evidence to support the routine use of endovascular AAA repair for those with small AAAs. The appropriate threshold for intervention should be individualized based on each patient's rupture risk (of which diameter is one component), operative risk (which is modified by endovascular repair), life expectancy, and the durability of repair (which for endovascular repair remains to be seen) as well as each patient's preference for immediate versus deferred risk. Finlayson's analysis suggested that endovascular repair should not change the threshold for repair compared to open surgery except in elderly patients in poor health in whom any repair is of questionable value. Subsequent data suggest that outcomes with endovascular repair may be improved in smaller diameter aortas, although this may simply represent selection bias and the natural history of small AAAs. At the current time, it seems most appropriate to enroll willing patients with small aneurysms in randomized trials to determine whether early endovascular intervention will ultimately improve outcomes.

## REFERENCES

1. The United Kingdom Small Aneurysm Trial Participants. 1998. Mortality results for randomized controlled trial of early elective surgery or ultrasonographic surveillance for small abdominal aortic aneurysms. Lancet **352:** 1649–1655.
2. LEDERLE, F.A., S.E. WILSON, G.R. JOHNSON, et al. 2002. Immediate repair compared with surveillance of small abdominal aortic aneurysms. N. Engl. J. Med. **346:** 1437–1444.
3. The United Kingdom Small Aneurysm Trial Participants. 2002. Long-term outcomes of immediate repair compared with surveillance of small abdominal aortic aneurysms. N. Engl. J. Med. **346:** 1445–1452.

4. VALENTINE, R.J., J.D. DECAPRIO, J.M. CASTILLO, *et al.* 2000. Watchful waiting in cases of small abdominal aortic aneurysms- appropriate for all patients? J. Vasc. Surg. **32:** 441–448; Discussion 448–450.

5. BROWN, L.C. & J.T. POWELL. 1999. Risk factors for aneurysm rupture in patients kept under ultrasound surveillance. UK Small Aneurysm Trial Participants. Ann. Surg. **230:** 289–296; Discussion 296–297.

6. CRONENWETT, J.L., T.F. MURPHY & G.B. ZELENOCK, *et al.* 1985. Actuarial analysis of variables associated with rupture of small abdominal aortic aneurysms. Surgery **98:** 472–483.

7. STERPETTI, A.V., A. CAVALLARO, N. CAVALLARI, *et al.* 1991. Factors influencing the rupture of abdominal aortic aneurysms. Surg. Gynecol. Obstet. **173:** 175–178.

8. DARLING, R.C., III, D.C. BREWSTER, R.C. DARLING, *et al.* 1989. Are familial abdominal aortic aneurysms different? J. Vasc. Surg. **10:** 39–43.

9. VERLOES, A., N. SAKALIHASAN, L. KOULISCHER, *et al.* 1995. Aneurysms of the abdominal aorta: familial and genetic aspects in three hundred thirteen pedigrees. J. Vasc. Surg. **21:** 646–655.

10. LIMET, R., N. SAKALIHASSAN & A. ALBERT. 1991. Determination of the expansion rate and incidence of rupture of abdominal aortic aneurysms. J. Vasc. Surg. **14:** 540–548.

11. SCHEWE, C.K., H.P. SCHWEIKART, G. HAMMEL, *et al.* 1994. Influence of selective management on the prognosis and the risk of rupture of abdominal aortic aneurysms. Clin. Investig. **72:** 585–591.

12. FILLINGER, M.F., S.P. MARRA, M.L. RAGHAVAN, *et al.* 2003. Prediction of rupture risk in abdominal aortic aneurysm during observation: wall stress versus diameter. J. Vasc. Surg. **37:** 724–732.

13. FILLINGER, M.F., M.L. RAGHAVAN, S.P. MARRA, *et al.* 2002. In vivo analysis of mechanical wall stress and abdominal aortic aneurysm rupture risk. J. Vasc. Surg. **36:** 589–597.

14. KATZ, D.A., B. LITTENBERG & J.L. CRONENWETT. 1992. Management of small abdominal aortic aneurysms. Early surgery vs. watchful waiting. JAMA **268:** 2678–2686.

15. SCHERMERHORN, M.L., J.D. BIRKMEYER & D.A. GOULD, *et al.* 2000. Cost-effectiveness of surgery for small abdominal aortic aneurysms on the basis of data from the United Kingdom small aneurysm trial. J. Vasc. Surg. **31:** 217–226.

16. PRINSSEN, M., E.L. VERHOEVEN, J. BETH, *et al.* 2004. A randomized trial comparing conventional and endovascular repair of abdominal aortic aneurysms. N. Engl. J. Med. **351:** 1607–1618.

17. GREENHALGH, R.M., L.C. BROWN, G.P. KWONG, *et al.* 2004. Comparison of endovascular aneurysm repair with open repair in patients with abdominal aortic aneurysms (EVAR trail 1), 30-day operative mortality results: randomised controlled trial. Lancet **364:** 843–848.

18. LEE, W.A., J.W. CARTER, G. UPCHURCH, *et al.* 2004. Perioperative outcomes after open and endovascular repair of intact abdominal aortic aneurysms in the United States during 2001. J. Vasc. Surg. **39:** 491–496.

19. BIANCARI, F., R. HOBO & T. JUVONEN. 2006. Glasgow Aneurysm Score predicts survival after endovascular stenting of abdominal aortic aneurysm in patients from the EUROSTAR registry. Br. J. Surg. **93:** 191–194.

20. Lifeline Registry of EVAR Publications Committee. 2005. Lifeline registry of endovascular aneurysm repair: long-term primary outcome measures. J. Vasc. Surg. **42:** 1–10.

21. EVAR trial participants. 2005. Endovascular aneurysm repair versus open repair in patients with abdominal aortic aneurysm (EVAR trial 1): randomised controlled trial. Lancet **365:** 2179–2186.
22. BLANKENSTEIJN, J.D., S.E. DE JONG, M. PRINSSEN, *et al.* 2005. Two-year outcomes after conventional or endovascular repair of abdominal aortic aneurysms. N. Engl. J. Med. **352:** 2398–2405.
23. FRANSEN, G.A., S.R. VALLABHANENI, C.J. VAN MARREWIJK, *et al.* 2003. Rupture of infra-renal aortic aneurysm after endovascular repair: a series from EUROSTAR registry. Eur. J. Vasc. Endovasc. Surg. **26:** 487–493.
24. HARRIS, P.L., S.R. VALLABHANENI, P. DESGRANGES, *et al.* 2000. Incidence and risk factors of late rupture, conversion, and death after endovascular repair of infrarenal aortic aneurysms: the EUROSTAR experience. European collaborators on stent/graft techniques for aortic aneurysm repair. J. Vasc. Surg. **32:** 739–749.
25. LAHEIJ, R.J., J. BUTH, P.L. HARRIS, *et al.* 2000. Need for secondary interventions after endovascular repair of abdominal aortic aneurysms. Intermediate-term follow-up results of a European collaborative registry (EUROSTAR). Br. J. Surg. **87:** 1666–1673.
26. VERHOEVEN, E.L., I.F. TIELLIU, T.R. PRINS, *et al.* 2004. Frequency and outcome of re-interventions after endovascular repair for abdominal aortic aneurysm: a prospective cohort study. Eur. J. Vasc. Endovasc. Surg. **28:** 357–364.
27. HALLETT, J.W. JR., D.M. MARSHALL, T.M. PETTERSON, *et al.* 1997. Graft-related complications after abdominal aortic aneurysm repair: reassurance from a 36-year population-based experience. J. Vasc. Surg. **25:** 277–284; Discussion 285–286.
28. BIANCARI, F., K. YLONEN, V. ANTTILA, *et al.* 2002. Durability of open repair of infrarenal abdominal aortic aneurysm: a 15-year follow-up study. J. Vasc. Surg. **35:** 87–93.
29. FINLAYSON, S.R., J.D. BIRKMEYER, M.F. FILLINGER, *et al.* 1999. Should endovascular surgery lower the threshold for repair of abdominal aortic aneurysms? J. Vasc. Surg. **29:** 973–985.
30. ARMON, M.P., S.W. YUSUF, S.C. WHITAKER, *et al.* 1997. Influence of abdominal aortic aneurysm size on the feasibility of endovascular repair. J. Endovasc. Surg. **4:** 279–283.
31. SCHERMERHORN, M.L., S.R. FINLAYSON, M.F. FILLINGER, *et al.* Life expectancy after endovascular versus open abdominal aortic aneurysm repair: results of a decision analysis model on the basis of data form EUROSTAR. J. Vasc. Surg. **36:** 1112–1120.
32. EVAR trial participants. 2005. Endovascular aneurysm repair and outcome in patients unfit for open repair of abdominal aortic aneurysm (EVAR trial 2): randomised controlled trial. Lancet **365:** 2187–2192.
33. ROCKMAN, C.B., P.J. LAMPARELLO, M.A. ADELMAN, *et al.* 2002. Aneurysm morphology as a predictor of endoleak following endovascular aortic aneurysm repair: do smaller aneurysms have better outcomes? Ann. Vasc. Surg. **16:** 644–651.
34. OURIEL, K., S.D. SRIVASTAVA, T.P. SARAC, *et al.* 2003. Disparate outcome after endovascular treatment of small versus large abdominal aortic aneurysm. J. Vasc. Surg. **37:** 1206–1212.
35. PEPPELENBOSCH, N., J. BUTH, P.L. HARRIS, *et al.* 2004. Diameter of abdominal aortic aneurysm and outcome of endovascular aneurysm repair: does size matter? A report from EUROSTAR. J. Vasc. Surg. **39:** 288–297.

36. WELBORN, M.B. III, F.S. YAU, J.G. MODRALL, *et al.* 2005. Endovascular repair of small abdominal aortic aneurysms: a paradigm shift? Vasc. Endovasc. Surg. **39:** 381–391.
37. WOLF, Y.G., T.J. FOGARTY, C.I. OLCOTT, *et al.* 2000. Endovascular repair of abdominal aortic aneurysms: eligibility rate and impact on the rate of open repair. J. Vasc. Surg. **32:** 519–523.
38. ARKO, F.R., K.A. FILIS, S.A. SEIDEL, *et al.* 2004. How many patients with infrarenal aneurysms are candidates for endovascular repair? The Northern California experience. J. Endovasc. Ther. **11:** 33–40.
39. RESCH, T., K. IVANCEV, M. LINDH, *et al.* 1999. Abdominal aortic aneurysm morphology in candidates for endovascular repair evaluated with spiral computed tomography and digital subtraction angiography. J. Endovasc. Surg. **6:** 227–232.
40. LEE, W.A., T.S. HUBER, C.M. HIRNEISE, *et al.* 2002. Eligibility rates of ruptured and symptomatic AAA for endovascular repair. J. Endovasc. Surg. **9:** 436–442.
41. WILSON, W.R., G. FISHWICK, R.F.B. SIR PETER, *et al.* 2004. Suitability of ruptured AAA for endovascular repair. J. Endovasc. Ther. **11:** 635–640.
42. HINCHLIFFE, R.J., P. ALRIC, D. ROSE, *et al.* 2003. Comparison of morphologic features of intact and ruptured aneurysms of infrarenal abdominal aortia. J. Vasc. Surg. **38:** 88–92.
43. STERNBERGH, W.C., III, S.R. MONEY, R.K. GREENBERG, *et al.* 2004. Influence of endograft oversizing on device migration, endoleak, aneurysm shrinkage, and aortic neck dilation: results from the Zenith Multicenter Trial. J. Vasc. Surg. **39:** 20–26.
44. CONNERS, M.S., III, W.C. STERNBERGH, III, G. CARTER, *et al.* 2002. Endograft migration one to four years after endovascular abdominal aortic aneurysm repair with the AneuRx device: a cautionary note. J. Vasc. Surg. **36:** 476–484.
45. MOHAN, I.V., R.J. LAHEIJ & P.L. HARRIS. 2001. Risk factors for endoleak and the evidence for stent-graft oversizing in patients undergoing endovascular aneurysm repair. Eur. J. Vasc. Endovasc. Surg. **21:** 344–349.
46. ALBERTINI, J., S. KALLIAFAS, S. TRAVIS, *et al.* 2000. Anatomical risk factors for proximal perigraft endoleak and graft migration following endovascular repair of abdominal aortic aneurysms. Eur. J. Vasc. Endovasc. Surg. **19:** 308–312.
47. ZARINS, C.K., D.A. BLOCH, T. CRABTREE, *et al.* 2003. Stent graft migration after endovascular aneurysm repair: importance of proximal fixation. J. Vasc. Surg. **38:** 1264–1272.
48. ZARINS, C.K., R.A. WHITE & T.J. FOGARTY. 2000. Aneurysm rupture after endovascular repair using the AneuRx stent graft. J. Vasc. Surg. **31:** 960–970.
49. AZIZZADEH, A., L.A. SANCHEZ, B.G. RUBIN, *et al.* 2005. Aortic neck attachment failure and the AneuRx graft: incidence, treatment options, and early results. Ann. Vasc. Surg. **19:** 516–521.
50. CAO, P. 2005. Comparison of surveillance vs. aortic endografting for small aneurysm repair (CEASAR) trial: study, design and progress. Eur. J. Vasc. Endovasc. Surg. **30:** 245–251.

# Pathophysiology of Abdominal Aortic Aneurysms

## Insights from the Elastase-Induced Model in Mice with Different Genetic Backgrounds

ROBERT W. THOMPSON, JOHN A. CURCI, TERRI L. ENNIS, DONGLI MAO, MONICA B. PAGANO, AND CHRISTINE T.N. PHAM

*Departments of Surgery (Section of Vascular Surgery), Radiology, Cell Biology and Physiology, Medicine, and Pathology and Immunology, Washington University School of Medicine, St. Louis, Missouri, USA*

ABSTRACT: Abdominal aortic aneurysms (AAAs) represent a complex degenerative disorder involving chronic aortic wall inflammation and destructive remodeling of structural connective tissue. Studies using human AAA tissues have helped identify a variety of molecular mediators and matrix-degrading proteinases, which contribute to aneurysm disease, thereby providing a sound foundation for understanding AAAs; however, these human tissue specimens represent only the "end stage" of a long and progressive disease process. Further progress in understanding the pathophysiology of AAAs is therefore dependent in part on the development and application of effective animal models that recapitulate key aspects of the disease. Based on original studies in rats, transient perfusion of the abdominal aorta with porcine pancreatic elastase has provided a reproducible and robust model of AAAs. More recent applications of this model to mice have also opened new avenues for investigation. In this review, we summarize investigations using the elastase-induced mouse model of AAAs including results in animals with targeted deletion of specific genes and more general differences in mice on different genetic backgrounds. These studies have helped us identify genes that are essential to the development of AAAs (such as MMP9, IL6, and AT1R) and to reveal other genes that may be dispensable in aneurysm formation. Investigations on mice from different genetic backgrounds are also beginning to offer a novel approach to evaluate the genetic basis for susceptibility to aneurysm development.

KEYWORDS: abdominal aortic aneurysm; animal models of disease; genetically altered mice; elastase; inflammation; extracellular matrix; proteinases; cytokines; genetic susceptibility

Address for correspondence: Robert W. Thompson, M.D., Section of Vascular Surgery, Department of Surgery, Washington University School of Medicine, 5101 Queeny Tower, One Barnes-Jewish Hospital Plaza, St. Louis, Missouri, 63110. Voice: 314-362-7410; fax: 314-747-3548.
e-mail: thompson@wudosis.wustl.edu

Ann. N.Y. Acad. Sci. 1085: 59–73 (2006). © 2006 New York Academy of Sciences.
doi: 10.1196/annals.1383.029

## INTRODUCTION

Abdominal aortic aneurysms (AAAs) are a common and life-threatening degenerative disease.[1] AAAs occur in 5–9% of the population over the age of 65 years and are most frequently associated with cigarette smoking, pulmonary emphysema, coronary artery disease, and peripheral (occlusive) atherosclerosis.[2–6] AAAs arise over a period of years and most tend to gradually expand with time, and the risk of aortic rupture increases steadily with progressive aneurysm growth. Although AAAs can be readily detected in asymptomatic individuals by abdominal imaging studies, there are currently no specific therapies known to alter the natural history of small asymptomatic AAAs. Better understanding of the fundamental pathologic mechanisms that contribute to aneurysmal degeneration is therefore critical toward the development of new therapeutic approaches.

Aneurysmal degeneration is a complex process involving destructive remodeling of connective tissue throughout the affected segment of aortic wall. Four interrelated factors have been implicated in this pathological remodeling: (a) chronic inflammation within the outer aortic wall accompanied by neovascularization and elevated production of proinflammatory cytokines; (b) excessive local production and dysregulation of matrix-degrading proteinases; (c) progressive destruction of structural matrix proteins, particularly elastin and collagen, which leads to weakening and dilatation of the aortic wall; and (d) depletion of medial smooth muscle cells (SMC), which may result in an impaired capacity for connective tissue repair.[7] Structural and hemodynamic conditions unique to the human infrarenal aorta may explain the propensity for AAAs to form in this region, but the recruitment of inflammatory cells into the elastic media and adventitia appears to be an early and crucial step.[8] The factors involved in this process likely include oxidized lipoproteins,[9,10] localized tissue hypoxia,[11,12] reactive oxygen and nitrogen species,[13,14] prostanoids and leukotrienes,[15–18] and microbial infection[19] as well as elevated local expression of specific cytokines and chemokines associated with an immunoinflammatory response.[20–25] Matrix degradation may also release chemoattractant molecules that serve to amplify and localize inflammatory cells to the outer aortic wall. One example of this is the release of elastin-degradation peptides (EDPs) within aneurysm tissue, which can stimulate monocyte chemotaxis through interaction with a 67-kDa cell surface elastin-binding protein.[26–28] Indeed, the generation of high local concentrations of EDPs is thought to be one of the mechanisms underlying the development of experimental AAAs induced by transient aortic perfusion with pancreatic elastase.

Although studies of human aortic tissue procured during surgical AAA repair have provided valuable clues to pathogenesis, these specimens of "end-stage" disease give limited information on the dynamic changes involved in progressive aneurysmal degeneration. The development of small animal models of AAAs has therefore been a significant advance, allowing more detailed investigations on the cellular and molecular mechanisms of disease in a temporally controlled manner.[29–31] The purpose of this review is to summarize findings with one particular mouse model of AAAs; however, it is emphasized that different models of aneurysm disease have unique strengths and weaknesses, but none reproduce all aspects of human AAAs.

## GENERAL CHARACTERISTICS OF THE ELASTASE-INDUCED AAAS IN MICE

Transient intraluminal perfusion of the abdominal aorta with porcine pancreatic elastase has provided the most widely used animal model of AAAs ever since it was first described in rats by Anidjar and colleagues.[32–34] Under the experimental conditions used in our laboratory to adapt this model to mice, only mild aortic dilatation is observed immediately after elastase perfusion and there is initially little evidence of elastin degradation by light microscopy.[35] Aortic wall diameter and structure remain stable for up to 7 days, after which a rapid and significant increase in aortic diameter (AD) begins to occur. Aneurysms typically develop by day 14, defined by an increase in diameter to at least 100% greater than the normal (pre-perfusion) aorta (FIG. 1). The delayed onset of aortic dilatation in this model is temporally and spatially associated with transmural aortic wall infiltration by mononuclear phagocytes, increased local expression of elastolytic matrix metalloproteinases (MMPs), and pronounced destruction of the medial elastic lamellae. The elastase-induced model of AAAs has therefore been fruitful to examine the role of chronic inflammation and specific matrix-degrading enzymes in aortic degeneration and to test the effects of different pharmacological agents or genetic alterations on aneurysm formation. Based on a series of studies conducted over the past several years, FIGURE 2 illustrates a general scheme of molecular, cellular, and tissue changes thought to occur during the development of elastase-induced AAAs and how these events are temporally related to aneurysm formation. The results of experiments involving different genetically altered mice and various *in vivo* treatments are also summarized in TABLES 1 and 2.

## ELASTASE-INDUCED AAAs IN GENETICALLY ALTERED MICE

Proteolytic degradation of medial elastin is considered one of the key features of aneurysm formation. Studies using the elastase-induced rat model of AAAs provided the first experimental evidence that pharmacological MMP inhibitors can suppress aneurysmal degeneration along with preservation of medial elastin.[36] Although these initial experiments involved the use of the tetracycline antibiotic doxycycline as a broad-spectrum MMP

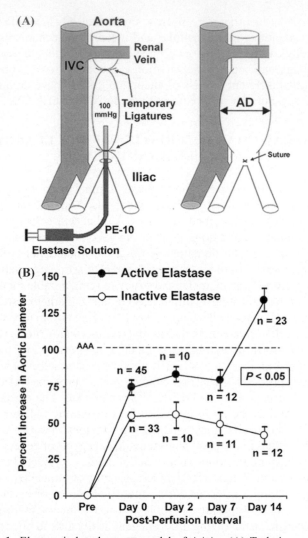

**FIGURE 1.** Elastase-induced mouse model of AAAs. (**A**) Technique used for transient intraluminal perfusion of the abdominal aorta with porcine pancreatic elastase. After measurement of the pre-perfusion AD, a dilute solution of porcine pancreatic elastase is instilled into the isolated segment of infrarenal abdominal aorta for 5 min at 100 mmHg pressure. The perfusion catheter is removed and flow is restored to the lower extremities and the immediate postperfusion AD is measured 5 min later. Final AD measurements are obtained during a repeat laparotomy at various intervals up to 14 days, immediately prior to euthanasia and tissue procurement. (**B**) Aortic dilatation at various intervals after aortic perfusion with either elastase or heat-inactivated elastase as a control. The initial dilatation (approximately 50–70%) is observed regardless of the perfusion solution with stabilization of AD up to day 7. Rapid secondary dilatation occurs between day 7 and 14 in mice perfused with elastase, but not in controls. AAAs are defined as an overall extent of aortic dilatation greater than 100% (*dashed horizontal line*). Data from Pyo et al.[35]

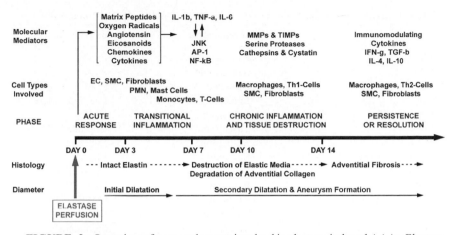

**FIGURE 2.** Overview of temporal events involved in elastase-induced AAAs. Elastase perfusion injury initially induces local expression and release of numerous molecular mediators of acute inflammation through its effects on resident aortic wall cells (EC, SMC, fibroblasts) and initial recruitment of inflammatory cells (PMN). Transition to a chronic inflammatory response involves recruitment of monocyte/macrophages and T cells along with increased local activity of several different types of matrix-degrading proteinases. The effects of these enzymes on structural aortic wall proteins (elastin and collagen) result in rapid secondary dilatation and aneurysm formation by day 14. Later events involving adaptive immune responses and connective tissue repair may act to stabilize the aortic wall, but failure of these processes may result in progressive dilatation.

inhibitor, similar results were obtained using nonantimicrobial tetracycline derivatives and hydroxamate-based MMP antagonists.[37–39]

The aneurysm-suppressing effects of doxycycline were confirmed following development and initial characterization of the elastase-induced mouse model of AAAs.[35] The response to elastase perfusion was subsequently examined in mice with targeted disruption of the MMP-9 or MMP-12 genes to discern if either of these elastolytic proteinases is specifically required for the development of experimental AAAs. These experiments revealed that the extent of aneurysmal dilatation and the incidence of AAAs were both substantially reduced in MMP-9 (−/−) mice, but that aneurysm development was unaffected in mice with isolated deficiency of MMP-12. The reduction in aneurysmal dilatation in MMP-9 (−/−) mice was associated with preservation of medial elastin and collagenous fibrosis in the adventitia, but there was no detectable suppression of elastase-induced inflammation. Additional studies in mice deficient in tissue inhibitor of metalloproteinases-1 (TIMP-1), the principal endogenous inhibitor of MMPs, revealed significant enhancement of elastase-induced AAAs.[40,41] These observations thereby demonstrate that expression of a single metalloproteinase (MMP-9) is required for the development of elastase-induced AAAs, helping

**TABLE 1. Genetically altered mice tested in the elastase-induced mouse model of AAAs**

| Gene targeted | AAA phenotype | Author (reference) |
|---|---|---|
| MMP-9 | Resistant | Pyo[35] |
| MMP-12 | Susceptible | Pyo[35] |
| MMP-9/MMP-12 | Resistant | Pyo[35] |
| TIMP-1 | Enhanced | Lee, Eskandari[40,41] |
| MMP-9/TIMP-1 | Enhanced | Lee[40] |
| MMP-2 | Susceptible | Unpublished |
| MMP-8 | Susceptible | Eliason[57] |
| Neutrophil elastase | Susceptible | Eliason[57] |
| Urokinase-PA | Susceptible | Unpublished |
| Cat-S | Resistant | Bartoli[48] |
| Cat-C (DPP-I) | Resistant | Unpublished |
| NOS-2 (iNOS) | Susceptible | Lee[50] |
| Apo-E | Susceptible | Steinmetz[51] |
| IL-1R | Resistant | Unpublished |
| TNFR | Resistant | Unpublished |
| IL-6 | Resistant | Unpublished |
| IL-10 | Enhanced | Geraghty[58] |
| B cells | Susceptible | Unpublished |
| CD8 (T cells) | Susceptible | Unpublished |
| CD4 (T cells) | Enhanced | Unpublished |
| AT1 (Ang II receptor) | Resistant | Unpublished |
| AT2 (Ang II receptor) | Susceptible | Unpublished |
| ALOX5 (5-Lipoxygenase) | Susceptible | Unpublished |
| FLAP | Susceptible | Unpublished |

support the possibility that treatment with MMP inhibitors might have utility in patients with small AAAs.[42–46]

The elastase-induced mouse model of AAAs has provided the opportunity to examine the role of several additional proteinases in aneurysmal degeneration. For example, studies in mice lacking expression of MMP-2, MMP-8, or urokinase-plasminogen activator (u-PA) revealed no suppression of elastase-induced AAAs. In contrast, recent experiments have revealed novel functions for cysteine proteases of the cathepsin family in AAAs such as cathepsin-S (Cat-S), a protease secreted by macrophages and SMC that has potent elastin-degrading activity. Gene expression profiling studies revealed that aortic wall expression of Cat-S, Cat-K, and Cat-C is markedly increased early after elastase perfusion (day 3), whereas expression of the endogenous cathepsin antagonist, cystatin-C, is actually diminished.[47] Treatment of mice with E-64, a broad-spectrum inhibitor of cysteine proteases, resulted in suppression of AAAs with preservation of aortic elastin.[48] In mice with targeted gene deletion of Cat-S, there was a significant reduction in the incidence of AAAs and a 55% reduction in the extent of aortic dilatation compared to wild-type controls. Cat-S ($-/-$) mice also exhibited a minimal postelastase aortic wall

TABLE 2. Treatments tested in the elastase-induced mouse model of AAAs

| Agent (route) | Effects on AAAs | Author/reference |
|---|---|---|
| Doxycycline (oral) | Suppression | Pyo[35] |
| Doxycycline (local) | Suppression | Bartoli[59] |
| Cigarette smoking | Enhanced | Buckley[60] |
| Simvastatin (ip) | Suppression | Steinmetz[51] |
| Enalapril, lisinopril (oral) | Suppression | Borhani[61] |
| Losartan (oral) | Suppression | Borhani[61] |
| PDTC (ip) | Suppression | Parodi[62] |
| Curcumin (oral) | Suppression | Parodi[63] |
| E-64 (Cathepsin inhibitor) | Suppression | Bartoli[48] |
| Ang II (sc) | No Effect | Unpublished |
| Anti-PMN antibody (iv) | Suppression | Eliason[57] |
| Anti-IL-6 antibody (ip) | Suppression | Unpublished |
| MK886 (FLAP antagonist) | No Effect | Unpublished |

inflammatory response and striking preservation of medial elastin, but gelatin zymography of aortic tissue extracts revealed no associated reduction in MMP-9 activity. These findings demonstrated for the first time that Cat-S plays a functionally important and necessary role in the development of aneurysmal degeneration and that the contributions of Cat-S to AAAs are independent of MMP-9. Additional studies have revealed a similarly crucial but distinct role for Cat-C, also known as dipeptidyl peptidase-I (DPP-I). DPP-I is a lysosomal enzyme required for activation of granule-associated proteases such as neutrophil elastase, Cat-G, and granzymes as well as mast cell chymases. The finding that mice deficient in DPP-I exhibit suppression of elastase-induced AAAs indicates that DDP-I (or one of its "downstream" proteases) plays a pivotal role in the transition from acute to chronic inflammation during the development of aneurysmal lesions.

The schematic diagram shown in FIGURE 2 illustrates that the early events in development of elastase-induced AAAs involve numerous molecular mediators including cellular signaling molecules, proinflammatory cytokines, and chemoattractants. It has therefore been of interest to examine mice with targeted deficiencies in genes involved in these processes to determine which mediators might be most important in the unique vascular response to injury that results in aneurysm formation. For example, previous studies in rats with pharmacological inhibitors of inducible nitric oxide synthase (iNOS) led to the prediction that nitric oxide produced by this enzyme is critical in the inflammatory response associated with aneurysm formation,[49] yet mice lacking expression of iNOS were found to exhibit no resistance to aneurysm formation despite evidence of increased nitric oxide production.[50] In other experiments it was found that mice with genetically determined hypercholesterolemia (due to deficiency in apolipoprotein-E) are also fully susceptible to

**TABLE 3. AD measurements in different inbred strains of laboratory mice**

| Strain | n | AD pre, mm | AD post, mm | AD final, mm |
|---|---|---|---|---|
| 129/SvEv | 41 | 0.54 ± 0.01 | 0.85 ± 0.02 | 0.98 ± 0.02 |
| 129/SvJ | 6 | 0.59 ± 0.03 | 0.92 ± 0.03 | 1.16 ± 0.08 |
| CBA/CaJ | 8 | 0.54 ± 0.01 | 0.88 ± 0.02 | 1.10 ± 0.08 |
| Balb/cJ | 4 | 0.53 ± 0.00 | 0.88 ± 0.01 | 1.08 ± 0.19 |
| C3H/HeJ | 7 | 0.56 ± 0.03 | 0.90 ± 0.03 | 1.22 ± 0.16 |
| C57BL/10SnJ | 6 | 0.52 ± 0.01 | 0.88 ± 0.02 | 1.18 ± 0.11 |
| FVB/N | 5 | 0.53 ± 0.00 | 0.88 ± 0.02 | 1.39 ± 0.08† |
| C57BL/6J | 66 | 0.53 ± 0.00 | 0.91 ± 0.01 | 1.38 ± 0.03† |
| Analysis of variance (ANOVA)* | | NS | NS | $P \leq 0$. |

Adult male mice from a series of eight different inbred strains underwent transient aortic perfusion with elastase to induce aneurysmal degeneration. AD measurements were obtained before (AD pre-) and immediately after (AD post-) elastase perfusion with final measurements obtained at 14 days (AD final). Data shown represent the mean ± SEM. *One-way ANOVA with Student-Newman-Keuls *post hoc* multiple comparisons test ($†P < 0.001$ vs. 129/SvEv).

elastase-induced AAAs, but that aneurysm development is suppressed by treatment with statins in both normal and Apo-E $(-/-)$ mice.[51] This finding likely reflects the pleiotropic effects of statins acting to interfere with key inflammatory signaling pathways as a mechanism of suppressing aneurysmal degeneration. Recent clinical studies have also highlighted the potential benefits of treatment with statins in patients with AAAs.[52,53]

Given the acute inflammatory response that follows elastase-induced aortic injury, it is not surprising that there is a significant increase in mouse aortic wall production of proinflammatory cytokines early in the development of elastase-induced AAAs such as IL-1β, TNF-α, and IL-6.[47] The roles of IL-1β and TNF-α in this response have been examined in rats, where treatment with cytokine-specific inhibitors suppresses elastase-induced AAAs.[54] Preliminary work in our laboratory has also led to the observation that elastase-induced AAAs are suppressed in mice lacking expression of the cell-surface receptors for IL-1β and TNF-α along with limited development of the aortic wall inflammatory response. In other studies we have examined a potential functional role for IL-6 in AAAs. This is of particular interest because IL-6 is prominently expressed in explant cultures of human AAA tissue and is significantly elevated in the circulating plasma of patients with AAAs, suggesting that circulating IL-6 levels reflect inflammatory processes involved in the early stages of aneurysm formation.[16,25,55,56] We have observed that elastase perfusion leads to early increases in IL-6 production within mouse aortic tissue (days 3 to 7) along with elevated circulating IL-6 concentrations. In mice with targeted deletion of IL-6, however, there is a significant suppression of elastase-induced AAAs along with a diminished inflammatory response and preservation of aortic elastin. Similar findings were observed in wild-type mice

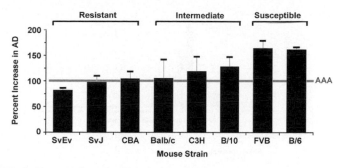

**FIGURE 3.** Extent of aortic dilatation in different inbred strains of laboratory mice. Adult male mice from a series of eight different inbred strains underwent transient aortic perfusion with elastase to induce aneurysmal degeneration and AD measurements were obtained (see TABLE 3). The overall extent of aortic dilatation was calculated as the percentage increase between pre-perfusion AD and final AD on day 14 with the data shown representing the mean ± SEM. Each strain was defined as resistant, intermediate, or susceptible to the development of elastase-induced AAAs.

treated with an anti-IL-6-neutralizing antibody. Taken together, these findings demonstrate that elevated production of IL-6 within the elastase-injured aortic tissue may play a crucial role in macrophage recruitment and activation, secretion of matrix-degrading proteinases, apoptosis of medial SMC, and other aspects of aneurysmal degeneration. Application of the elastase-induced model of AAAs to genetically altered mice has therefore been especially valuable in establishing the temporal and cellular expression of proinflammatory cytokines as well as the hierarchy of cytokine-driven aortic wall inflammatory responses in aneurysm development.

## INHERITED VARIATION IN SUSCEPTIBILITY TO ELASTASE-INDUCED AAAs

During investigations on elastase-induced AAAs in genetically altered mice, it has become increasingly evident that the extent of aneurysmal dilatation varies considerably between the different inbred laboratory strains used as background controls. For example, the mean extent of aortic dilatation in C57BL/6J background controls used for experiments on IL-6-deficient mice was approximately 150% as compared to only 75% for the 129/SvEv background controls used in experiments on TIMP-1-deficient mice. This observation is important from a practical point of view, emphasizing that it is critical to use control animals on the same genetic background when conducting experiments with gene-targeted animals. Furthermore, these observations suggest that the susceptibility to form AAAs following elastase perfusion is associated, at least in part, with genetically determined inherited traits.

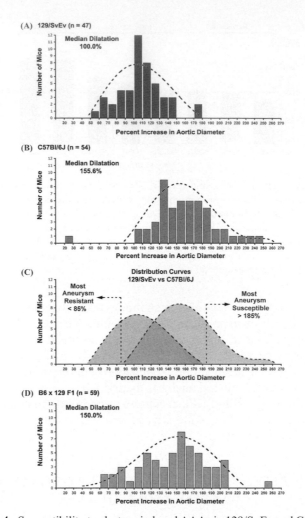

**FIGURE 4.** Susceptibility to elastase-induced AAAs in 129/SvEv and C57Bl/6J mice. A series of mice underwent transient aortic perfusion with elastase to induce aneurysmal degeneration and the overall extent of aortic dilatation was calculated as the percentage increase on day 14 (see FIG. 3). (**A** and **B**) Population distributions for the overall extent of aortic dilatation in 47 male 129/SvEv mice (mean ± SEM, 104.9 ± 3.8%; median, 100.0%) and 54 male C57Bl/6J mice (mean ± SEM, 158.8 ± 4.4%; median, 155.6%), demonstrating a significant difference in susceptibility to AAAs ($P < 0.001$). (**C**) Comparison of distribution curves for 129/SvEv and C57Bl/6J mice indicating that animals exhibiting less than 85% dilatation can be considered highly resistant and those with more than 185% dilatation can be considered highly susceptible. (**D**) Population distribution for the overall extent of aortic dilatation in 59 male F1 mice derived from an outcross between 129/SvEv and C57Bl/6J mice demonstrating a degree of susceptibility to AAAs intermediate to that observed in the two parental strains (mean ± SEM, 153.1 ± 4.2%; median, 150.0%).

To address this question in more depth we examined the extent of aneurysmal dilatation following elastase perfusion in six additional inbred strains of laboratory mice along with data accumulated from different experiments on 129/SvEv and C57BL/6J mice. As shown in TABLE 3, there were no differences in either pre-perfusion AD or immediate postperfusion AD between these eight strains; however, there were significant differences in final AD 14 days after elastase perfusion (ranging from $0.98 \pm 0.02$ mm in 129/SvEv to $1.44 \pm 0.04$ mm in C57BL/6J). As shown in FIGURE 3, there were also significant differences between these strains with respect to the overall extent of aneurysmal dilatation. Indeed, using the overall extent of aneurysmal dilatation as the basis for phenotypic characterization, these different laboratory strains can be designated as "AAA resistant," "AAA intermediate," or "AAA susceptible."

Because the widest divergence in susceptibility to aneurysmal dilatation occurred between 129/SvEv and C57BL/6J mice, these strains were further examined to determine if these differences would provide a suitable basis for investigations on genetic susceptibility. Following elastase perfusion in approximately 50 mice from each strain, the population distributions of values for overall percentage aortic dilatation in each strain were found to follow near-normal (Gaussian) distributions (FIG. 4). The 129/SvEv mice exhibited a median overall extent of dilatation of 100.0% whereas the C57BL/6J mice had a median overall extent of dilatation of 155.6%. These population distributions are sufficiently distinct that animals with dilatation less than 85% can be considered to be highly AAA resistant and those with dilatation greater than 185% can be considered to be highly AAA susceptible (FIG. 4C); thus, use of these phenotypic definitions will be helpful in studies aimed at defining the genetic susceptibility toward AAA development including the mode of inheritance, phenotypic penetrance, and the potential identification and mapping of quantitative trait loci (QTL). Indeed, in an initial study of mice derived from an outcross between 129/SvEv and C57BL/6J animals (i.e., B6xSvEv F1 heterozygotes), the distribution of values for aortic dilatation was somewhat broader and intermediate between the values observed for either of the two parental strains with a median overall extent of dilatation of 150.0% (FIG. 4D). This finding is therefore consistent with an inherited, genetically determined susceptibility to the development of elastase-induced AAAs. It is expected that future investigations based on this information will help define the inherited genetic elements that might influence aneurysmal dilatation in this experimental model.

## ACKNOWLEDGMENTS

This study was supported by grant R01 HL56701 from the National Heart, Lung, and Blood Institute (RWT).

## REFERENCES

1. THOMPSON, R.W., P.J. GERAGHTY & J.K. LEE. 2002. Abdominal aortic aneurysms: basic mechanisms and clinical implications. Curr. Prob. Surg. **39:** 110–230.
2. ALCORN, H.G., S.K. WOLFSON, JR., K. SUTTON-TYRRELL, et al. 1996. Risk factors for abdominal aortic aneurysms in older adults enrolled in The Cardiovascular Health Study. Arterioscler. Thromb. Vasc. Biol. **16:** 963–970.
3. LEDERLE, F.A., G.R. JOHNSON, S.E. WILSON, et al. 1997. Prevalence and associations of abdominal aortic aneurysm detected through screening. Aneurysm Detection and Management (ADAM) Veterans Affairs Cooperative Study Group. Ann. Intern. Med. **126:** 441–449.
4. BLANCHARD, J.F. 1999. Epidemiology of abdominal aortic aneurysms. Epidemiol. Rev. **21:** 207–221.
5. BLANCHARD, J.F., H.K. ARMENIAN & P.P. FRIESEN. 2000. Risk factors for abdominal aortic aneurysm: results of a case-control study. Am. J. Epidemiol. **151:** 575–583.
6. LEDERLE, F.A., D.B. NELSON & A.M. JOSEPH. 2003. Smokers' relative risk for aortic aneurysm compared with other smoking-related diseases: a systematic review. J. Vasc. Surg. **38:** 329–334.
7. THOMPSON, R.W. 1996. Basic science of abdominal aortic aneurysms: emerging therapeutic strategies for an unresolved clinical problem. Curr. Opin. Cardiol. **11:** 504–518.
8. KOCH, A.E., G.K. HAINES, R.J. RIZZO, et al. 1990. Human abdominal aortic aneurysms. Immunophenotypic analysis suggesting an immune-mediated response. Am. J. Pathol. **137:** 1199–1213.
9. PAPAGRIGORAKIS, E., D. ILIOPOULOS, P.J. ASIMACOPOULOS, et al. 1997. Lipoprotein(a) in plasma, arterial wall, and thrombus from patients with aortic aneurysm. Clin. Genet. **52:** 262–271.
10. SCHILLINGER, M., H. DOMANOVITS, M. IGNATESCU, et al. 2002. Lipoprotein (a) in patients with aortic aneurysmal disease. J. Vasc. Surg. **36:** 25–30.
11. VORP, D.A., P.C. LEE, D.H. WANG, et al. 2001. Association of intraluminal thrombus in abdominal aortic aneurysm with local hypoxia and wall weakening. J. Vasc. Surg. **34:** 291–299.
12. SCHILLINGER, M., M. EXNER, W. MLEKUSCH, et al. 2002. Heme oxygenase-1 gene promoter polymorphism is associated with abdominal aortic aneurysm. Thromb. Res. **106:** 131–136.
13. MILLER, F.J., JR., W.J. SHARP, X. FANG, et al. 2002. Oxidative stress in human abdominal aortic aneurysms: a potential mediator of aneurysmal remodeling. Arterioscler. Thromb. Vasc. Biol. **22:** 560–565.
14. DALMAN, R.L. 2003. Oxidative stress and abdominal aneurysms: how aortic hemodynamic conditions may influence AAA disease. Cardiovasc. Surg. **11:** 417–419.
15. HOLMES, D.R., W. WESTER, R.W. THOMPSON, et al. 1997. Prostaglandin E2 synthesis and cyclooxygenase expression in abdominal aortic aneurysms. J. Vasc. Surg. **25:** 810–815.
16. WALTON, L.J., I.J. FRANKLIN, T. BAYSTON, et al. 1999. Inhibition of prostaglandin E2 synthesis in abdominal aortic aneurysms: implications for smooth muscle cell viability, inflammatory processes, and the expansion of abdominal aortic aneurysms. Circulation. **100:** 48–54.
17. BAYSTON, T., S. RAMESSUR, J. REISE, et al. 2003. Prostaglandin E2 receptors in abdominal aortic aneurysm and human aortic smooth muscle cells. J. Vasc. Surg. **38:** 354–359.

18. ZHAO, L., M.P. MOOS, R. GRABNER, *et al.* 2004. The 5-lipoxygenase pathway promotes pathogenesis of hyperlipidemia-dependent aortic aneurysm. Nat. Med. **10:** 966–973.
19. LINDHOLT, J.S., H.A. ASHTON & R.A. SCOTT. 2001. Indicators of infection with Chlamydia pneumoniae are associated with expansion of abdominal aortic aneurysms. J. Vasc. Surg. **34:** 212–215.
20. PEARCE, W.H., I. SWEIS, J.S. YAO, *et al.* 1992. Interleukin-1 beta and tumor necrosis factor-alpha release in normal and diseased human infrarenal aortas. J. Vasc. Surg. **16:** 784–789.
21. KOCH, A., S. KUNKEL, W. PEARCE, *et al.* 1993. Enhanced production of the chemotactic cytokines interleukin-8 and monocyte chemoattractant protein-1 in human abdominal aortic aneurysms. Am. J. Pathol. **142:** 1423–1431.
22. SZEKANECZ, Z., M.R. SHAH, W.H. PEARCE, *et al.* 1994. Human atherosclerotic abdominal aortic aneurysms produce interleukin (IL)-6 and interferon-gamma but not IL-2 and IL-4: the possible role for IL-6 and interferon-gamma in vascular inflammation. Agents Actions. **42:** 159–162.
23. NEWMAN, K.M., J. JEAN-Claude, H. LI, *et al.* 1994. Cytokines that activate proteolysis are increased in abdominal aortic aneurysms. Circulation **90:** II224–II227.
24. MCMILLAN, W.D. & W.H. PEARCE. 1997. Inflammation and cytokine signaling in aneurysms. Ann. Vasc. Surg. **11:** 540–545.
25. JONES, K.G., D.J. BRULL, L.C. BROWN, *et al.* 2001. Interleukin-6 (IL-6) and the prognosis of abdominal aortic aneurysms. Circulation **103:** 2260–2265.
26. SENIOR, R.M., G.L. GRIFFIN & R.P. MECHAM. 1980. Chemotactic activity of elastin-derived peptides. J. Clin. Invest. **66:** 859–862.
27. HINEK, A. 1994. Nature and the multiple functions of the 67-kD elastin-/laminin binding protein. Cell. Adhes. Commun. **2:** 185–193.
28. HANCE, K.A., M. TATARIA, S.J. ZIPORIN, *et al.* 2002. Monocyte chemotactic activity in human abdominal aortic aneurysms: role of elastin degradation peptides and the 67-kD cell surface elastin receptor. J. Vasc. Surg. **35:** 254–261.
29. DOBRIN, P.B. 1999. Animal models of aneurysms. Ann. Vasc. Surg. **13:** 641–648.
30. CARRELL, T.W., A. SMITH & K.G. BURNAND. 1999. Experimental techniques and models in the study of the development and treatment of abdominal aortic aneurysm. Br. J. Surg. **86:** 305–312.
31. DAUGHERTY, A. & L.A. CASSIS. 2004. Mouse models of abdominal aortic aneurysms. Arterioscler. Thromb. Vasc. Biol. **24:** 429–434.
32. ANIDJAR, S., J.L. SALZMANN, D. GENTRIC, *et al.* 1990. Elastase-induced experimental aneurysms in rats. Circulation **82:** 973–981.
33. ANIDJAR, S., P.B. DOBRIN, M. EICHORST, *et al.* 1992. Correlation of inflammatory infiltrate with the enlargement of experimental aortic aneurysm. J. Vasc. Surg. **16:** 139–147.
34. ANIDJAR, S., P.B. DOBRIN, G. CHEJFEC, *et al.* 1994. Experimental study of determinants of aneurysmal expansion of the abdominal aorta. Ann. Vasc. Surg. **8:** 127–136.
35. PYO, R., J.K. LEE, J.M. SHIPLEY, *et al.* 2000. Targeted gene disruption of matrix metalloproteinase-9 (gelatinase B) suppresses development of experimental abdominal aortic aneurysms. J. Clin. Invest. **105:** 1641–1649.
36. PETRINEC, D., S. LIAO, D.R. HOLMES, *et al.* 1996. Doxycycline inhibition of aneurysmal degeneration in an elastase-induced rat model of abdominal aortic aneurysm: preservation of aortic elastin associated with suppressed production of 92 kD gelatinase. J. Vasc. Surg. **23:** 336–346.

37. CURCI, J.A., D. PETRINEC, S.X. LIAO, *et al.* 1998. Pharmacologic suppression of experimental abdominal aortic aneurysms: a comparison of doxycycline and four chemically modified tetracyclines. J. Vasc. Surg. **28:** 1082–1093.
38. MOORE, G., S. LIAO, J.A. CURCI, *et al.* 1999. Suppression of experimental abdominal aortic aneurysms by systemic treatment with a hydroxamate-based matrix metalloproteinase inhibitor (RS 132908). J. Vasc. Surg. **29:** 522–532.
39. BIGATEL, D.A., J.R. ELMORE, D.J. CAREY, *et al.* 1999. The matrix metalloproteinase inhibitor BB-94 limits expansion of experimental abdominal aortic aneurysms. J. Vasc. Surg. **29:** 130–138.
40. LEE, J.K., C. BUCKLEY, M. BORHANI, *et al.* 2003. Endogenous expression of TIMP-1 regulates development of experimental abdominal aortic aneurysms independent of interactions with gelatinase B (abstract). Circulation (Suppl IV) **108:** 166.
41. ESKANDARI, M.K., J.D. VIJUNGCO, A. FLORES, *et al.* 2005. Enhanced abdominal aortic aneurysm in TIMP-1-deficient mice. J. Surg. Res. **123:** 289–293.
42. THOMPSON, R.W., S. LIAO & J.A. CURCI. 1998. Therapeutic potential of tetracycline derivatives to suppress the growth of abdominal aortic aneurysms. Adv. Dent. Res. **12:** 159–165.
43. THOMPSON, R.W. & B.T. BAXTER. 1999. MMP inhibition in abdominal aortic aneurysms: rationale for a prospective randomized clinical trial. Ann. N.Y. Acad. Sci. **878:** 159–178.
44. CURCI, J.A., D. MAO, D.G. BOHNER, *et al.* 2000. Preoperative treatment with doxycycline reduces aortic wall expression and activation of matrix metallo-proteinases in patients with abdominal aortic aneurysms. J. Vasc. Surg. **31:** 325–342.
45. PRALL, A.K., G.M. LONGO, W.G. MAYHAN, *et al.* 2002. Doxycycline in patients with abdominal aortic aneurysms and in mice: comparison of serum levels and effect on aneurysm growth in mice. J. Vasc. Surg. **35:** 923–929.
46. BAXTER, B.T., W.H. PEARCE, E.A. WALTKE, *et al.* 2002. Prolonged administration of doxycycline in patients with small asymptomatic abdominal aortic aneurysms: report of a prospective (Phase II) multicenter study. J. Vasc. Surg. **36:** 1–12.
47. VANVICKLE-CHAVEZ, S. J., W.S. TUNG, T.S. ABSI, *et al.* 2006. Temporal changes in mouse aortic wall gene expression during the development of elastase-induced abdominal aortic aneurysms. J. Vasc. Surg. **43(5):** 1010–1020.
48. BARTOLI, M.A., G.-P. SHI, T.L. ENNIS, *et al.* 2004. Role of cathepsin S in de-velopment of experimental abdominal aortic aneurysms (abstract). Arterioscler. Thromb. Vasc. Biol. **24:** e64.
49. JOHANNING, J.M., D.P. FRANKLIN, D.C. HAN, *et al.* 2001. Inhibition of inducible nitric oxide synthase limits nitric oxide production and experimental aneurysm expansion. J. Vasc. Surg. **33:** 579–586.
50. LEE, J.K., M. BORHANI, T.L. ENNIS, *et al.* 2001. Experimental abdominal aortic aneurysms in mice lacking expression of inducible nitric oxide synthase. Arte-rioscler. Thromb. Vasc. Biol. **21:** 1393–1401.
51. STEINMETZ, E.F., C. BUCKLEY, M.L. SHAMES, *et al.* 2005. Treatment with simvas-tatin suppresses the development of experimental abdominal aortic aneurysms in normal and hypercholesterolemic mice. Ann. Surg. **241:** 92–101.
52. NAGASHIMA, H., Y. AOKA, Y. SAKOMURA, *et al.* 2002. A 3-hydroxy-3-methylglutaryl coenzyme A reductase inhibitor, cerivastatin, suppresses production of matrix metalloproteinase-9 in human abdominal aortic aneurysm wall. J. Vasc. Surg. **36:** 158–163.

53. SUKHIJA, R., W.S. ARONOW, R. SANDHU, *et al.* 2006. Mortality and size of abdominal aortic aneurysm at long-term follow-up of patients not treated surgically and treated with and without statins. Am. J. Cardiol. **97:** 279–280.
54. HINGORANI, A., E. ASCHER, M. SCHEINMAN, *et al.* 1998. The effect of tumor necrosis factor binding protein and interleukin-1 receptor antagonist on the development of abdominal aortic aneurysms in a rat model. J. Vasc. Surg. **28:** 522–526.
55. JUVONEN, J., H.M. SURCEL, J. SATTA, *et al.* 1997. Elevated circulating levels of inflammatory cytokines in patients with abdominal aortic aneurysm. Arterioscler. Thromb. Vasc. Biol. **17:** 2843–2847.
56. ROHDE, L.E., L.H. ARROYO, N. RIFAI, *et al.* 1999. Plasma concentrations of interleukin-6 and abdominal aortic diameter among subjects without aortic dilatation. Arterioscler. Thromb. Vasc. Biol. **19:** 1695–1699.
57. ELIASON, J.L., K.K. HANNAWA, G. AILAWADI, *et al.* 2005. Neutrophil depletion inhibits experimental abdominal aortic aneurysm formation. Circulation **112:** 232–240.
58. GERAGHTY, P.J., B.C. STARCHER, M. BORHANI, *et al.* 2001. Interleukin-10 deficiency potentiates aortic collagen and elastin degradation in elastase-induced murine aortic aneurysm formation (abstract). Arterioscler. Thromb. Vasc. Biol. **21:** 676.
59. BARTOLI, M.A., F. PARODI, J. CHU, *et al.* 2006. Localized administration of doxycycline suppresses development of experimental abdominal aortic aneurysms. Ann. Vasc. Surg. **20(2):** 228–236.
60. BUCKLEY, C., C.W. WYBLE, M. BORHANI, *et al.* 2004. Accelerated enlargement of experimental abdominal aortic aneurysms in a mouse model of chronic cigarette smoke exposure. J. Am. Coll. Surg. **199:** 896–903.
61. BORHANI, M., J.K. LEE, T.L. ENNIS, *et al.* 2000. Enalapril suppresses experimental aortic aneurysm formation in mice: evidence for a novel molecular mechanism distinct from angiotensin converting enzyme inhibition. Surg. Forum. **51:** 397–399.
62. PARODI, F.E., D. MAO, T.L. ENNIS, *et al.* 2005. Suppression of experimental abdominal aortic aneurysms in mice by treatment with pyrrolidine dithiocarbamate, an antioxidant inhibitor of nuclear factor-kappaB. J. Vasc. Surg. **41:** 479–489.
63. PARODI, F.E., D. MAO, T.L. ENNIS, *et al.* 2005. Oral administration of diferuloylmethane (curcumin) suppresses proinflammatory cytokines and destructive connective tissue remodeling in experimental abdominal aortic aneurysms. Ann. Vasc. Surg. **41(3):** 479–489.

# Regression of Abdominal Aortic Aneurysm by Inhibition of c-Jun N-Terminal Kinase in Mice

KOICHI YOSHIMURA,[a] HIROKI AOKI,[a] YASUHIRO IKEDA,[a]
AKIRA FURUTANI, [b] KIMIKAZU HAMANO,[b]
AND MASUNORI MATSUZAKI[a,c]

[a]*Department of Molecular Cardiovascular Biology, Yamaguchi University School of Medicine, 1-1-1 Minami Kogushi, Ube, Yamaguchi 755-8505, Japan*

[b]*Department of Surgery and Clinical Science, Yamaguchi University School of Medicine, 1-1-1 Minami Kogushi, Ube, Yamaguchi 755-8505, Japan*

[c]*Department of Cardiovascular Medicine, Yamaguchi University School of Medicine, 1-1-1 Minami Kogushi, Ube, Yamaguchi 755-8505, Japan*

ABSTRACT: Abdominal aortic aneurysm (AAA) is a common disease that, when surgical treatment is inapplicable, results in rupture of the aorta with high mortality. Although nonsurgical treatment for AAA is eagerly awaited, the destruction of the aortic walls in AAA has been considered an irreversible process. We found that c-Jun N-terminal kinase (JNK) is highly activated in human AAA walls. We also found that JNK activity is essential for the expression of matrix metalloproteinase (MMP)-9 and, concurrently, suppression of the extracellular matrix (ECM) biosynthesis. We therefore investigated the role of JNK in the pathogenesis of AAA *in vivo*. We created a mouse AAA model by periaortic application of $CaCl_2$, which was accompanied by activation of JNK and MMPs, and suppression of lysyl oxidase (LOX), which is an essential biosynthetic enzyme for collagen and elastin fibers. Our data indicate that, in addition to MMP activities, suppression of ECM biosynthesis may contribute to the AAA pathogenesis because local LOX gene delivery prevented AAA formation. Treatment of mice with SP600125, a specific JNK inhibitor, completely abrogated the formation of $CaCl_2$-induced AAA. Furthermore, SP600125 treatment after the establishment of AAA caused a reduction in the aortic diameters with normalized tissue architecture. SP600125 treatment also caused significant regression of angiotensin II-induced AAA in ApoE-null mice after its establishment, as demonstrated by serial ultrasonographic studies in live animals. These data demonstrate that JNK dictates the abnormal ECM metabolism in

Address for correspondence: Koichi Yoshimura, M.D., Ph.D., Department of Molecular Cardiovascular Biology, Yamaguchi University School of Medicine, 1-1-1 Minami Kogushi, Ube, Yamaguchi 755-8505, Japan. Voice: +81-836-22-2361; fax: +81-836-22-2362.
e-mail: yoshimko@yamaguchi-u.ac.jp

Ann. N.Y. Acad. Sci. 1085: 74–81 (2006). © 2006 New York Academy of Sciences.
doi: 10.1196/annals.1383.031

AAA pathogenesis by enhancing tissue degradation and suppressing tissue repair. Therefore, inhibition of JNK may provide a novel therapeutic option for AAA.

KEYWORDS: abdominal aortic aneurysm; regression; pharmacological therapy; c-Jun N-terminal kinase; matrix metalloproteinase; extracellular matrix

## INTRODUCTION

Abdominal aortic aneurysm (AAA) is a common disease among elderly people and eventually progresses to rupture with a high mortality when surgical treatment is inapplicable. Because many patients are already at a high risk of rupture at the point of initial diagnosis, a nonsurgical therapy that reduces AAA diameter would provide a therapeutic option to reduce the rupture risk. Unfortunately, an effective reduction in AAA size by nonsurgical therapy has not been achieved and therapeutic options are currently limited to open aneurysm repair or endovascular repair.

It is widely accepted that matrix metalloproteinases (MMPs), particularly MMP-9 and MMP-2, cause the loss of critical extracellular matrix (ECM) components, including collagen and elastin, thereby leading to AAA development.[1-4] In fact, pharmacological inhibition of MMPs has been shown to reduce the expansion rate of AAA in animal models[5-7] and in early clinical trials.[8,9] MMP inhibition, however, does not cause effective reduction in AAA size. It has been assumed that the destruction of the wall structure and the enlargement of aneurysmal diameter are progressive and irreversible in AAA. Interestingly, successful endovascular stent grafting results in the regression of AAA diameter in human patients,[10] suggesting that the aneurysmal wall has the potential to regress if exacerbating factors are eliminated and/or tissue repair is reinforced.

Here we demonstrate that pharmacological inhibition of c-Jun N-terminal kinase (JNK) restores the aortic tissue architecture and causes regression of established AAA in mice.[11]

## PREVENTION OF AAA DEVELOPMENT
## BY JNK INHIBITION

Recent studies indicate that JNK is involved in a number of cellular stress responses and also in the signaling of inflammation.[12] We previously found that JNK is highly activated in human AAA walls and that specific inhibition of JNK significantly suppressed the secretion of MMP-9 and prevented collagen degradation in human AAA walls in *ex vivo* culture.[11,13] To gain further insight into the role of JNK in AAA, we screened for JNK-dependent genes in vascular smooth muscle cells using JNK pathway-oriented transcriptome analyses. Interestingly, 5 of the top 20 JNK-induced genes were genes for positive regulators of MMP-9 activity (TABLE 1). These findings led us to hypothesize that JNK is essential for the development of AAA *in vivo*. To test this hypothesis, we created AAA in mice using periaortic application of 0.5 M $CaCl_2$.[2] Following the application of $CaCl_2$, mice were treated with SP600125, a specific JNK inhibitor,[14] or vehicle for 10 weeks. We chose pharmacological inhibition of JNK because of the practical relevance of a pharmacological approach in humans with AAA. Treatment of mice with SP600125 completely abrogated the increase in aortic outer diameter induced by $CaCl_2$ (FIG. 1A). An angiographic study also demonstrated the inhibitory effect of SP600125 on dilation of the aortic inner diameter by $CaCl_2$. Treatment with SP600125 prevented the destruction of the aortic tissue architecture such as thinning of the medial layer and disruption of the elastic lamellae, which are hallmarks of human AAA. SP600125 reduced phospho-c-Jun, a marker of JNK activity, and MMP-9 levels. In addition, SP600125 reduced macrophage infiltration in the periaortic tissue, suggesting that chronic JNK inhibition abrogates proinflammatory signaling in AAA. These findings demonstrate that inhibition of JNK is an effective therapeutic option to prevent the development of AAA.


## ROLE OF ECM BIOSYNTHESIS IN AAA

It has been suggested that not only ECM degradation but also connective tissue repair is involved in the destruction of the aneurysmal wall during the development of AAA.[3,6] We investigated the role of ECM biosynthesis in a mouse AAA model induced by $CaCl_2$. The local activity of lysyl oxidase

TABLE 1. Selected JNK-dependent genes in vascular smooth muscle cells

| Accession# | Description | JNK-dependence index |
|---|---|---|
| **Selected JNK-induced genes** | | |
| Genes involved in proinflammatory signaling and MMP-9 activation | | |
| D00403 | interleukin-1 alpha | 3.892 |
| S62933 | TrkC | 3.533 |
| U16359 | inducible nitric oxide synthase | 3.327 |
| U24441 | matrix metallopeptidase 9 | 2.931 |
| AA946503 | lipocalin 2 | 2.660 |
| **Selected JNK-suppressed genes** | | |
| Genes encoding biosynthetic enzymes for collagen and elastin | | |
| L25331 | lysyl hydroxylase | −0.215 |
| AI102814 | lysyl oxidase | −0.375 |
| X78949 | prolyl 4-hydroxylase | −0.461 |

Highly JNK-dependent genes in vascular smooth muscle cells were identified by our JNK pathway-oriented transcriptome analyses. Five genes involved in proinflammatory signaling and MMP-9 activation were ranked within the top 20 JNK-induced genes. Three biosynthetic enzymes for collagen and elastin were identified as JNK-suppressed genes. (Modified from Yoshimura et al.[11])

(LOX), which is a cross-linking enzyme essential for stabilization of collagen and elastin fibers,[15] was decreased below the basal level by 3 weeks and continuing to up to 5 weeks after $CaCl_2$ treatment. The serum level of MMP-9 was elevated for up to 5 weeks, suggesting that the ECM metabolism was shifted to degradation during AAA development. To enhance the ECM biosynthesis, we performed local gene delivery of LOX by abluminal application of adenoviral vector at 3 weeks after $CaCl_2$ treatment. Angiographic and macroscopic analyses demonstrated that the inner and outer diameters of aortae in the LOX group were significantly smaller than those in the LacZ group at 6 weeks after $CaCl_2$ treatment (FIG. 1B). Since a transient enhancement of LOX prevented AAA formation *in vivo*, a continuous suppression of LOX activity appears to be crucial in the pathogenesis of AAA. Because we found that JNK activation suppresses expression of ECM biosynthetic enzymes including LOX (TABLE 1), JNK may enhance AAA formation by attenuating connective tissue repair.

## REGRESSION OF AAA BY JNK INHIBITION

Our *in vitro* data suggested that inhibition of JNK not only suppresses a degradation pathway, but also restores a biosynthetic pathway of ECM.[11,13] Therefore, we hypothesized that JNK inhibition might cause regression of already established AAA, which presumably requires active ECM biosynthesis and connective tissue repair. We tested this hypothesis in a $CaCl_2$-induced AAA model in mice. Periaortic application of $CaCl_2$ caused significant dilation of the aorta after 6 weeks. We started SP600125 or vehicle treatment at 6 weeks after $CaCl_2$ treatment and continued for an additional 6 weeks. Vehicle treatment resulted in no significant changes in aortic diameters, indicating that $CaCl_2$-induced AAA was fully established at 6 weeks and maintained for an additional 6 weeks. Treatment with SP600125 caused a striking reduction in aneurysmal diameter compared with vehicle treatment as well as before starting the treatment with SP600125 (FIG. 2A). Histologically, disruption and flattening of elastic lamellae were observed in the aneurysmal wall 6 weeks after $CaCl_2$ treatment and persisted for an additional 6 weeks with vehicle treatment. In contrast, the SP600125-treated aortic wall showed a wavy morphology with less disruption of the elastic lamellae, indicating that JNK inhibition enhances the repair of tissue architecture (FIG. 2B). These data demonstrated that JNK inhibition causes regression of established AAA induced by $CaCl_2$.

We tested the effect of JNK inhibition in another AAA model created by continuous infusion of angiotensin II in apolipoprotein E-null mice.[16] This AAA model is advantageous because AAA develops in the suprarenal aorta, allowing us to monitor the aneurysmal diameter by ultrasonography repeatedly. After angiotensin II infusion, we divided these mice into two groups with equivalent aortic diameters as assessed by ultrasonography and initiated a

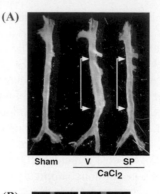

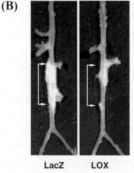

**FIGURE 1.** Prevention of AAA development. **(A)** Prevention of AAA development by JNK inhibition. Aortic morphometry was performed after perfusion fixation of the aortae at the physiological perfusion pressure. A representative photograph is shown for aortae 10 weeks after periaortic application of saline (Sham) or $CaCl_2$ followed by the treatment with vehicle (V) or a specific JNK inhibitor, SP600125 (SP). **(B)** Prevention of AAA development by reinforced ECM biosynthesis. A representative photograph is shown for aortae 6 weeks after periaortic application of $CaCl_2$. Local gene delivery of LOX by adenoviral vector was performed 3 weeks after $CaCl_2$ treatment. LacZ gene transfer was used as a negative control. (Modified from Yoshimura et al.[11])

treatment with vehicle or SP600125 for an additional 8 weeks. The vehicle-treated group showed no significant change in aneurysmal diameter, indicating that this AAA was established during the 4 weeks of angiotensin II infusion. Notably, the SP600125 group showed a reduction in the aortic diameter during the 8 weeks of treatment (FIG. 2C). These data demonstrated that JNK inhibition causes regression of angiotensin II-induced AAA after its establishment.

## CONCLUSIONS

We found that inhibition of JNK causes a significant regression of AAA in mice. This finding has two important implications. First, we indicated that

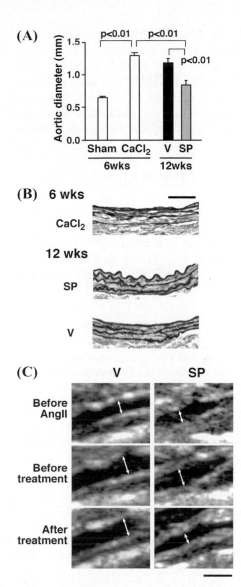

**FIGURE 2.** Regression of established AAA in mice. **(A)** AAA was established 6 weeks after the CaCl$_2$ treatment (6 weeks). Treatment with a specific JNK inhibitor, SP600125 (SP) or vehicle (V), was continued from 6 to 12 weeks after the CaCl$_2$ treatment. Maximal aortic diameters were determined 6 weeks after the CaCl$_2$ treatment or sham operation (open columns), and after an additional 6 weeks of vehicle (*closed columns*) or SP600125 (*shaded columns*) treatment. **(B)** Representative images are shown for elastica van Gieson staining. Bars indicate 40 μm. **(C)** Representative images of serial ultrasonographic studies are shown for the same regions in ApoE–/– mice before and after angiotensin II (Ang II) infusion (before treatment) and after treatment with vehicle (V) or SP600125 (SP). *Arrows* indicate the lumen of aortae. A *bar* indicates 2 mm. (Modified from Yoshimura *et al.*[11])

the walls of established AAA still have the potential to recover from a catastrophic state and that pharmacological treatments could potentially induce the regression of AAA. Secondly, we identified JNK as a critical factor causing abnormal ECM metabolism in the pathogenesis of AAA and also as a therapeutic target for both prevention and regression of AAA. We hope that a JNK-inhibition strategy would help to improve the overall survival of AAA patients by expanding the nonsurgical therapeutic options.

## ACKNOWLEDGMENTS

This work was supported in part by Grants-in-aid for Scientific Research (KAKENHI 12770651, 14657284, and 17591337 to KY; 12670673, 12204081, 14370229, and 16390365 to HA; and 16209026 to MM) from MEXT Japan and a Grant from the Sankyo Company to the Department of Molecular Cardiovascular Biology, Yamaguchi University School of Medicine.

## REFERENCES

1. PYO, R. *et al*. 2000. Targeted gene disruption of matrix metalloproteinase-9 (gelatinase B) suppresses development of experimental abdominal aortic aneurysms. J. Clin. Invest. **105:** 1641–1649.
2. LONGO, G.M. *et al*. 2002. Matrix metalloproteinases 2 and 9 work in concert to produce aortic aneurysms. J. Clin. Invest. **110:** 625–632.
3. THOMPSON, R.W., P.J. GERAGHTY & J.K. LEE. 2002. Abdominal aortic aneurysms: basic mechanisms and clinical implications. Curr. Probl. Surg. **39:** 110–230.
4. BAXTER, B.T. 2004. Could medical intervention work for aortic aneurysms? Am. J. Surg. **188:** 628–632.
5. PETRINEC, D. *et al*. 1996. Doxycycline inhibition of aneurysmal degeneration in an elastase-induced rat model of abdominal aortic aneurysm: preservation of aortic elastin associated with suppressed production of 92 kD gelatinase. J. Vasc. Surg. **23:** 336–346.
6. HUFFMAN, M.D. *et al*. 2000. Functional importance of connective tissue repair during the development of experimental abdominal aortic aneurysms. Surgery **128:** 429–438.
7. PRALL, A.K. *et al*. 2002. Doxycycline in patients with abdominal aortic aneurysms and in mice: comparison of serum levels and effect on aneurysm growth in mice. J. Vasc. Surg. **35:** 923–929.
8. MOSORIN, M. *et al*. 2001. Use of doxycycline to decrease the growth rate of abdominal aortic aneurysms: a randomized, double-blind, placebo-controlled pilot study. J. Vasc. Surg. **34:** 606–610.
9. BAXTER, B.T. *et al*. 2002. Prolonged administration of doxycycline in patients with small asymptomatic abdominal aortic aneurysms: report of a prospective (Phase II) multicenter study. J. Vasc. Surg. **36:** 1–12.
10. BUTH, J. & P. HARRIS. 2005. Endovascular Treatment of Aortic Aneurysms. *In* Vascular Surgery, R.B. Rutherford, ED.: 1452–1475. Elsevier. Philadelphia.

11. YOSHIMURA, K. *et al*. 2005. Regression of abdominal aortic aneurysm by inhibition of c-Jun N-terminal kinase. Nat. Med. **11:** 1330–1338.
12. MANNING, A.M. & R.J. DAVIS. 2003. Targeting JNK for therapeutic benefit: from junk to gold? Nat. Rev. Drug Discov. **2:** 554–565.
13. YOSHIMURA, K. *et al*. Identification of c-Jun N-terminal kinase as a therapeutic target for abdominal aortic aneurysm. Ann. N. Y. Acad. Sci. This volume.
14. BENNETT, B.L. *et al*. 2001. SP600125, an anthrapyrazolone inhibitor of Jun N-terminal kinase. Proc. Natl. Acad. Sci. USA **98:** 13681–13686.
15. KAGAN, H.M. & W. LI. 2003. Lysyl oxidase: properties, specificity, and biological roles inside and outside of the cell. J. Cell. Biochem. **88:** 660–672.
16. DAUGHERTY, A., M.W. MANNING & L.A. CASSIS. 2000. Angiotensin II promotes atherosclerotic lesions and aneurysms in apolipoprotein E-deficient mice. J. Clin. Invest. **105:** 1605–1612.

# Role of the Renin-Angiotensin System in the Development of Abdominal Aortic Aneurysms in Animals and Humans

ALAN DAUGHERTY, DEBRA L. RATERI, AND LISA A. CASSIS

*Cardiovascular Research Center, Graduate Center for Nutritional Sciences, University of Kentucky, Lexington, Kentucky, USA*

ABSTRACT: The mediators for the initiation, progression, and rupture of abdominal aortic aneurysms (AAAs) have not been defined. Recent evidence has demonstrated that chronic infusion of angiotensin II via subcutaneously placed osmotic pumps can reproducibly form AAAs in mice. The evolution of AngII-induced AAAs in these mice is complex. Rapid medial macrophage accumulation precedes transmedial breaks and large lumen expansion, which are restricted to the suprarenal aorta. After this initial phase, there is a more gradual rate of lumen expansion that is progressive with continued AngII exposure. There is extensive aortic remodeling during this gradual expansion phase. An initial prominent thrombus gradually resolves and is replaced by fibrous tissue containing several types of inflammatory cells. At prolonged intervals of AngII infusion, internal aortic diameters of the suprarenal aorta can increase up to fourfold compared to the same region in saline-infused mice. The extrapolation of these data in mice to the development of human AAAs remains to be determined. However, there are a considerable number of drugs available to potentially test the efficacy of inhibiting the renin-angiotensin system on the progression of the human disease.

KEYWORDS: aortic aneurysms; angiotensin; animal models

## INTRODUCTION

Biochemical and cellular processes involved in the initiation, progression, and eventual rupture of human abdominal aortic aneurysms (AAAs) are poorly understood. Definitions of the natural history of the disease and the mediators responsible for the progressive pathology will be needed to design potential therapies for retarding AAA expansion and preventing rupture. Although there are likely to be multiple pathways to provoke the formation of AAAs, the

Address for correspondence: Alan Daugherty, Cardiovascular Research Center, Wethington Building, room 521, University of Kentucky, Lexington, KY 40536-0200. Voice: 859-323-4933 × 81389; fax: 859-257-3646.

e-mail: Alan.Daugherty@uky.edu

Ann. N.Y. Acad. Sci. 1085: 82–91 (2006). © 2006 New York Academy of Sciences.
doi: 10.1196/annals.1383.035

octapeptide, angiotensin II (AngII) has recently emerged as a candidate that could have a pivotal role in this disease.[1] This premise is primarily based on the reproducible formation of AAAs during infusion of AngII into mice. The evidence of a role of AngII in the formation of human AAAs is not so direct and is also under-researched. This article will overview the role of AngII in the formation of AAAs in both animal models and human disease.

### *AngII as a Direct Stimulant of Experimental AAAs*

AngII was initially demonstrated to promote the development of AAAs when infused into LDL receptor –/– mice via subcutaneously implanted osmotic pumps.[2] Subsequently, many labs have demonstrated that the infusion of AngII into apolipoprotein E –/– mice also generates AAAs.[3 8] Also, there has been a report that AngII infusion promotes the development of AAAs in a small percentage of normolipidemic mice.[9] As in humans, there is a greater incidence and severity of AAAs in male compared to female mice.[10,11] The location of the AAAs has been similar in all mouse studies with an easily discernable bulge in the suprarenal area immediately distal to the branch of the right renal artery. Interestingly, this is also the location of AAAs that form in long-term hyperlipidemic mice in the absence of AngII-infusion or when compounded with deficiency of iNOS.[12–15] TABLE 1 summarizes the multiple publications in which pharmacological, surgical, and genetic manipulations have been used to garner mechanistic insight into the formation of AngII-induced AAAs.

The basis for the localization of AngII-induced AAAs forming in the suprarenal region has not been elucidated. It appears to be unrelated to changes in hemodynamic pressure since AAAs can form in the absence of measurable changes in blood pressure.[3] In addition, a decrease in AngII-induced AAA incidence and severity has been noted by interventions that did not affect blood pressure.[11,16] The formation of AAAs in the suprarenal aorta is consistent with specific differences in this region of the aorta contributing to the formation of the disease.

The natural history of the cellular changes in AngII-induced AAAs has been discerned by the acquisition and characterization of suprarenal aortas following selected intervals of AngII infusion.[17] The initial cellular change was an infiltration of macrophages into the media of the aneurysm-prone area. Soon after, a transmedial break was detected that caused luminal expansion. A rapid expansion of the lumen diameter of the suprarenal aorta can be detected within days of AngII infusion.[18] In the majority of mice, the patency of the aorta was retained by the adventitia. Complex inflammatory processes ensue in response to the intramural thrombus that develops in the region of the medial damage. After the initial rapid lumen expansion, there is a more gradual rate of expansion. Although the dimensions of the aorta only change modestly during

**TABLE 1. Effect of pharmacological, surgical, and genetic interventions on the development of AAAs in AngII-infused mice**

| | Approach | Result | References |
|---|---|---|---|
| Pharmacological | AT1 receptor antagonist: losartan | Complete ablation of AAAs | 34 |
| | AT2 receptor antagonist: PD123319 | Increased severity of AAAs | 34 |
| | Doxycycline | Decreased incidence and severity | 16 |
| | 17 beta-estradiol | Decreased incidence and severity | 35 |
| | Mineralocortcoid receptor antagonist: spironolactone | No effect | 36 |
| | Rho-kinase inhibition: fasudil | Decreased incidence and severity | 37 |
| | JNK inhibitor: SP600125 | Decreased size and caused regression | 38 |
| | Antioxidant: vitamin E | Decreased size and rupture rate | 7 |
| | Cyclooxygenase 2 inhibition: celecoxib | Decreased incidence and severity | 39 |
| | Cyclooxygenase 1 inhibition: SC-560 | No effect | 39 |
| Surgical | Ovariectomy | No effect | 11 |
| | Orchidectomy | Decreased incidence and severity | 11 |
| Genetic | Urokinase deficiency | Decreased incidence | 9 |
| | Osteopontin deficiency | Decreased incidence | 5 |
| | CCR2 deficiency on bone marrow-derived cells | Decreased incidence | 6 |

this phase, there is profound remodeling in which the thrombus is typically resorbed and replaced by fibrous tissue that is intermeshed with several leukocytes types, including macrophages, T and B lymphocytes. Interestingly, the region becomes re-endothelialized and a "neomedia" may form throughout the entire lumen.

In recent studies, we have prolonged the duration of AngII to determine whether there are progressive changes in the size and characteristics of AAAs. ApoE–/– mice were implanted with Alzet pumps infusing AngII at a rate of 1,000 ng/kg/min. Pumps were replaced every 28 days for an 84-day duration. During the infusion interval, the lumen diameter and area of the suprarenal aorta were monitored noninvasively using a high-frequency Visualsonics ultrasound machine.[19] Systolic blood pressure was monitored on conscious mice using a tail cuff method (Visitech Systems, Inc., Apex, NC). As can be seen in FIGURE 1A, a rapid (within 7–14 days) increase in lumen area of the suprarenal aorta is followed by a more gradual increase (28–84 days), which continues throughout AngII infusion. Blood pressure was maintained at a constant elevated level during the entire infusion interval. After 84 days of infusion, mice were perfusion fixed at physiological pressures and aortas were dissected free. While most aortas exhibited extensive expansion, there was considerable heterogeneity in gross appearance. FIGURE 1B shows an example of an AAA that had an external diameter of 4.55 mm. This contrasts to a normal aorta with an external diameter of ~ 0.8 mm. Also, there was considerable remodeling of aneursymal tissue with regions of thinning (FIG. 1C). These changes were not noted in the AAAs formed in response to 28 days of AngII infusion. Therefore, aneurysms generated during AngII infusion have large changes in their histological characteristics as a function of the duration of infusion.

### Renin-Angiotensin System in Other Models of the Disease

In addition to the infusion of AngII as a stimulus to promote the development and maturation of AAAs, there is evidence for a role of the renin-angiotensin system in other models of the disease. A common animal model of AAA is the intraluminal infusion of elastase. This model was originally developed in rats and subsequently used in mice.[20,21] Angiotensin-converting enzyme (ACE) immunostaining is present in the AAAs that form in elastase-infused rats.[22] This increase in ACE within the aneurysmal tissue may have pathological consequences since three ACE inhibitors (captopril, lisinopril, and enalapril) prevented AAA development in this model. This ability of ACE inhibitors to prevent elastase-induced AAAs was not associated with hemodynamic effects. The AT1 receptor antagonist, losartan, had no effect on the formation of AAAs.[23] Similarly, the aortic aneurysms formed by the administration of beta-aminopropionitrile to rats are inhibited by the ACE inhibitor, temocapril,

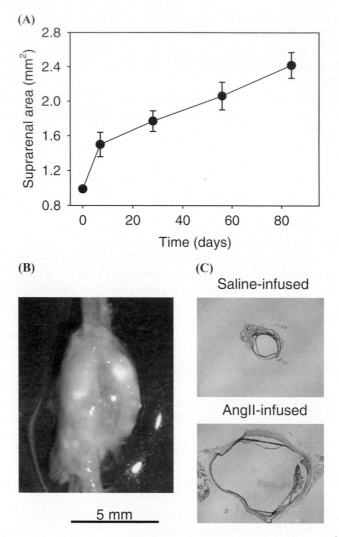

**FIGURE 1.** Characteristics of AngII-induced AAAs in apolipoprotein $E^{-/-}$ mice infused with AngII for prolonged intervals. **(A)** Sequential measurements of suprarenal aortic lumen area of apolipoprotein $E^{-/-}$ mice ($n = 16$) infused with AngII (1000 ng/kg/min) acquired noninvasively by high-frequency ultrasound. **(B)** An example of a large dilated suprarenal aorta after 84 days of AngII infusion. **(C)** Tissue sections from apolipoprotein $E^{-/-}$ mice infused with either saline (upper) or AngII (lower) for 84 days.

but not by the AT1 receptor antagonist, CS866.[24] Finally, Brown Norway rats have spontaneous breaks in aortic elastin fibers as seen in AAAs, which are prevented by the administration of either an ACE inhibitor, enalapril, or the AT1 receptor antagonist, losartan.[25]

## *Evidence for AngII as a Factor in the Development of Human AAAs*

Currently, there is not extensive literature elucidating the role of the renin-angiotensin system in the development of human AAAs. There are relatively few gene association studies in AAA research that specifically relate to the renin-angiotensin system. One study has examined the relationship of the A1166C polymorphism in the AT1 receptor gene and found a significantly greater incidence in patients afflicted with AAA compared to an age- and gender-matched control group.[26] Several gene association studies have been performed on polymorphisms of ACE and their relationship to AAAs. These have all focused on the relative presence of the DD or II genotype. This polymorphism is created by the insertion (I allele) or deletion (D allele) of a 287-bp sequence in intron 16 of the ACE gene. The DD genotype is associated with an increased plasma activity of ACE. The presence of the DD genotype has been demonstrated to be independently related to the disease.[26,27] However, two other studies failed to positively associate DD genotype with AAA.[28,29] A common shortcoming of all these studies is the use of relatively small numbers of subjects. This deficiency is combined with a disease that has a high inter-individual variability in its expansion rates and an accuracy of ultrasonic measurements that are large relative to the expansion rates. Therefore, meaningful gene association studies will probably require large numbers of subjects and would be assisted by use of modalities with enhanced resolution such as computed tomography.

Concentrations of plasma constituents are common in determining their role in disease. However, there are substantial technical problems in measuring plasma concentrations of AngII. These issues include the very low plasma concentrations and the short half-life of the peptide. Also, since AngII is one of a family of closely related peptides with distinct biological activity, the commonly used immunologically based measurements of AngII require the tedious resolution of peptides by high-performance liquid chromatography prior to performing an assay that would reliably quantify plasma concentrations. Even if plasma concentrations are accurately determined, these may be of little predictive value since the generation of AngII locally at the site of AAA formation could be the primary determinant of disease progression.

The presence of some components of the classic renin-angiotensin pathway has been detected in human AAA tissue. This includes ACE, which has been detected in human AAA tissue by immunocytochemistry in association with macrophages.[30] Chymase, which has the ability to convert AngI to AngII, is also present in AAA, but in the mast cells of the adventitia. Furthermore, extracts of AAA tissue form angiotensin peptides.[30,31] These reports note that the role of chymase predominates over ACE in these extracts. However, this may not reflect its relative importance in intact tissue since the preparation of the extract may result in the release of intracellular stores of chymase. Although details of the synthetic pathway need to be fully described, AngII formed in AAA tissue exerts biological effects. This has been shown recently in a study demonstrating that the AT1 receptor antagonist, irbesartan, decreased the production of osteoprotegrin from AAA explants.[32]

There are multiple drugs used clinically in the treatment of different cardiovascular diseases that effectively inhibit ACE or antagonize AT1 receptors. These drugs could be used to directly test the hypothesis that the inhibition of the renin-angiotensin system would retard expansion, or even cause regression, of human AAAs. However, since drugs of these classes are considered within the standards of care for individuals with cardiovascular disease that commonly coexists in patients with AAAs, it is unlikely that clinical trials with placebo group comparisons would be performed. One approach that may be useful in the future is the use of renin inhibitors that are currently under development.[33] These compounds would effectively inhibit the synthesis of all bioactive angiotensin peptides and could be used as adjuncts to ACE inhibitors and AT1 receptor antagonists.

## CONCLUSIONS

The reproducibility with which AngII promotes the formation of AAAs in mice is consistent with an imbalance in the renin-angiotensin system being a pathogenic mechanism of this disease. The potential applicability of these findings in animal models combined with the wide range of drugs to inhibit the renin-angiotensin system may provide a basis for a therapy to treat human AAA.

## ACKNOWLEDGMENTS

Work performed in the authors' laboratory was supported by the National Institutes of Health (HL62846 and HL70239) and the American Heart Association.

## REFERENCES

1. DAUGHERTY, A. & L. CASSIS. 2004. Angiotensin II and abdominal aortic aneurysms. Curr. Hypertens. Rep. **6:** 442–446.
2. DAUGHERTY, A. & L. CASSIS. 1999. Chronic angiotensin II infusion promotes atherogenesis in low density lipoprotein receptor −/− mice. Ann. N. Y. Acad. Sci. **892:** 108–118.
3. DAUGHERTY, A., M.W. MANNING, & L.A. CASSIS. 2000. Angiotensin II promotes atherosclerotic lesions and aneurysms in apolipoprotein E-deficient mice. J. Clin. Invest. **105:** 1605–1612.
4. WANG, Y.X., B. MARTIN MCNULTY, A.D. FREAY, et al. 2001. Angiotensin II increases urokinase-type plasminogen activator expression and induces aneurysm in the abdominal aorta of apolipoprotein E-deficient mice. Am. J. Pathol. **159:** 1455–1464.

5. BRUEMMER, D., A.R. COLLINS, G. NOH, *et al.* 2003. Angiotensin II-accelerated atherosclerosis and aneurysm formation is attenuated in osteopontin-deficient mice. J. Clin. Invest. **112:** 1318–1331.
6. ISHIBASHI, M., K. EGASHIRA, Q. ZHAO, *et al.* 2004. Bone marrow-derived monocyte chemoattractant protein-1 receptor CCR2 is critical in angiotensin II-induced acceleration of atherosclerosis and aneurysm formation in hypercholesterolemic mice. Arterioscler. Thromb. Vasc. Biol. **24:** e174–e178.
7. GAVRILA, D., W.G. LI, M.L. MCCORMICK, *et al.* 2005. Vitamin E inhibits abdominal aortic aneurysm formation in angiotensin ii-infused, apolipoprotein E-deficient mice. Arterioscler. Thromb. Vasc. Biol. **25:** 1671–1677.
8. AYABE, N., V.R. BABAEV, Y. TANG, *et al.* 2005. Transiently heightened angiotensin II has distinct effects on atherosclerosis and aneurysm formation in hyperlipidemic mice. Atherosclerosis **184:** 312–321.
9. DENG, G.G., B. MARTIN-MCNULTY, D.A. SUKOVICH, *et al.* 2003. Urokinase-type plasminogen activator plays a critical role in angiotensin II-induced abdominal aortic aneurysm. Circ. Res. **92:** 510–517.
10. MANNING, M.W., L.A. CASSIS, J. HUANG, *et al.* 2002. Abdominal aortic aneurysms: fresh insights from a novel animal model of the disease. Vasc. Med. **7:** 45–54.
11. HENRIQUES, T.A., J. HUANG, S.S. D'SOUZA, *et al.* 2004. Orchiectomy, but not ovariectomy, regulates angiotensin ii-induced vascular diseases in apolipoprotein E deficient mice. Endocrinology **145:** 3866–3872.
12. TANGIRALA, R.K., E.M. RUBIN & W. PALINSKI. 1995. Quantitation of atherosclerosis in murine models: correlation between lesions in the aortic origin and in the entire aorta, and differences in the extent of lesions between sexes in LDL receptor-deficient and apolipoprotein E-deficient mice. J. Lipid Res. **36:** 2320–2328.
13. CARMELIET, P., L. MOONS, R. LIJNEN, *et al.* 1997. Urokinase-generated plasmin activates matrix metalloproteinases during aneurysm formation. Nature Genet. **17:** 439–444.
14. DAUGHERTY, A. & L.A. CASSIS. 2004. Mouse models of abdominal aortic aneurysms. Arterioscler. Thromb. Vasc. Biol. **24:** 429–434.
15. KUHLENCORDT, P.J., R. GYURKO, F. HAN, *et al.* 2001. Accelerated atherosclerosis, aortic aneurysm formation, and ischemic heart disease in apolipoprotein E/endothelial nitric oxide synthase double-knockout mice. Circulation **104:** 448–454.
16. MANNING, M.W., L.A. CASSIS, & A. DAUGHERTY. 2003. Differential effects of doxycycline, a broad-spectrum matrix metalloproteinase inhibitor, on angiotensin II-induced atherosclerosis and abdominal aortic aneurysms. Arterioscler. Thromb. Vasc. Biol. **23:** 483–488.
17. SARAFF, K., F. BABAMUSTA, L.A. CASSIS & A. DAUGHERTY. 2003. Aortic dissection precedes formation of aneurysms and atherosclerosis in angiotensin II-infused, apolipoprotein E-deficient mice. Arterioscler. Thromb. Vasc. Biol. **23:** 1621–1626.
18. BARISIONE, C., R.J. CHARNIGO, D.A. HOWATT, *et al.* 2006. Rapid dilation of the abdominal aorta during infusion of angiotensin II detected by noninvasive high frequency ultrasound. J. Vasc. Surg. **44:** 372–376.
19. MARTIN-MCNULTY, B., J. VINCELETTE, R. VERGONA, *et al.* 2005. Noninvasive measurement of abdominal aortic aneurysms in intact mice by a high frequency ultrasound imaging system. Ultrasound Med. Biol. **31:** 746–749.

20. ANIDJAR, S., P.B. DOBRIN, M. EICHORST, *et al.* 1992. Correlation of inflammatory infiltrate with the enlargement of experimental aortic aneurysms. J. Vasc. Surg. **16:** 139–147.

21. PYO, R., J.K. LEE, J.M. SHIPLEY, *et al.* 2000. Targeted gene disruption of matrix metalloproteinase-9 (gelatinase B) suppresses development of experimental abdominal aortic aneurysms. J. Clin. Invest. **105:** 1641–1649.

22. SINHA, I., K.K. HANNAWA, G. AILAWADI, *et al.* 2006. The nitric oxide donor DETA-NONOate decreases matrix metalloproteinase-9 expression and activity in rat aortic smooth muscle and abdominal aortic explants. Ann. Vasc. Surg. **20:** 92–98.

23. LIAO, S., M. MIRALLES, B.J. KELLEY, *et al.* 2001. Suppression of experimental abdominal aortic aneurysms in the rat by treatment with angiotensin-converting enzyme inhibitors. J. Vasc. Surg. **33:** 1057–1064.

24. NAGASHIMA, H., K. UTO, Y. SAKOMURA, *et al.* 2002. An angiotensin-converting enzyme inhibitor, not an angiotensin II type-1 receptor blocker, prevents beta-aminopropionitrile monofumarate-induced aortic dissection in rats. J. Vasc. Surg. **36:** 818–823.

25. HUANG, W., F. ALHENC GELAS & M.J. OSBORNE-PELLEGRIN. 1998. Protection of the arterial internal elastic lamina by inhibition of the renin-angiotensin system in the rat. Circ. Res. **82:** 879–890.

26. FATINI, C., G. PRATESI, F. SOFI, *et al.* 2005. ACE DD genotype: a predisposing factor for abdominal aortic aneurysm. Eur. J. Vasc. Endovasc. Surg. **29:** 227–232.

27. POLA, R., E. GAETANI, A. SANTOLIQUIDO, *et al.* 2001. Abdominal aortic aneurysm in normotensive patients: association with angiotensin-converting enzyme gene polymorphism. Eur. J. Vasc. Endovasc. Surg. **21:** 445–449.

28. HAMANO, K., M. OHISHI, M. UEDA, *et al.* 1999. Deletion polymorphism in the gene for angiotensin-converting enzyme is not a risk factor predisposing to abdominal aortic aneurysm. Eur. J. Vasc. Endovasc. Surg. **18:** 158–161.

29. YEUNG, J.M., M. HEELEY, S. GRAY, *et al.* 2002. Does the angiotensin-converting enzyme (ACE) gene polymorphism affect rate of abdominal aortic aneurysm expansion? Eur. J. Vasc. Endovasc. Surg. **24:** 69–71.

30. IHARA, M., H. URATA, A. KINOSHITA, *et al.* 1999. Increased chymase-dependent angiotensin II formation in human atherosclerotic aorta. Hypertension **33:** 1399–1405.

31. NISHIMOTO, M., S. TAKAI, H. FUKUMOTO, *et al.* 2002. Increased local angiotensin II formation in aneurysmal aorta. Life Sciences **71:** 2195–2205.

32. MORAN, C.S., M. MCCANN, M. KARAN, *et al.* 2005. Association of osteoprotegerin with human abdominal aortic aneurysm progression. Circulation **111:** 3119–3125.

33. AZIZI, M., R. WEBB, J. NUSSBERGER & N.K. HOLLENBERG. 2006. Renin inhibition with aliskiren: where are we now, and where are we going? J. Hypertens. **24:** 243–256.

34. DAUGHERTY, A., M.W. MANNING & L.A. CASSIS. 2001. Antagonism of AT2 receptors augments Angiotensin II-induced abdominal aortic aneurysms and atherosclerosis. Br. J. Pharmacol. **134:** 865–870.

35. MARTIN-MCNULTY, B., D.M. THAM, V. DA CUNHA, *et al.* 2003. 17 beta-estradiol attenuates development of angiotensin II induced aortic abdominal aneurysm in apolipoprotein E deficient mice. Arterioscler. Thromb. Vasc. Biol. **23:** 1627–1632.

36. CASSIS, L.A., M.J. HELTON, D.A. HOWATT, *et al.* 2005. Aldosterone does not mediate angiotensin II-induced atherosclerosis and abdominal aortic aneurysms. Br. J. Pharmacol. **144:** 443–448.
37. WANG, Y.X., B. MARTIN-MCNULTY, V. DA CUNHA, *et al.* 2005. Fasudil, a Rho-kinase inhibitor, attenuates angiotensin II-induced abdominal aortic aneurysm in apolipoprotein E-deficient mice by inhibiting apoptosis and proteolysis. Circulation **111:** 2219–2226.
38. YOSHIMURA, K., H. AOKI, Y. IKEDA, *et al.* 2005. Regression of abdominal aortic aneurysm by inhibition of c-Jun N-terminal kinase. Nat. Med. **11:** 1330–1338.
39. KING, V.L., D. TRIVEDI, J.M. GITLIN, & C.D. LOFTIN. 2006. Selective cyclooxygenase-2 inhibition with celecoxib decreases angiotensin II-induced abdominal aortic aneurysm formation in mice. Arterioscler Thromb. Vasc. Biol. **26:** 1137–1143.

# AAA Disease

## Mechanism, Stratification, and Treatment

RONALD L. DALMAN,[a] MAUREEN M. TEDESCO,[a] JONATHON MYERS,[b] AND CHARLES A. TAYLOR[c]

[a]Department of Surgery, Stanford University Medical Center, Stanford, CA, USA

[b]Palo Alto Institute for Research and Education, Palo Alto, CA, USA

[c]Department of Bioengineering, Stanford University, Stanford, CA, USA

ABSTRACT: Abdominal aortic aneurysm (AAA) is a common and frequently lethal disease of older Americans. No medical therapy has been proven effective in retarding progression of small AAAs prior to surgical repair. With the emerging ability of magnetic resonance (MR) flow imaging and MR-based computational analysis to define aortic hemodynamic conditions, and bio-imaging strategies to monitor aortic inflammation real time *in vivo*, the opportunity now exists to confirm the potential value of medical interventions such as supervised exercise training as first line therapy for small AAA disease.

KEYWORDS: abdominal aortic aneurysm; exercise; hemodynamics

## INTRODUCTION

Advanced age, a history of cigarette smoking, male gender, and family history have traditionally been recognized as significant risk factors for abdominal aortic aneurysm (AAA) disease. Of these, smoking is the most significant; after adjustment for confounding risks, smoking is associated with a fivefold increase in AAA risk in men.[1] The incidence of unsuspected, asymptomatic AAA in men and women over 60 years of age is 4% to 8% and 0.5% to 1.5%, respectively.[1–7] Risks of rupture and sudden death are most closely related to diameter. AAAs $\geq$ 6 cm have a 10% to 20% chance of rupture within 12 months.[8–10] One-third of all AAAs eventually rupture if left untreated.

While more is being learned about AAA biology and behavior,[11] aneurysm diameter remains the most important clinical determinant for risk of rupture.[12] Typically identified as an incidental finding on abdominal imaging studies,

Address for correspondence: Ronald L. Dalman, M.D., F.A.C.S., F.A.H.A., Division of Vascular Surgery, Stanford University Medical Center, 300 Pasteur Dr. Suite H3642, Stanford, CA 94305-5642. Voice: 650-723-2031; fax: 650-498-6044.
e-mail: rld@stanford.edu

Ann. N.Y. Acad. Sci. 1085: 92–109 (2006). © 2006 New York Academy of Sciences.
doi: 10.1196/annals.1383.008

the mean growth rate of small AAAs ($\leq 5.5$ cm) is 2.6 mm/y, increasing with aneurysm diameter.[13,14] Surgical repair is currently the only effective method of AAA treatment. Despite numerous advances in surgical techniques and perioperative management, operative mortality for open elective and ruptured AAA repair has remained stable at 5.6% and 45.7%, respectively, for more than 20 years.[15] Postoperative survival has also not improved over the past two decades, perhaps due to more aggressive indications for repair offsetting improvements in surgical, medical, and anesthetic perioperative management. While newer endovascular exclusion strategies and devices limit the operative morbidity associated with open surgical repair in patients with suitable anatomy, these "endografts" have their own limitations, namely late migration, endoleak formation, and continued aneurysm expansion that mandate continued surveillance and frequent reintervention following initial technical success.[8]

The United States Preventative Services Task Force (USPSTF) recently updated its recommendations regarding the potential utility of screening ultrasound examinations to detect AAA disease. In 1996 the USPSTF had found insufficient evidence to recommend for or against routine AAA screening of asymptomatic adults. On the basis of a systematic re-review of updated information, including the results from four population-based, randomized, controlled screening trials, the Task Force recently concluded that AAA screening may reduce AAA-related mortality by 43% in men aged 65 to 75 years. Although surgical repair, as the only effective treatment, is associated with significant risks, the natural history of the disease outweighs these risks for men with AAAs greater than 5.5 cm. The potential utility of intervention for smaller AAA was also considered, but the risks of surgical repair greatly outweighed the potential benefit of reduced AAA rupture, even taking into account the likelihood that widespread screening will identify tens of thousands of new patients with smaller AAAs.[16]

The high prevalence and lethality of AAA disease stimulated the NIH-HLBI to issue a disease-specific request for applications (RFA) in December 1998. This RFA succeeded in generating considerable new knowledge regarding aneurysm pathogenesis and increased public awareness about AAAs. Despite these accomplishments, however, no potential therapeutic strategy has been demonstrated to improve clinical outcome in "worried well" patients with small, preclinical AAAs. Reducing the expansion rate of small AAAs by 50% would effectively eliminate the need for surgery in many older patients.[8] Strategies that have proven effective in limiting rodent AAA progression in biologically relevant models[17] have included matrix metalloproteinase (MMP) inhibition (doxycycline[18] and hydroxamic acids[19]), reduction of mural inflammation (angiotensin-converting enzyme (ACE) inhibitors,[20] suppression of NF-κB expression,[21,22] statins,[23,24] antioxidants,[25] osteopontin inhibition[26]) as well as hemodynamic conditioning[25,27,28] and medial smooth muscle cell augmentation.[29] Despite these promising results, there has been only one adequately powered, randomized, clinical trial of medical therapy (propranolol) for small AAA disease. Beta-blockade was found to have no effect on the expansion rate of small AAA.[30] An additional trial testing doxycycline is ongoing.[31]

A major translational hurdle is the lack of direct indicators of aneurysm inflammation or inflammatory tone in models as well as patients. External aneurysm diameter, while of demonstrated value in predicting aneurysm rupture and patient survival in natural history studies, is less useful as the sole end point for validation or optimization of medical intervention strategies. This is true because expansion rate as the final common denominator of the degenerative process is likely to be relatively insensitive to more subtle but significant changes in AAA cellularity and pro- and anti-inflammatory mediator expression. Recently described analytical methods to estimate aortic wall strain from cross-sectional image data sets improve prediction of impending symptomatic evolution or rupture of large AAA but offer little additional insight regarding monitoring of less advanced disease. Circulating MMP-9 and hsCRP levels, while correlated with AAA status (present or absent, likelihood of clinical events, etc.) are not likely to be sufficiently disease specific to guide therapy for small aneurysm management; for example, reductions may not correlate with reduced AAA progression. We and others are currently working to identify and validate methods of directly assessing mural cellularity and inflammation *in vivo* to facilitate translation of promising therapies such as those described in the previous paragraph from bench to bedside.

Aneurysms occur with greatest frequency in the distal aorta. Although many theories have been advanced to explain this tendency, differential hemodynamic influences present along the length of the thoracic and abdominal aortas are potentially the most significant. Compared with the suprarenal aorta, the infrarenal environment in resting subjects is characterized by increased peripheral resistance, increased oscillatory wall shear stress (WSS), and reduced flow. These "resistive" hemodynamic conditions predispose arteries to degenerative diseases.[32] Infrarenal aortic MMP-9 expression is significantly greater than that present in the thoracic aorta during resting conditions. Transposition of the abdominal aorta to the thoracic position, however, reduces mural protease expression while reciprocal transposition of the thoracic aorta to the abdominal position increases levels to those seen in the infrarenal aorta *in situ*.[33] Major limb amputation,[34] chronic spinal cord injury,[35] and severe peripheral vascular disease[36] have recently been recognized as potential new risk factors for AAA disease, associations that highlight the pathogenic significance of resistive hemodynamic conditions. We have accumulated evidence over the last several years demonstrating that these high-risk sedentary hemodynamic conditions are completely obliterated with moderate levels of exercise.

In addition to directly modulating mural MMP-9 expression, luminal hemodynamic conditions may also significantly influence underlying aortic inflammatory tone.[37] Resistive aortic hemodynamics such as those found in the infrarenal aorta under sedentary conditions promote aortic inflammation and the production of reactive oxygen species (ROS).[38,39] ROS in turn promote the upregulation and activation of proteolytic MMPs implicated in human AAA pathogenesis,[40-42] inactivate endogenous antiproteases, increase expression of proinflammatory transcription factors, chemokines and cytokines, and stimulate apoptosis.[43] The antioxidative[44] and antiapoptotic[45] influences of increased antegrade flow as is present in the aorta following lower extremity exercise may reduce aortic inflammation, maintain or improve intimal and medial vascular cell populations, and ultimately attenuate AAA progression.[25,46-51]

Aortic hemodynamic conditions directly reflect daily and lifelong patterns of lower extremity activity and exercise.[52-54] Despite considerable indirect evidence that aortic hemodynamic conditions influence AAA risk, the association between physical activity levels and disease progression has not been tested in a scientifically rigorous fashion. Coupled with the lack of effective treatment options for patients diagnosed with small AAAs, the significant disease-related anxiety present in patients who understand they have a life-threatening illness that carries a small chance of sudden death in the months or years prior to eligibility for surgical repair,[16,55] and the well-demonstrated benefits of exercise capacity for predicting cardiovascular and all-cause mortality,[56] confirming the relationship between activity level and disease risk may guide development of innovative new therapies while substantially improving the health of small AAA patients.

To confirm the degree to which aortic hemodynamic conditions influence human AAA disease progression, we recently conducted a prevalence survey in the "ultimate" sedentary patient population, spinal cord injury (SCI) patients. This population-based, controlled study included SCI patients $\geq$ 55 years old who had been injured and unable to walk for $\geq$ 5 years. Aortic and iliac artery diameters in SCI patients ($n = 123$) were compared to those of control patients ($n = 129$) without known abdominal or iliac aneurysms recruited from an age and risk–factor-matched ambulatory patient database prospectively maintained for the express purpose of examining SCI-related medical conditions. Aortic and iliac diameters were determined via transabdominal ultrasound. Normal aortic diameter (D) was defined as 2.0 cm (range 1.8–2.4); D $\leq$ 1.8 cm were "small," $2.5 \geq D \leq 3.0$ "enlarged," and D $\geq$ 3.0 were defined as AAAs.[57] When grouped by 0.1 cm increments, aortic diameters in SCI patients trended higher than control, while iliac arteries were smaller. Overall there were significantly more AAAs, enlarged aortas, and small iliac arteries in SCI patients (all $P < 0.05$, TABLE 1). The prevalence of larger aortas in the SCI cohort was not explained by differences noted in traditional risk factors[58]

Diminished iliac artery diameter is expected in SCI patients as a result of the known propensity of arteries to remodel inward in response to sustained blood flow reductions. The paradoxical presence of increased aortic diameter and AAA prevalence in SCI patients is not consistent with known flow/remodeling relationships and supports the growing body of evidence that sedentary existence and chronically reduced/asymmetric aortic flow represent independent

**TABLE 1. Aortic and iliac artery diameter in SCI and control subjects**

| Diameter | SCI (%) | Control (%) | $P$-value |
|---|---|---|---|
| Aorta (cm $\pm$ SD) | $2.3 \pm 0.9$ | $2.0 \pm 0.4$ | <0.01 |
| $\geq 3.0$ cm (AAA) | 11 (8.9) | 4 (3.1) | 0.04 |
| $\geq 2.5$ cm (AAA + enlarged) | 31 (25.2) | 15 (11.6) | <0.01 |
| Common iliac(s) | $1.1 \pm 0.3$ | $1.1 \pm 0.2$ | ns |
| $\geq 1.5$ cm (aneurysm) | 9 (5.4) | 12 (5.3) | ns |
| $\geq 1.25$ (aneurysm + enlarged) | 26 (15.5) | 44 (19.4) | ns |
| <1.0 cm (small) | 80 (47.6) | 59 (26.0) | <0.01 |

Reprinted with permission from the Society of Vascular Surgery.[58]

risk factors for AAA disease.[34–36] Considered another way, normal aortic flow associated with ambulation reduces AAA disease risk in otherwise comparable patient groups. MR arteriography demonstrated increased aortic contours in SCI compared to control patients. The SCI patients were chosen at random for MR flow analysis from the larger SCI patient cohort after being demonstrated to have aortic diameters < 3 cm (did not meet AAA criteria) by ultrasound. Despite the absence of a formal aneurysm, we found a predilection for infrarenal aneurysmal degeneration despite diminutive iliac artery diameter present in the setting of spinal cord injury.

MR flow imaging and computational flow methods confirm the ability of lower extremity exercise to reduce proinflammatory hemodynamic conditions in the infrarenal aorta. In additional experiments we measured aortic flow in healthy subjects aged 20–30 and 50–70 years,[53,54,59] and atherosclerotic patients suffering from intermittent claudication (unpublished data) at rest and following lower extremity exercise. For these experiments we constructed a custom MR-compatible exercise cycle for the GE 0.5T open magnet.[60] Each subject was positioned such that his/her abdominal aorta was centered in the magnet. The cycle was then adjusted for subject size and strength. Cine phase-contrast MRI (PC-MRI) was performed to acquire time-resolved anatomic and through-plane velocity maps[61–63] perpendicular to the abdominal aorta at supraceliac and infrarenal levels at rest and during steady-state exercise conditions (150% of resting heart rate). The cine acquisitions were gated to the cardiac cycle using a plethysmograph, and images were reconstructed to 16 time points over the cardiac cycle.

We applied a level set segmentation method[64,65] to identify the flow lumen using cross-sectional aortic images for each time step. From these time-resolved segmentations and the associated velocity data we computed blood flow rate[63] and WSS.[66] Temporal oscillations of flow and shear were quantified by oscillatory flow (OFI)[60] and shear (OSI)[67] indices, respectively. In the older, healthy subjects, wall shear stress increased from $2.0 \pm 0.7$ to $7.3 \pm 2.4$ dynes/cm$^2$ in the supraceliac aorta and $1.4 \pm 0.8$ to $16.5 \pm 5.1$ dynes/cm$^2$ at the infrarenal level (both $P < 0.001$) from rest to exercise. Blood velocity surface plots for peak systole, end systole, and end diastole at the supraceliac and infrarenal levels at rest and during exercise for a healthy 20-year-old subject were constructed. These plots illustrated increased blood velocities at peak systole, end systole, and end diastole from rest to exercise for both the supraceliac and infrarenal locations. Moderate exercise increased infrarenal more than supraceliac flow, suggesting that lower extremity hyperemia occurs in part at the expense of mesenteric flow. Proinflammatory infrarenal aortic hemodynamic conditions present at rest (retrograde and oscillating diastolic flow) were obliterated during exercise. Aortic WSS increased during the entire cardiac cycle at all levels.

Although lower extremity exercise increases aortic flow and WSS, until recently little evidence was available to suggest that intermittent exercise produces sustained cardiovascular benefits. The exercise literature clearly demonstrates, however, that daily exercise periods are associated with marked reductions in all cause mortality and vascular-related complications in patients with cardiovascular disease.[68] Single episodes also produce sustained increases in human circulating progenitor cells,[69] redox-related gene expression, and when repeated over long intervals, conduit artery remodeling and disease resistance.[70] Similar shear-mediated effects present in our high-flow AAA models are associated with reduced aneurysm progression, albeit in a greatly truncated time frame due to continuously increased flow. It is likely, however, that gene expression and protein phosphorylation triggered by episodic increases in WSS modify arterial structure and function for sustained intervals following frequent intermittent exercise episodes.

We also developed and validated three-dimensional finite element methods for modeling blood flow[64,65,71–79] and applied these methods to computing flow in subject-specific models from CT and MRI data sets.[64,65,71,74,77–80] FIGURE 1 depicts velocity profiles computed for the abdominal aorta of a 19-year-old subject. The anatomic model was constructed from contrast-enhanced MR angiography data. Boundary conditions were specified on the basis of flow velocities measured at two discrete locations (supraceliac and immediately infrarenal aorta) at rest and during exercise using cine phase-contrast (PC)-MRI. The aorta demonstrates exceptionally complex flow patterns over the cardiac cycle under resting conditions, and the flow velocity field becomes more unidirectional and ordered under exercise conditions. While the blood flow in the abdominal aorta is still laminar (the solutions retain periodicity and do not exhibit random behavior associated with turbulent flow), it is clearly highly complex, particularly in the lower abdominal aorta in diastole.

Using updated finite element methods for solving nonlinear one-dimensional equations of blood flow that enforce pressure continuity and mass conservation at branch points as well as flow rate, pressure resistance, and impedance boundary conditions,[81–83] we modeled blood flow and pressure in the abdominal aorta of an SCI patient as well as an ambulatory control patient and AAA geometric model to analyze flow and WSS relationships in more

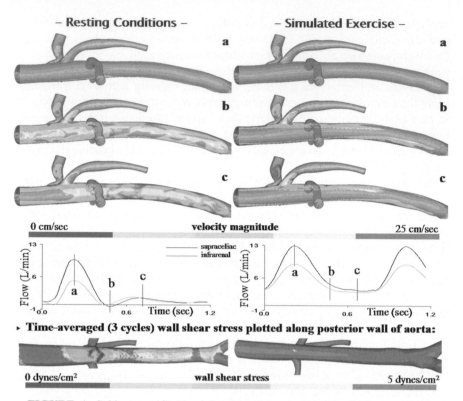

**FIGURE 1.** Subject-specific blood flow simulation in the abdominal aorta. The geometric model was constructed from MRA data and flow boundary conditions were based on PC-MRI data. (Adapted from B.T. Tang, C.P. Cheng, M.T. Draney, N.M. Wilson, P.S. Tsao, R.J. Herfkens, C.A. Taylor. Abdominal Aortic Hemodynamics in Young Healthy Adults at Rest and During Lower Limb Exercise: Quantification Using Image-based Computer Modeling. To appear in *American Journal of Physiology–Heart and Circulatory Physiology*.)

detail (FIG. 2). Models were constructed on the basis of MRA anatomic data. A fractal tree bifurcation model was generated for SCI vascular beds.[84] Starting with the common iliac arteries, this continued (using known diameter relationships) to the diameter of precapillary arterioles (10 μm). For the SCI patient with smaller common iliac arteries the peripheral resistance was increased. If the infrarenal flow was similar between SCI and ambulatory patients, this would be expected to result in higher pulse pressures in SCI patients, but this proved not to be the case. This can be explained by the long wavelengths (meters) of pressure wave travel in the arterial system. We did note a slower decay of the pressure pulse in SCI patients as compared to the normal subjects in our models. This can be understood by noting that the pressure decay time constant is related to the product of the proximal arterial compliance and the distal vascular resistance, the latter of which increases considerably in the SCI

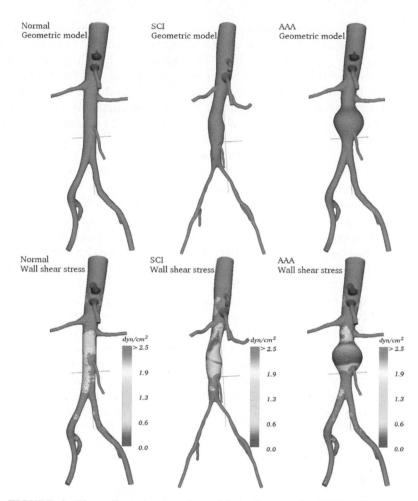

**FIGURE 2.** Three-dimensional aortic models (top) and resting WSS estimates at peak systole (below) of normal and SCI aorta and 4cm AAA, respectively.

patients. Furthermore, resting WSS differed significantly between conditions; roughly twofold lower in SCI and fivefold lower in AAA than in normal aorta. These data support our overall contention that SCI hemodynamic conditions accurately represent an extreme example of the consequences of sedentary existence and that proinflammatory hemodynamic conditions (e.g., reduced antegrade WSS) increase AAA risk in SCI patients. Beyond resting differences, however, SCI is unique in that no increase in aortic WSS occurs on the basis of ambulation. Considering that modest lower extremity exercise in older individuals increases resting aortic WSS approximately 16-fold, and that even sedentary, obese individuals walk on average 80 min/day or 2 km at

5 km/h in "displacement activities,"[85] even minimally active individuals generate at least $2\times$ the total time-averaged WSS experienced by immobile SCI patients during a 24-h period. ($1.3$ h $\times$ $16$ dynes/cm$^2$ + $22.7$ h $\times$ $1$dyne/cm$^2$ vs. $24$ h $\times$ $1$dyne/cm$^2$.) Therefore, we estimate at a minimum a fourfold time-averaged aortic WSS difference occurs between SCI and sedentary patients with even a minimum amount of activity. Pending investigations will confirm whether increasing activity levels confer similar levels of protection against AAA degeneration in ambulatory patients.

Higher levels of physical activity are associated with lower risks of death and cardiovascular disease morbidity. The long-term physiologic consequences of supervised exercise training include decreased resting heart rate, decreased heart rate, and systolic blood pressure at any matched submaximal workload, an increase in work capacity and maximal oxygen uptake as well as a faster return to resting hemodynamic conditions following cessation of activity. These responses may be due to peripheral or cardiac adaptations or both, but peripheral adaptations clearly become more significant with age. In 1984 Froelicher and Myers evaluated exercise conditions using maximal oxygen uptake treadmill and supine bicycle radionuclide testing.[86] Patients in the exercise group (72) underwent 1 year of supervised exercise sessions with exercise intensity progressing in standard fashion throughout the year. As compared to the control group, a significant training effect after 12 months was demonstrated by reduced resting and submaximal heart rates and increased measured and estimated maximal oxygen uptake. No changes were observed in maximal perceived exertion, respiratory exchange ratio, or systolic blood pressure between the two groups initially or at 1 year, or between the initial and 1-year tests within the exercise group. Analysis of variance confirmed that the training effect, including an increase in peak $VO_2$, occurred in subgroups of the exercise intervention patients relative to controls. However, no changes were noted in ECG or cardiac radionucleotide tests, suggesting that most of the beneficial changes associated with exercise occurred in the periphery.[86]

In addition to improving exercise capacity, exercise training significantly improves patient survival. In a meta-analysis of 48 scientifically valid, randomized trials including 8,940 patients undergoing cardiac rehabilitation compared to usual care, exercise training was associated with reduced all-cause mortality (odds ratio (OR = 0.80) and cardiac mortality (OR = 0.74). In addition, exercise training was associated with greater reductions in cholesterol, triglycerides, and systolic blood pressure.[87] Benefits of increased activity are also noted outside the supervised training scenarios: a meta-analysis of 30 cohort studies involving more than 2 million person-years of observation demonstrated a nearly linear decline in the risk of coronary heart disease with increasing levels of physical activity.[88] Both measured fitness level and self-reported physical activity confer protection. Of 6,213 men referred for exercise testing between 1987 and 2000, 842 also underwent assessment of self-reported adulthood activity patterns. The predictive power of exercise capacity and activity patterns along with clinical and exercise test data were assessed for all-cause mortality during a mean of 5 years of follow-up. Considering clinical characteristics such as history of cardiovascular disease, smoking, hypertension, diabetes, obesity, and elevated cholesterol levels, exercise test data and self-reported activity patterns, expressing data by age-adjusted quartiles, exercise capacity HR (hazard ratio) per quartile = 0.72; 95% CI: 0.58 to 0.89, $P = 0.002$) and energy expenditure from self-reported activity during adulthood (HR per quartile = 0.72, 95% CI: 0.58 to 0.89, $P = 0.002$) were the only significant predictors of mortality. Age-adjusted mortality decreased per quartile increase in exercise capacity (HR for very low capacity = 1.0, HR for low = 0.59, HR for moderate = 0.46, HR for high = 0.28) and physical activity (HRs 1.0, 0.63, 0.42, and 0.38, respectively, $P < 0.001$). A 1,000-kcal/week increase in activity was approximately similar to a 1 metabolic equivalent (MET) increase in fitness; both conferred a mortality benefit of 20%.[89]

Although most such survival data have been obtained from cardiac rehabilitation studies, exercise capacity predicts mortality equally well in patients without coronary disease. Examining the same cohort of patients (as in Ref. 89), Drs. Myers and Froelicher classified their patients into two groups: 3,679 with an abnormal exercise test result or a history of cardiovascular disease or both, and 2,534 with a normal exercise test result and no history of cardiovascular disease.[56] After adjustment for age, the peak exercise capacity measured in METs was the strongest predictor of the risk of death among both normal subjects and those with cardiovascular disease. Absolute peak exercise capacity was a stronger predictor of the risk of death than the percentage of the age-predicted value achieved, and there was no interaction between the use or nonuse of beta blockers and the predictive power of exercise capacity. Each 1-MET increase in exercise capacity conferred a 12% improvement in survival,[56] and in a related study, health care costs were incrementally lower by an average of 5.4% per MET increase.[90]

Exercise training and increased levels of physical fitness are also highly effective in reducing systemic markers of inflammation relevant to AAAs. Serum high-sensitivity C-reactive protein (hsCRP) levels are increased in patients with AAA disease,[91] correlate in a stepwise fashion to increasing aneurysm diameter,[93] and apparently originate in part from within aneurysm tissue itself.[92] Exercise training reduces a wide range of serum inflammatory markers including hsCRP level: 2.5 h/week for 6 months reduced mononuclear production of atherogenic cytokines by 58% ($P < 0.001$), while production of atheroprotective cytokines rose by 36% (P < 0.001). Changes in cytokine production were proportionate to the time spent performing repetitive lower-body motion exercises (P < 0.02), suggesting a dose-response relationship. Serum hsCRP levels dropped by 35% with exercise training.[93]

Beyond the direct effects of training, self-reported physical activity shows a significant and inverse dose-response relationship with C-reactive protein and other serum indicators of inflammation, even after adjustment for the confounding effects of traditional atherosclerotic risk factors. These effects are present in men with and without evidence of preexisting coronary disease.[94] Analyzing data from the > 13,000 participants ≥ 20 years old in the National Health and Nutrition examination survey (1988–1994) adjusted for age, sex, ethnicity, work status, education, cotinine concentration, hypertension, body mass index (BMI), waist-to-hip ratio, high-density lipoprotein cholesterol concentration, and aspirin use, the odds ratios for elevated C-reactive protein concentration were 0.98 (95% CI = 0.78–1.23), 0.85 (0.70–1.02), and 0.53 (0.40–0.71) for participants engaged in light, moderate, and vigorous physical activity, respectively, during the previous month compared to participants who did not engage in any leisure-time physical activity.[94] Similar results were obtained in an analysis of self-reported activity from 5,888 men and women ≥ 65 years of age in the Cardiovascular Health Study, although in that study multivariate regression analysis suggested that the association of higher levels of physical activity with lower hsCRP levels may be mediated by body mass index.[95] This is relevant in that the arterial wall is only one potential source of cytokines, which induce C-reactive protein production. Adipose cells also produce cytokines including IL-6, which induces hepatic CRP synthesis. Similar to the effects of exercise, caloric restriction and weight loss also lower IL-6 and CRP and may reduce overall systemic inflammatory tone.

This uncertainty regarding the mechanism by which exercise and activity level reduce inflammation (local aortic hemodynamic vs. metabolic response) highlights the critical need for the identification and validation of methods to directly quantify aortic inflammation or AAA-specific systemic disease markers. Even though CRP levels generally correlate with AAA size, elevated levels do not accurately identify subsets of small AAA patients who will ultimately demonstrate aneurysm enlargement.[92] This uncertainty is not limited to the role of CRP alone. Given the significance of inducible nitric oxide synthase (iNOS) activity and nitric oxide generation in human AAA pathogenesis,[96] and the potent efficacy of selective iNOS inhibition in limiting progression of experimental AAA at all stages of development,[97,98] the ability of exercise to reduce aortic iNOS and adhesion molecule expression and activity in hypercholesterolemic animal models[99] and TNF-α 1, IL-1, IL-6, and iNOS in lower extremity skeletal muscle (but not serum) of patients with congestive heart failure[100] suggests that direct aortic responses play a significant role in the ability of exercise training to reduce AAA progression.

## SUMMARY

Despite intense public interest in AAA disease, the list of promising therapies as identified by experimental modeling is growing much more rapidly than is evidence supporting their efficacy in human disease. This "translational bottleneck" is accentuated by the lack of recognition of direct indicators of aneurysm inflammation, inflammatory tone, and disease progression at the cellular level. The current standard for determination of AAA disease progression is external aneurysm diameter measurement.[93] This metric, while of demonstrated value in predicting aneurysm rupture or patient survival in natural history studies, is not well suited to the purpose of validating or optimizing medical intervention. Diameter enlargement is an indirect cumulative indicator of disease progression, relatively insensitive to more primary and fundamental changes in mural inflammation and remodeling. These fundamental molecular processes, the targets of experimental therapeutic strategies, are not quantifiable using current imaging or monitoring modalities.

Patients with reduced activity levels are at higher risk of AAA disease. Hyperemic luminal conditions present following exercise effectively reduce aortic inflammation, serum CRP levels, and progression of experimental AAAs. We are initiating a multicenter trial to compare exercise capacity and self-reported activity levels between patients with AAA of various sizes and to study the potential role of supervised exercise training to limit progression of small AAA disease. Our hypothesis, based on the exercise literature noted in the preceding paragraphs, is that increased activity reduces the incidence and progression of small AAA disease. These studies are also designed to identify novel bioimaging strategies to quantify and track aortic inflammation, providing new methods of monitoring disease progression and helping to eliminate the translational bottleneck that currently impedes progress in AAA research.

## REFERENCES

1. LEDERLE, F.A., G.R. JOHNSON, S.E. WILSON, *et al.* 2000. The aneurysm detection and management study screening program: validation cohort and final results. Aneurysm Detection and Management Veterans Affairs Cooperative Study Investigators. Arch. Intern. Med. **160:** 1425–1430.
2. ASHTON, H.A., M.J. BUXTON, N.E. DAY, *et al.* 2002. Multicentre Aneurysm Screening Study Group. The Multicentre Aneurysm Screening Study (MASS) into the effect of abdominal aortic aneurysm screening on mortality in men: a randomized controlled trial. Lancet **360:** 1531–1539.
3. LAWRENCE-BROWN, M.M., P.E. NORMAN, K. JAMROZIK, *et al.* 2001. Initial results of ultrasound screening for aneurysm of the abdominal aorta in Western Australia: relevance for endoluminal treatment of aneurysm disease. Cardiovasc. Surg. **9:** 234–240.
4. WILMINK, T.B. & C.R. QUICK. 1998. Epidemiology and potential for prevention of abdominal aortic aneurysm. Br. J. Surg. **85:** 155–162.
5. WILMINK, T.B., C.R. QUICK, C.S. HUBBARD, *et al.* 1999. The influence of screening on the incidence of ruptured abdominal aortic aneurysms. J. Vasc. Surg. **30:** 203–208.
6. LINDHOLT, J.S., S. JUUL, H. FASTING, *et al.* 2002. Hospital costs and benefits of screening for abdominal aortic aneurysms. Results from a randomized population screening trial. Eur. J. Vasc. Endovasc. Surg. **23:** 55–60.

7. KENT, K.C., R.M. ZWOLAK, M.R. JAFF, *et al.* 2004. Screening for abdominal aortic aneurysm: a consensus statement. J. Vasc. Surg. **39:** 267–269.

8. BREWSTER, D.C., J.L. CRONENWETT, J.W. HALLETT, *et al.* 2003. Guidelines for the treatment of abdominal aortic aneurysms. Report of a subcommittee of the Joint Council of the American Association for Vascular Surgery and Society for Vascular Surgery. J. Vasc. Surg. **37:** 1106–1117.

9. WILMINK, A.B., M. FORSHAW, C.R. QUICK, *et al.* 2002. Accuracy of serial screening for abdominal aortic aneurysms by ultrasound. J. Med. Screen **9:** 125–127.

10. WILMINK, A.B., C.S. HUBBARD & C.R. QUICK. 1997. Quality of the measurement of the infrarenal aortic diameter by ultrasound. J. Med. Screen **4:** 49–53.

11. WASSEF, M., B.T. BAXTER, R. CHISHOLM, *et al.* 2001. Pathogenesis of abdominal aortic aneurysms: a multidisciplinary research program supported by the National Heart, Lung and Blood Institute. J. Vasc. Surg. **34:** 730–738.

12. FILLINGER, M.F., M.L. RAGHAVAN, S.P. MARRA, *et al.* 2002. *In vivo* analysis of mechanical wall stress and abdominal aortic aneurysm rupture risk. J. Vasc. Surg. **36:** 589–597.

13. LEDERLE, F.A., G.R. JOHNSON, S.E. WILSON, *et al.* 2002. Rupture rate of large abdominal aortic aneurysms in patients refusing or unfit for elective repair. JAMA **287:** 2968–2972.

14. BRADY, A.R., S.G. THOMPSON, R.M. GREENHALGH & J.T. POWELL, FOR THE UK SMALL ANEURYSM TRIAL PARTICIPANTS. 2003. Cardiovascular risk factors and abdominal aortic aneurysm expansion: only smoking counts. Br. J. Surg. **90:** 491–492.

15. HELLER, J.A., A. WEINBERG, R. ARONS, *et al.* 2000. Two decades of abdominal aortic aneurysm repair: have we made any progress? J. Vasc. Surg. **32:** 1091–1100.

16. FLEMING, C., E.P. WHITLOCK, T.L. BELL, *et al.* 2005. Screening for abdominal aortic aneurysm: a best-evidence systemic review for the U. S. Preventative Services Task Force. Ann. Intern. Med. **142:** 203–211.

17. DAUGHERTY, A. & L.A. CASSIS. 2004. Mouse models of abdominal aortic aneurysm disease. Arteriosclero. Thromb. Vasc. Biol. **24:** 1–6.

18. PETRINEC, D., S. LIAO, D.R. HOLMES, *et al.* 1996. Doxycycline inhibition of aneurysmal degeneration in an elastase-induced rat model of abdominal aortic aneurysm; preservation of aortic elastin associated with suppressed production of 92 kD gelatinase. J. Vasc. Surg. **23:** 336–346.

19. BIGATEL, D.A., J.R. ELMORE, D.J. CAREY, *et al.* 1999. The matrix metalloproteinase inhibitor BB-94 limits expansion of experimental abdominal aortic aneurysms. J. Vasc. Surg. **29:** 130–138.

20. LIAO, S., M. MIRALLES, B.J. KELLEY, *et al.* 2001. Suppression of experimental abdominal aortic aneurysms in the rat by treatment with angiotensin-converting enzyme inhibitors. J. Vasc. Surg. **33:** 1057–1064.

21. NAKASHIMA, H., M. AOKI, T. MIYAKE, *et al.* 2004. Inhibition of experimental abdominal aortic aneurysm in the rat by use of decoy oligodeoxynucleotides suppressing activity of nuclear factor kappaB and its transcription factors. Circulation **109:** 132–138.

22. LAWRENCE, D.M., R.S. SINGH, D.P. FRANKLIN, *et al.* 2004. Rapamycin suppresses experimental aneurysm growth. J. Vasc. Surg. **40:** 334–338.

23. NAGASHIMA, H., Y. AOKA, Y. SAKOMURA, *et al.* 2002. A 3-hydroxy-3-methylglutaryl coenzyme A reductase inhibitor, cerivastatin, suppresses

production of matrix metalloproteinase-9 in the human abdominal aortic aneurysm wall. J. Vasc. Surg. **36:** 158–163.

24. STEINMETZ, E.F., C. BUCKLEY, M. SHAMES, *et al.* 2005. Treatment with simvastatin suppresses the development of experimental abdominal aortic aneurysms in normal and hypercholesterolemic mice. Ann. Surg. **241:** 92–101.

25. DALMAN, R.L. 2006. Vitamin E limits AAA. Arterioscler. Thromb. Vasc. Biol. **26:** e21.

26. BRUEMMER, D., A.R. COLLINS, G. NOH, *et al.* 2003. Angiotensin II-accelerated atherosclerosis and aneurysm formation is attenuated in osteopontin-deficient mice. J. Clin. Invest. **112:** 1318–1331.

27. SHO, E., M. SHO, K. HOSHINA, *et al.* 2004. Hemodynamic forces regulate mural macrophage infiltration in experimental aortic aneurysms. Exp. Mol. Pathol. **76:** 108–116.

28. SHO, E., M. SHO, H. NANJO, *et al.* 2004. Hemodynamic regulation of CD34$^+$ cell localization and differentiation in experimental aneurysms. Arteriosclero. Thomb. Vasc. Biol. **24:** 1916–1921.

29. HOSHINA, K., H. KOYAMA, T. MIYATA, *et al.* 2004. Aortic wall cell proliferation via basic fibroblast growth factor gene transfer limits progression of experimental aortic aneurysm. J. Vasc. Surg. **40:** 512–518.

30. POWELL, J.T. & A.R. BRADY. 2004. Detection, management and prospects for the medical treatment of small abdominal aortic aneurysms. Arterioscler. Thomb. Vasc. Biol. **24:** 241–245.

31. BAXTER, B.T., W.H. PEARCE, E.A. WALTKE, *et al.* 2002. Prolonged administration of doxycycline in patients with small asymptomatic abdominal aortic aneurysms: report of a prospective (phase II) multicenter study. J. Vasc. Surg. **36:** 1–12.

32. TAYLOR, C.A., T.J. HUGHES & C.K. ZARINS. 1999. Effects of exercise on hemodynamic conditions in the abdominal aorta. J. Vasc. Surg. **29:** 1077–1089.

33. ALIWADI, G., B.S. KNIPP, G. LU, *et al.* 2003. A non-intrinsic regional basis for increased infrarenal aortic MMP-9 expression and activity. J. Vasc. Surg. **37:** 1059–1066.

34. VOLLMAR, J.F., F. PAES, P. PAUSCHINGER, *et al.* 1989. Aortic aneurysms as late sequela of above knee amputation. Lancet **7:** 834–835.

35. GORDON, I.L., C.A. KOHL, M. AREFI, *et al.* 1996. Spinal cord injury increases the risk of abdominal aortic aneurysm. Am. Surg. **62:** 249–252.

36. SANDGREN, T., B. SONESSON, A.R. AHLGREN, *et al.* 2001. Arterial dimensions in the lower extremities of patients with abdominal aortic aneurysm disease: no evidence of a generalizing dilating diathesis. J. Vasc. Surg. **34:** 730–738.

37. GIMBRONE, M.A., JR., K.R. ANDERSON, J.N. TOPPER, *et al.* 1999. Special communication: the critical role of mechanical forces in blood vessel development, physiology and pathology. J. Vasc. Surg. **29:** 1104–1151.

38. KUNSCH, C. & R.M. MEDFORD. 1999. Oxidative stress as a regulator of gene expression. Circ. Res. **82:** 753–766.

39. BERK, B.C. 1999. Redox signals that regulate the vascular response to injury. Thromb. Haemost. **82:** 753–766.

40. MCMILLAN, W.D. & W.H. PEARCE. 1999. Increased levels of metalloproteinase-9 are associated with abdominal aortic aneurysms. J. Vasc. Surg. **29:** 122–127.

41. PYO, R., J.K. LEE, J.M. SHIPLEY, *et al.* 2000. Targeted gene disruption of matrix metalloproteinase-9 (gelatinase B) suppresses development of experimental abdominal aortic aneurysms. J. Clin. Invest. **105:** 1641–1649.

42. PARKS, W.C. 2002. A confederacy of proteinases. J. Clin. Invest. **110:** 613–614.
43. LUM, H. & K.A. ROEBUCK. 2001. Oxidant stress and endothelial cell dysfunction. Am. J. Physiol. Cell. Physiol. **280:** C719–C741.
44. DE KEULENAER, G.W., R.W. ALEXANDER, M. USHIO-FUKAI, *et al.* 1998. Oscillatory and steady laminar shear stress differentially effect human endothelial redox state: the role of a superoxide-producing NADH oxidase. Circ. Res. **82:** 1094–1101.
45. MASUDA, H., Y.J. ZHUANG, T.M. SINGH, *et al.* 1999. Adaptive remodeling on internal elastic lamina and endothelial lining during flow-induced arterial enlargement. Arteriosclero. Thromb. Vasc. Biol. **19:** 2298–2307.
46. TOBIASCH, E., I. GUNTHER & F.H. BACH. 2001. Heme oxygenase protects pancreatic beta cells from apoptosis caused by various stimuli. J. Invest. Med. **49:** 566–571.
47. TULIS, D.A., W. DURANTE, X. LIU, *et al.* 2001. Adenovirus-mediated heme-oxygenase gene delivery inhibits injury-induced vascular neointimal formation. Circulation **104:** 2710–2715.
48. SUTTNER, D.M. & P.A. DENNERY. 1999. Reversal of HO-1 related cytoprotection with increased expression is due to reactive iron. FASEB J. **13:** 1800–1808.
49. SCHILLINGER, M., M. EXNER, W. MIEKUSCH, *et al.* 2002. Heme oxygenase 1 gene promoter polymorphism is associated with abdominal aortic aneurysm. Thromb. Res. **106:** 131–136.
50. NAKAHASHI, T.K., K. HOSHINA, P.S. TSAO, *et al.* 2002. Flow loading induces macrophage antioxidative gene expression in experimental aneurysms. Arterioscler. Thromb. Vasc. Biol. **22:** 2017–2022.
51. MILLER, F.J., JR. 2002. Aortic aneurysms: It's all about the stress. Arteriosclero. Thromb. Vasc. Biol. **22:** 1948–1949.
52. TAYLOR, C.A., C.P. CHENG, L.A. ESPINOSA, *et al.* 2002. *In vivo* quantification of blood flow and wall shear stress in the human abdominal aorta during lower limb exercise. Ann. Biomed. Eng. **30:** 402–408.
53. CHENG, C.P., R.J. HERFKENS & C.A. TAYLOR. 2003. Comparison of abdominal aortic hemodynamics between men and women at rest and during lower limb exercise. J. Vasc. Surg. **37:** 118–123.
54. CHENG, C.P., R.J. HERFKENS & C.A. TAYLOR. 2003. Abdominal aortic hemodynamic conditions in healthy subjects aged 50–70 at rest and during lower limb exercise: *in vivo* quantification using MRI. Atherosclerosis **168:** 223–231.
55. LEDERLE, F.A., G.R. JOHNSON, S.E. WILSON, *et al.* FOR THE ADAM VA CSP PROGRAM. 2003. Quality of life, impotence, and activity level in a randomized trial of immediate repair vs. surveillance of small abdominal aortic aneurysms. J. Vasc. Surg. **38:** 745–752.
56. MYERS, J., M. PRAKASH, V. FROELICHER, *et al.* 2002. Exercise capacity and mortality among men referred for exercise testing. N. Engl. J. Med. **346:** 793–801.
57. LEDERLE, F.A., G.R. JOHNSON, S.E. WILSON, *et al.* 1997. Prevalence and associations of abdominal aortic aneurysm detected through screening. Aneurysm Detection and Management (ADAM) Veterans Affairs Cooperative Study Group. Ann. Intern. Med. **15:** 441–449.
58. YEUNG, J.J., H.J. KIM, T.A. ABBRUZZESE, *et al.* 2006. Aortoiliac hemodynamic and morphologic adaptation to chronic spinal cord injury. J.Vasc. Surg. In press.
59. TAYLOR, C.A., C.P. CHENG, L.A. ESPINOSA, *et al.* 2002. *In vivo* quantification of blood flow and wall shear stress in the human abdominal aorta during lower limb exercise. Ann. Biomed. Eng. **30:** 402–408.

60. CHENG, C.P., D.F. SCHWANDT, E.L. TOPP, *et al.* 2003. Dynamic exercise imaging with an MR-compatible stationary cycle within the general electric open magnet. Magn. Reson. Med. **49:** 581–585.

61. PELC, N.J., M.A. BERNSTEIN, A. SHIMAKAWA, *et al.* 1991. Encoding strategies for three-direction phase-contrast MR imaging of flow. J. Magn. Reson. Imaging **1:** 405–413.

62. PELC, N.J., R.J. HERFKENS, A. SHIMAKAWA, *et al.* 1991. Phase contrast cine magnetic resonance imaging. Magn. Reson. Q. **7:** 229–254.

63. PELC, N.J., F.G. SOMMER, K.C. LI, *et al.* 1994. Quantitative magnetic resonance flow imaging. Magn. Reson. Q. **10:** 125–147.

64. WANG, K., R. DUTTON & C.A. TAYLOR. 1999. Geometric image segmentation and image-based model construction for computational hemodynamics. IEEE Eng. Med. Biol. **18:** 33–39.

65. WANG, K.C. 2001. Level set methods for computational prototyping with application to hemodynamic modeling. Department of Electrical Engineering, Stanford University, Stanford, CA.

66. CHENG, C.P., D. PARKER & C.A. TAYLOR. 2002. Quantification of wall shear stress in large blood vessels using Lagrangian interpolation functions with cine phase-contrast magnetic resonance imaging. Ann. Biomed. Eng. **30:** 1020–1032.

67. HE, X. & D. KU. 1996. Pulsatile flow in the human left coronary artery bifurcation: average conditions. J. Biomech. Eng. **118:** 74–82.

68. SASSUK, S.S. & J.E. MANSON. 2003. Physical activity and the prevention of cardiovascular disease. Curr. Athero. Reports **5:** 299–307.

69. REHMAN, J., J. LI, L. PARVATHANENI, *et al.* 2004. Exercise acutely increases circulation progenitor cells and monocyte-macrophage-derived angiogenic cells. J. Am. Coll. Cardiol. **43:** 2314–2318.

70. GREEN, D., A. MAIORANA, G. O'DRISCOLL, *et al.* Effect of exercise training on endothelium-derived nitric oxide function in humans. J. Physiol. (London) 9/16/04, epub ahead of print.

71. TAYLOR, C.A., T.J.R. HUGHES & C.K. ZARINS. 1996. Computational investigations in vascular disease. Comp. Phys. **10:** 224–232.

72. TAYLOR, C.A., T.J.R. HUGHES & C.K. ZARINS. 1998. Finite element modeling of blood flow in arteries. Comp. Meth. Appl. Mech. Eng. **158:** 155–196.

73. TAYLOR, C.A., T.J.R. HUGHES, C.K. ZARINS. 1998. Finite element modeling of three-dimensional pulsatile flow in the abdominal aorta: relevance to atherosclerosis. Ann. Biomed. Eng. **26:** 1–14.

74. TAYLOR, C.A., M.T. DRANEY, J.P. KU, *et al.* 1999. Predictive medicine: computation techniques in therapeutic decision-making. Comp. Aided Surg. **4:** 231–247.

75. KU, J.P., M.T. DRANEY, F.R. ARKO, *et al.* 2002. *In vivo* validation of numerical predications of blood flow in arterial bypass grafts. Ann. Biomed. Eng. **30:** 743–752.

76. KU, J.P., C.J. ELKINS & C.A. TAYLOR. 2005. Comparison of CFD and MRI flow and velocities in an in vitro large artery bypass graft model. Ann. Biomed. Eng. **33:** 257–269.

77. WANG, K. 1998. Level set methods and MR image segmentation for geometric modeling in computational hemodynamics. Presented at the IEEE Biomedical Engineering in Medicine and Biology Society. Hong Kong, China.

78. WILSON, N.M., R. DUTTON & C.A. TAYLOR. 2001. A software framework for creating patient specific geometric models from medical imaging data for

simulation-based medical planning of vascular surgery. Lecture Notes Comp. Sci. **2208:** 449–456.

79. WILSON, N.M. Geometric algorithms and software architecture for computational prototyping: applications in vascular surgery and MEMS. In Mechanical Engineering 2002. Stanford University, Stanford, CA.

80. TAYLOR, C.A. 1997. Finite element analysis of pulsatile flow in the human abdominal aorta: geometric model construction from spiral CT data. Presented at ASME Bioengineering. Sunriver, OR.

81. WAN, J., B.N. STEELE, S.A. SPICER, et al. 2002. One-dimensional finite element method for simulation-based medical planning for cardiovascular disease. Comp. Meth. Biomech. Biomed. Engin. **5:** 195–206.

82. STEELE, B.N., J. WAN, J.P. KU, et al. 2003. In vivo validation of a one-dimensional finite element method for simulation-based medical planning for cardiovascular bypass surgery. IEEE Trans. Biomed. Engin. **50:** 649–656.

83. VIGNON, I. & C.A. TAYLOR. 2004. Outflow boundary conditions for one-dimensional finite element modeling of blood flow and pressure waves in arteries. Wave Motion **39:** 361–374.

84. OLUFSEN, M.S. 1999. A structured tree outflow condition for blood flow in the larger systemic arteries. Am. J. Physiol. **267:** H257–H268.

85. SCHUTZ, Y., S. WEINSIER, P. TERRIER, et al. 2002. A new accelerometric method to assess the daily walking practice. Int. J. Obes. Relat. Metab. Disord. **26:** 111–118.

86. FROELICHER, V.F., D. JENSEN, F. GENTER, et al. 1984. A randomized trial of exercise training in patients with coronary heart disease. JAMA **252:** 1291–1297.

87. TAYLOR, R.S., A. BROWN, S. EBRAHIM, et al. 2004. Exercise-based rehabilitation for patients with coronary heart disease: systematic review and meta-analysis of randomized controlled trails. Am. J. Med. **16:** 682–692.

88. THOMPSON, P.D. 2002. Additional steps for cardiovascular health. NEJM **347:** 755–756.

89. MYERS, J., A. KAYKHA, S. GEORGE, et al. 2004. Fitness versus physical activity patterns in predicting mortality in men. Am. J. Med. **117:** 912–918.

90. WEISS, J.P., V.F. FROELICHER, J. MYERS, et al. 2004. Health-care costs and exercise capacity. Chest **126:** 608–613.

91. POWELL, J.T., B.R. MULLER & R.M. GREENHALGH. 1987. Acute phase proteins in patients with abdominal aortic aneurysm disease. J. Cardiovasc. Surg. **28:** 528–530.

92. NORMAN, P., C.A. SPENCER, M.M. LAWRENCE-BROWN, et al. 2004. C-reactive protein levels and the expansion of screen-detected abdominal aortic aneurysms in men. Circulation **110:** 862–866.

93. VAINAS, T., T. LUBBERS, F.R.M. STASSEN, et al. 2003. Serum C-reactive protein level is associated with abdominal aortic aneurysm size and may be produced by aneurysmal tissue. Circulation **107:** 1103–1105.

94. FORD, E.S. 2002. Does exercise reduce inflammation? Physical activity and C-reactive protein among U.S. adults. Epidemiology **13:** 561–568.

95. GEFFKEN, D.F., M. CUSHMAN, G.L. BURKE, et al. 2001. Association between physical activity and markers on inflammation in an elderly health population. Am. J. Epidemiol. **153:** 242–250.

96. ZHANG, J., J. SCHMIDT, E. RYSCHICH, et al. 2003. Inducible nitric oxide synthase is present in human abdominal aortic aneurysm and promotes oxidative vascular injury. J. Vasc. Surg. **38:** 360–367.

97. ARMSTRONG, P.J., D.P. FRANKLIN, D.J. CAREY, *et al.* 2005. Suppression of experimental aortic aneurysms: comparison of inducible nitric oxide synthase and cyclooxygenase inhibitors. Ann. Vasc. Surg. **19(2):** 248–257.

98. JOHANNING, J.M., P.J. ARMSTRONG, D.P. FRANKLIN, *et al.* 2002. Nitric oxide in experimental aneurysm formation: early events and consequences of nitric oxide inhibition. Ann. Vasc. Surg. **16:** 65–72.

99. YANG, A.L. & H.I. CHEN. 2003. Chronic exercise reduces adhesion molecules/iNOS expression and partially reverses vascular responsiveness in hypercholesterolemic rabbit aortae. Atherosclerosis **169:** 11–17.

100. GIELEN, S., V. ADAMS, S. MOBIUS-WINKLER, *et al.* 2003. Anti-inflammatory effects of exercise training in the skeletal muscle of patients with chronic heart failure. J. Am. Coll. Cardiol. **42:** 861–868.

# Refinements in Mathematical Models to Predict Aneurysm Growth and Rupture

RAMON BERGUER,[a,b] JOSEPH L. BULL,[a,b] AND KHALIL KHANAFER[a]

[a] *Vascular Mechanics Laboratory, Department of Biomedical Engineering, University of Michigan, Ann Arbor, Michigan*

[b] *Vascular Mechanics Laboratory, Section of Vascular Surgery, University of Michigan, Ann Arbor, Michigan*

ABSTRACT: The growth of aneurysms and eventually their likelihood of rupture depend on the determination of the stress and strain within the aneurysm wall and the exact reproduction of its geometry. A numerical model is developed to analyze pulsatile flow in abdominal aortic aneurysm (AAA) models using real physiological resting and exercise waveforms. Both laminar and turbulent flows are considered. Interesting features of the flow field resulting from using realistic physiological waveforms are obtained for various parameters using finite element methods. Such parameters include Reynolds number, size of the aneurysm (D/d), and flexibility of the aneurysm wall. The effect of non-Newtonian behavior of blood on hemodynamic stresses is compared with Newtonian behavior, and the non-Newtonian effects are demonstrated to be significant in realistic flow situations. Our results show that maximum turbulent fluid shear stress occurs at the distal end of the AAA model. Furthermore, turbulence is found to have a significant effect on the pressure distribution along AAA wall for both physiological waveforms. Related experimental work in which a bench top aneurysm model is developed is also discussed. The experimental model provides a platform to validate the numerical model. This work is part of our ongoing development of a patient-specific tool to guide clinician decision making and to elucidate the contribution of blood flow-induced stresses to aneurysm growth and eventual rupture. These studies indicate that accurately modeling the physiologic features of real aneurysms and blood is paramount to achieving our goal.

KEYWORDS: aneurysm; laminar; mechanical hinge; non-Newtonian; turbulent flow

Address for correspondence: Ramon Berguer, 2210 Taubman Health Center-0329, University of Michigan, Ann Arbor, MI, 48109-0329. Voice: 734-936-7301; fax: 734-647-9867.
e-mail: rberguer@umich.edu

Ann. N.Y. Acad. Sci. 1085: 110–116 (2006). © 2006 New York Academy of Sciences.
doi: 10.1196/annals.1383.033

## INTRODUCTION

Aortic aneurysms are responsible for more than 30,000 deaths yearly and diseases of the aorta are the 14th leading cause of death in the United States.[1,2] Most aortic aneurysms occur in the infrarenal abdominal aorta. Four principal causes of aortic aneurysms have been identified as follows: (1) proteolytic degradation of aortic wall connective tissue, (2) inflammation and immune responses, (3) mechanical wall stress, and (4) molecular genetics.[3] While the epidemiology and treatment of infrarenal abdominal aortic aneurysms (AAAs) have been well described, the mechanisms leading to accelerated aneurysm growth and eventual rupture remain poorly understood. From a flow mechanics standpoint, one can predict that changes in the geometry of an aneurysm will alter blood flow patterns and hemodynamic stresses within the aneurysm and aortic wall. Hemodynamic stresses associated with (or leading to) changes in the aortic wall, which affect its mechanical integrity, are important predictors of aneurysm dilation and the subsequent risk of rupture.

Intervention, either by direct surgical resection and grafting or by endovascular grafting, is indicated to treat AAAs when the maximum diameter exceeds 5 cm, although smaller aneurysms still have a significant risk of rupture. Previous research has identified the need to consider other predictors of AAAs rupture than the traditional measurement of aneurysm diameter such as thickness of its wall, herniation of soft plaque through the elastic coats of the aneurysm, magnitude and extension of the intraluminal thrombus, and local stress concentrators due to rigid calcium plaques. These material elements can be identified and measured by computational techniques from data obtained from standard computerized tomography (CT) scans of the aorta. The contribution of these elements to the pulsatile mechanics of the aneurysm wall can be simulated by numerical analysis (finite element method). The study of hemodynamic stresses acting on AAA walls to predict the likelihood of AAA rupture using computational techniques is better than the current practice of periodic measurement of the diameter changes in the AAA by ultrasound or CT. Numerical simulations allow for the study of conditions that are difficult or impossible to measure directly in humans or in animal models of AAA.

We propose that the stresses generated by the viscous and inertial forces associated with blood flow may be responsible for the changes in the wall that result in thrombus deposition and dilation. These flow-generated stresses can be modeled using fluid finite element analysis techniques. The much larger mechanical stresses imposed on the wall by the pulsatile pressure and the response of the wall—with areas of different elastic and deformation characteristics—determine the site of rupture. These larger stresses and the response of the wall to them can be modeled using solid mechanics numerical techniques. These numerical predictions of the risk of rupture of an AAA can provide invaluable clinical help: the mortality and severe complications attending the surgical or endovascular repair of certain types of aneurysms can be very high (30%) in patients with significant concomitant conditions such as emphysema or renal failure. The numerical analysis of the distribution of wall stresses within AAAs can assist in the clinical management of AAA patients by predicting the risk of rupture over time and permitting risk/benefit assessment for intervention or observation.

Addressing the smaller stresses derived from the viscous and inertial components of the flow of blood, we noted that the studies that have been published have used finite element analysis assuming laminar flows,[4–6] Newtonian behavior of blood, and idealized AAA geometries. Collectively, these studies demonstrated that increased fluid shear stress at various points along the aortic wall results in local changes in wall pressure and flow patterns that may result in dilation and deposition of thrombus. However, these published studies have not considered the effects of turbulence and non-Newtonian behavior of blood on the mechanics of the aneurysmal wall. Turbulence, induced by sudden expansion of the flow stream, generates additional stresses on the aneurysm wall. These additional stresses result in wall vibration and may be responsible for further wall dilation, and eventually greater turbulence, possibly a self-perpetuating mechanism for aneurysmal growth. Thus, turbulent flow should be considered in the study of aneurysms because it does exist in human aneurysms and by increasing mechanical wall stress, it would influence the rate of dilation of the wall.

Non-Newtonian blood characteristics should also be considered in the study of aneurysms: they exist in regions of low shear rates such as those of flow separation. Finally, patient-specific geometries of AAAs should be used for clinically meaningful and accurate results. The fact is that most physical and computational studies have been carried out in idealized models of AAAs that do not take into account real geometries and flow characteristics of human AAA.

## GOVERNING EQUATIONS AND BOUNDARY CONDITIONS

Incompressible, homogeneous, non-Newtonian flow in a rigid-walled aneurysm was considered as depicted in FIGURE 1. The boundary conditions for the velocity are: (1) no-slip at the walls, (2) zero radial velocity at the inlet, and (3) zero velocity gradients at the outlet. A waveform corresponding to resting and exercise flow conditions was used at the inlet to approximate *in vivo* measurements in the abdominal segment of the human aorta.[7,8] A finite element formulation based on the Galerkin method is employed to solve the governing equations using Fidap software (Fluent, Inc., Lebanon, NH) subject to the boundary and initial conditions for this study.

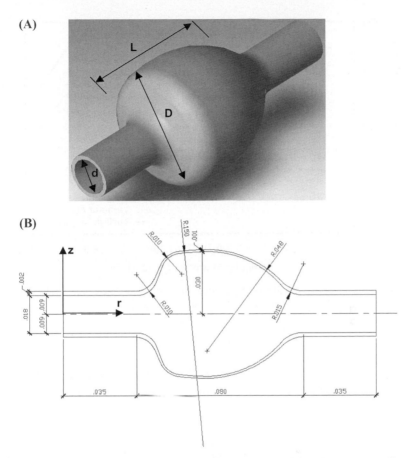

**FIGURE 1.** Aneurysm model and coordinate system ($d$ − 18 mm, $D$ = 60 mm, $L$ = 80 mm). r is the radial dimension, X is the axial position, and S is a position along the aneurysm wall length.

## METHODS

The combination of κ-ε model with specialized elements for near-wall modeling was used to simulate the turbulent characteristics of convective flow. The Boussinesq eddy–viscosity model was also imbedded. We accounted for the non-Newtonian behavior of blood by the Carreau equation for viscosity. The geometry of the flow mesh was modified to represent the shape of aneurysms more accurately as they occur in humans. To validate every operator imbedded in the model we constructed a flow rig with the same dimensions and operating parameters that are encountered in humans. In the testing segment of the rig we have the capability of collecting accurate data on pressure, flow velocity and

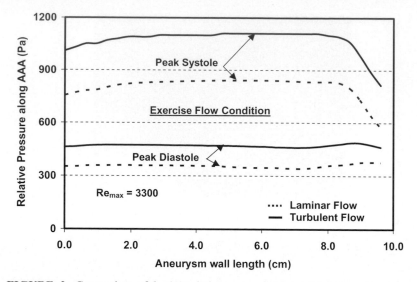

**FIGURE 2.** Comparison of the (**A**) relative pressure along AAA between laminar and turbulent flow conditions ($d = 18$ mm, $D = 80$ mm, $L = 80$ mm).

distribution, flow patterns (laser velocimetry); these have the same geometry as the aneurysm and operate according to the same numerical model. This permits a step-by-step validation of the assumptions imbedded in the numerical model.

## RESULTS AND DISCUSSION

The significance of turbulent flow on the relative pressure acting along the aneurysm compared with laminar flow using exercise flow condition is shown in FIGURE 2. Pressure values presented in this article are relative values (i.e., excess pressures) and correspond to the difference between the instantaneous pressure acting on the AAA wall and the instantaneous pressure at the exit of the computational model. This figure demonstrates that turbulent flow exhibits higher values of pressure acting on the AAA during peak systole and peak diastole than those seen with laminar flow. Turbulent flow, compared with laminar flow, increases the mechanical stress on the aneurysmal wall AAA that could mediate its further dilation and create conditions (flow separation) that enhance thrombus deposition. FIGURE 3 demonstrates the effect of resting and exercise flow conditions on the fluid shear stress on the aneurysm. Exercise waveforms generate larger fluid shear stresses than resting waveforms with peak values found at the distal half of the AAA. The rapid oscillating nature of the wall stresses over a long period of time

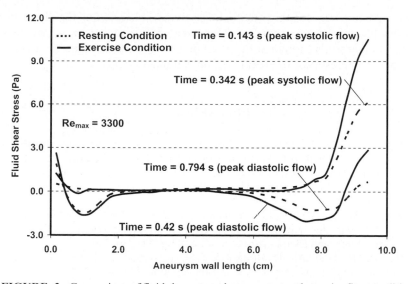

**FIGURE 3.** Comparison of fluid shear stress between rest and exercise flow conditions ($d = 18$ mm, $D = 80$ mm, $L = 80$ mm).

may alter the strength of the arterial wall and facilitate the growth of the aneurysm.

Solid mechanics analysis is carried out using ANSYS software to obtain the deformed shape and the stresses on the aneurysm subject to peak systolc pressure are shown in FIGURE 4. The analysis demonstrates a mechanical hinge

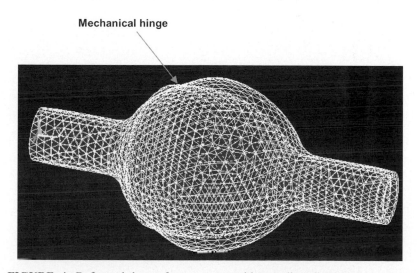

**FIGURE 4.** Deformed shape of an aneurysm with compliant distal end.

at the junction between the proximal, less distensible area and the distal, more distensible area of the aneurysm. This suggests a mechanism of mechanical stress similar to that found at the junction of a two-phase material. This area is where ruptures most frequently occur in human AAA.

## REFERENCES

1. WAINESS, R.M., J.B. DIMICK, J.A. COWAN, *et al.* 2004. Epidemiology of surgically treated abdominal aortic aneurysms in the United States. Vascular **12:** 218–224.
2. NATIONAL HOSPITAL DISCHARGE SURVEY. 2001. Annual Summary with Detailed Diagnosis and Procedure Data. Hyattsville, MD: National Center for Health Statistics; June 2004.
3. WASSEF, M., B.T. BAXTER, R.L. CHISHOLM, *et al.* 2001. Pathogenesis of abdominal aortic aneurysms: a multidisciplinary research program supported by the National Heart, Lung, and Blood Institute. J. Vasc. Surg. **34:** 730–738.
4. BUDWIG, R., D. ELGER, H. HOOPER & J. SLIPPY. 1993. Steady flow in abdominal aortic aneurysm models. ASME J. Biomech. Eng. **115:** 419–423.
5. ASBURY, C.L., J.W. RWBERTI, E.I. BLUTH & R.A. PEATTIE. 1995. Experimental investigation of steady flow in rigid models of abdominal aortic aneurysm. Annals. Biomed. Eng. **23:** 29–39.
6. FUKUSHIMA, T., T. MATSUZAWA & T. HOMMA. 1998. Visualization and finite element analysis of pulsatile flow in models of the abdominal aortic aneurysm. Biorheology **26:** 109–130.
7. MILLS, C., I. GABE, J. GAULT, *et al.* 1970. Pressure-flow relationships and vascular impedance in man, Cardiovasc. Res. **4:** 405–417.
8. PEDERSEN, E., H. SUNG, A. BURLSON & A. YOGANATHAN. 1993. Two-dimensional velocity measurements in a pulsatile flow model of the normal abdominal aorta simulating different hemodynamic conditions. J. Biomech. **26:** 1237–1247.

# Abdominal Aortic Aneurysm as a Complex Multifactorial Disease

## Interactions of Polymorphisms of Inflammatory Genes, Features of Autoimmunity, and Current Status of MMPs

WILLIAM H. PEARCE AND VERA P. SHIVELY[a]

[a]Department of Surgery, Division of Vascular Surgery, Northwestern University Feinberg School of Medicine, Chicago, IL, USA

ABSTRACT: The role of matrix metalloproteinases (MMPs) in the pathogenesis of abdominal aortic aneurysm (AAA) has focused on the degradation of the extracellular matrix (ECM). The new frontier of MMP biology involves the role of MMPs in releasing cryptic fragments and neoepitopes from the ECM and the impact of MMPs on the regulation of the inflammatory response. The ECM is a complex structure, much more important than an inert scaffold. Both MMP-2 and MMP-9 expose a cryptic epitope that controls angiogenesis. MMPs inhibit angiogenesis through the release of endostatin, endorepellin, arresten, canstatin, and tumstatin. Other breakdown products of the ECM include fragments of fragmin and elastin degradation products (EDPs). In addition, the ECM contains embedded vascular endothelial growth factor (VEGF) and transforming growth factor-beta (TGF-$\beta$). Inflammation is a complex, highly regulated system that involves the identification of injury or infection, response to the injury or infection, repair and healing, and return to normal homeostasis. In some instances, the inflammatory process leads to a pathologic process that is damaging to the host. MMPs play an important role in the control of the inflammatory response through the modification of proinflammatory cytokines, chemokines, and shedding of membrane receptors. Genetic association studies have been performed to help determine the genetic risk associated with certain single nucleotide polymorphisms (SNPs) However, because of the variability in the patient populations and the size of the population, it is difficult to draw any conclusions from these studies. While the etiology of AAA remains unknown, understanding of the inflammatory process and its regulatory points will develop new strategies for the treatment of AAA.

Address for correspondence: William H. Pearce, M.D., Department of Vascular Surgery, Northwestern University Feinberg School of Medicine, 201 E. Huron, #10-105, Chicago, IL 60611. Voice: 312-926-7775; fax: 312-695-4955.

e-mail: wpearce@nmh.org

Ann. N.Y. Acad. Sci. 1085: 117–132 (2006). © 2006 New York Academy of Sciences.
doi: 10.1196/annals.1383.025

**Perhaps one difficulty with understanding the pathogenesis of AAA is the lack of precise definition of the phenotype.**

KEYWORDS: aneurysm; MMPs; metalloproteinases; polymorphisms; inflammation

## INTRODUCTION

Abdominal aortic aneurysms (AAAs) are a complex multifactorial disease with an unknown etiology. In some individuals there is a clear genetic predisposition, while in others AAAs appear spontaneously. In the past 10 years since the first symposium on the pathogenesis of AAAs, we have developed a clearer understanding of the inflammatory nature of AAAs, the cells comprising the inflammatory infiltrate, the involvement of growth factors, cytokines, proteolytic enzymes, and their inhibitors. Matrix metalloproteinases (MMPs) appear to play a critical role in the pathogenesis of AAA. MMPs were first described more than 40 years ago in the developing tadpole.[1] Since then we have gained a greater understanding of the physiologic and biologic roles of these important enzymes. Until recently, it was generally held that the only function of MMPs was to degrade the extracellular matrix (ECM). However, current research has demonstrated a much broader role for MMPs including the control and regulation of the inflammatory response, wound healing, cancer metastasis, arthritis, and many other physiologic responses.[2–10] This review will briefly cover the biochemistry and molecular biology of MMPs and will focus on the role of MMPs in the control of inflammation and the release of cryptic neoepitopes from the ECM. The role of MMPs in the regulation of the inflammatory response may be a key factor in AAA development. In addition, the article will review the current status of studies on the polymorphisms of specific proinflammatory cytokines and MMPs.

## MATRIX METALLOPROTEINASES (MMPs)

MMPs were first described by Gross and colleagues in 1962 in studying the developing tadpole's tail.[1] Since then an entire area of biology has been devoted to MMPs and it is now recognized how important these enzymes are to normal and pathologic processes. MMPs are a subfamily of the metzincin superfamily of proteinases. There are four subfamilies including the serralysins, adamalysins, astracins, and matrixins. MMPs have been further subdivided according to their substrate specificity: collagenases, gelatinases, stromolysins, and matrilysins. This classification was later replaced by simply numbering the MMPs according to chronology of their identification. However, it is now recognized that MMPs have a wide range of substrate specificity including nonmatrix substrates with a great deal of overlap between MMPs

(TABLE 1). In addition, some MMPs are not secreted but membrane bound (MT-MMPs).

MMPs share a similar structure: (FIG. 1) a propeptide domain and a catalytic domain. Many MMPs also have a propeller domain connected by hinge region. Membrane-bound MMPs have cytoplasmic tails or glycosylphospatidyl anchors. The MMPs are recognized by their unique three-histadine catalytic domain that contains the zinc-binding site. Enzymatic activity is controlled by a conserved cysteine that acts as a "cysteine switch."[11] All MMPs except those that are membrane bound rely on this cysteine switch. The membrane-bound MMPs are activated by a separate mechanism. The only human disease associated with MMP (MMP-2) loss is the vanishing bone syndrome in which patients present with chronic arthritis and subcutaneous nodules.[12]

The cell surface plays an important role in the directional docking of MMPs to the cell surface. The MT-MMPs are differentially located on the cell membrane during migration.[7] Further, secreted MMPs may be docked at the leading edge of metastatic cells (invadopodia).[13] MMPs are regulated by transcription, activation of zymogen, and inhibition by α-2 macroglobulin and tissue inhibitors of metalloproteinases (TIMP) family. Transcription appears as the most important mechanism for regulation. However, MMP-2 is constitutively expressed and regulation occurs by either activation or inhibition. Some MMPs (−8, −9) are sequestered in Golgi vesicles and secreted. The promoters of MMP −1, −3, −7, −9, −10, and −13 share several elements that interact with either the FOS Jun or Ets, transcription factors. Variation in the promoter region has been associated with varying degrees of expression.[14] Polymorphisms of certain MMPs have been associated with several diseases including aortic aneurysms and coronary artery aneurysm (TABLE 2). Other molecules have been implicated in regulating the proteolytic activity of MMPs including chrondospondin, reversion-inducing cysteine-rich protein with kazal motifs (RECK), and neutrophil gelatinase-associated lipocalin (NGAL). The MMP-9–NGAL complex protects MMP-9 from degradation.

Activation and inhibition of MMPs is a highly complex process involving diverse interaction between multiple molecules. For example, TIMP-1/proMMP-9 complex interacts with MMP-3 to inactivate it. Thrombospondin, a cell surface receptor, is important in endocytosis and clearance of MMP-α2 macroglobulin complex. Activated MMPs are inhibited by the four TIMPs that show MMP specificity although some crossover exists. TIMP-3 is primarily bound to the ECM.

## MMPs IN AAA

In 1985 Busuttil first described the presence of collagenase-like activity in the aortic walls of patients with AAAs.[15] Since then many investigators have described the involvement of many members of the MMP family.[16–24] The

**TABLE 1. Selected human MMPs and their substrates**

| Protein name | Alternative name | Collagenous substrates | Noncollagenous ECM substrates | Nonstructural ECM component substrates |
|---|---|---|---|---|
| MMP-2 | Gelatinase-A | Collagen types I, IV, V, VII, X, XI, XIV, and gelatin | Aggrecan, elastin, fibronectin, laminin, nidogen, proteoglycan link protein, and versican | Active MMP-9, active MMP-13, FGF R1, IGF-BP3, IGF-BP5, IL-1β, recombinant TNF-α-peptide, and TGF-β |
| MMP-3 | Stromelysin-1 | Collagen types II, IV, IX, X, and gelatin | Aggrecan, casein, decorin, elastin, fibronectin, laminin, nidogen, perlecan, proteoglycan, proteoglycan link protein, and versican | α1-antichymotrypsin, α1-proteinase inhibitor, antithrombin III, E-cadherin, fibrinogen, IGF-BP3, L-selectin, ovostatin, pro-HB-EGF, pro-IL-1β, pro-MMP-1, pro-MMP8, pro-MMP-9, pro-TNF-α, and SDF-1 |
| MMP-7 | Matrilysin-1, neutrophil collagenase | Collagen types I, II, III, V, IV, and X | Aggrecan, casein, elastin, enactin, laminin, and proteoglycan link protein | B4 integrin, deconrin, defensin, E-cadherin, Fas-L, plasminogen, pro-MMP-2, pro-MMP-7, α2-antiplasmin, and pro-MMP-8 |
| MMP-8 | Collagenase-2 | Collagen types I, II, III, V, VII, VIII, X, and gelatin | Aggrecan, laminin, and nidogen | α2-antiplasmin and pro-MMP-8 |

*Continued.*

**TABLE 1. Continued**

| Protein name | Alternative name | Collagenous substrates | Noncollagenous ECM substrates | Nonstructural ECM component substrates |
|---|---|---|---|---|
| MMP-9 | Gelatinase-B | Collagen types IV, V, VII, X, and XIV | Fibronectin, laminin, nidogen, proteoglycan link protein, and versican | CXCL5, IL-1β, IL2-R, plasminogen, pro-TNF-α, SDF-1, and TGF-β |
| MMP-12 | Macrophage metalloelastase | | Elastin | Plasminogen |
| MMP-13 | Collagenase-3 | Collagen types I, II, III, IV, V, IX, X, XI, and gelatin | Aggrecan, fibronectin, laminin, perlecan, and tenascin | Plasminogen activator 2, pro-MMP-9, pro-MMP-13, and SDF-1 |
| MMP-14 | MT1-MMP | Collagen types I, II, III, and gelatin | Aggrecan, dermatan sulphate proteoglycan, fibrin, fibronectin, laminin, nidogen, perlecan, tenascin, and vitronectin | Pro-MMP-2, pro-MMP-13, and tissue transglutaminase |
| MMP-24 | MT5-MMP | Gelatin | Chondroitin sulfate, dermatin, sulfate, and fibronectin | Pro-MMP-2, and pro-MMP-13 |

*Although there are 23 human MMPs, 29 have been used in the literature. The symbols MMP-4, MMP-5, MMP-6, and MMP-29 are redundant in humans and are no longer in use. MMP-18 corresponds to a *Xenopus laevis* collagenase for which no human ortholog is known, and a human protein published as MMP-18 is now called MMP-19. Two nearly identical human genes found in a segment of chromosome 1 that is duplicated were called MMP-21 and MMP-22 but are now referred to as MMP-23A and MMP-23B.

Adapted with permission from Genome Biology 2003; 4:216.

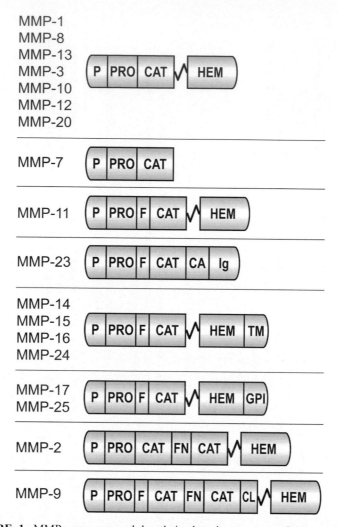

**FIGURE 1.** MMPs are grouped by their domain structure. CA, cysteine array; CAT, catalytic domain; CL collagen-like domain; F, furin-cleavage consensus sequence; FN, fibronectin-like repeats; GPI, glycosyl phosphatidylinositol linkage signal; HEM, hemopexin domain; Ig immunoglouline-like domain; P, leader sequence; PRO, pro-domain; TM, transmembrane domain. The hinge connects the CAT with the HEM domain.

MMPs that have been reported as important in AAAs include MMP-1, -2, -3, -8, -9, -10, -12, and -13. MMP-2 and MMP-9 appear to play a particularly important role in AAA formation and are referred to by Parks as the "confederacy of the proteinases" working in concert or alone.[25] The balance of MMPs and TIMPs has generally been thought to be in favor of degradation. In addition, even though collagen synthesis is increased, elastin synthesis is disorganized.

**TABLE 2. MMP polymorphisms and disease[a]**

| MMP Polymorphisms/Allele | Disease |
|---|---|
| MMP-3: 5A/5A | Coronary aneurysms |
| | AAA |
| 5A/6A | Coronary artery disease |
| MMP-9: C-1562T | Coronary artery disease |
| Microsatellite (CA)n | Intracranial aneurysm |
| | AAA |
| | Multiple sclerosis |
| MMP-12: A-82G | Coronary artery disease |

[a]Adapted from Ye, S. Matrix Biology 19 (2000) 623–629.

In knockout mice models of AAA, the absence of MMP-2 and MMP-9 is associated with a lower incidence of experimental AAAs. Whether one MMP plays a greater role in AAA formation is unclear. Circulating levels of MMP-9 have been used to follow aneurysms and postendovascular repair. The data are conflicting regarding the reliability of serum MMP-9 levels.

# ECM

The new frontier of MMP biology involves the role of MMPs in releasing cryptic fragments and neoepitopes from the ECM and the impact of MMPs on the regulation of the inflammatory response. The ECM is a complex structure, much more important than an inert scaffold. The ECM regulates cell migration, and contains embedded cytokines, growth factors, and inhibitors. The degradation of the ECM is important in a number of pathologic processes and plays an important role in angiogenesis. MMP-2 and MMP-9 expose cryptic epitopes that control angiogenesis (TABLE 3).[9] In addition, the MMPs inhibit angiogenesis through the release of endostatin by the direct cleavage of collagen XVIII by MMP-7. Other antiangiogenic proteins include endorepellin, derived from the C terminus of the protoglycan, perlecan, and three molecules with antiangiogenic and antitumor activities created by a cleavage of type IV collagen, arresten, canstatin, and tumstatin. Other breakdown products of the ECM include fragments of fragmin that induce cellular migration and elastin degradation products (EDPs) (chemotactic for macrophages). The ECM also

**TABLE 3. Cryptic fragments and growth factors released from the ECM by MMPs**

| | |
|---|---|
| TGF-β | NC1, endostatin |
| VEGF | C term, endorepellin |
| NC1-α1 arresten | Cryptic epitope |
| NC1-α 2 canstatin | TIMPs |
| NC1-α 3 tumstatin | MMPs |
| NC1, restin | EDPs |

contains embedded growth factors such as VEGF and TGF-β. In the mouse model of Marfan's Syndrome, TGF-β is increased due to the inability of the matrix to sequester the growth hormone.[26]

## MMPs' CONTROL OF INFLAMMATION

Inflammation is a complex, highly regulated system that involves the identification of injury or infection, response to the injury or infection, repair and healing, and return to normal homeostasis. However, in some instances the inflammatory process leads to a pathologic process that is damaging to the host. While an infectious etiology is clear in many cases, an unknown event may be responsible for the initiation of chronic diseases such as multiple sclerosis, rheumatoid arthritis, atherosclerosis, and even AAA. MMPs play an important role in the control of the inflammatory response through the modification of proinflammatory cytokines and chemokines, and shedding of membrane receptors.[27-29] The inflammatory substrates of MMPs include CXCL7, CXCL12, latent TGF-β, CXCL5, and many chemokine ligands (TABLE 1). An example of this regulatory system is the activation of IL-1β by MMP-2,-3, and -9 and its subsequent degradation by MMP-3. Although the phenotypes of most MMP knockout mice appear to be normal, many of these animals demonstrate abnormalities in their inflammatory response. For example, MMP-2 knockout mice demonstrate a decreased allergic inflammation and a more severe immune-mediated arthritis, while MMP-9 knockouts demonstrate prolonged contact hypersensitivity, less severe experimental arthritis, and protection against macrophage-induced aneurysm formation. MMP-12 knockouts are similarly protected from smoking-induced inflammation. This finding suggests a proinflammatory role for MMP-12.[30] Finally, MMPs may allow the entrance of infectious material to relatively inaccessible areas such as the media of the aorta. In summary, MMPs are not only responsible for the degradation of the structural integrity of the aorta, but are also important in the regulation of inflammatory response and the release of cryptic epitopes and growth factors.

## POLYMORPHISMS OF THE IMMUNE SYSTEM

Genetic studies of aortic aneurysms have generally focused on candidate genes encoding structural proteins (collagen, elastin, and fibrillin) and the MMPs and TIMPs. The genetics of inflammatory mediators in AAA is a more recent area of study. Numerous genetic association studies have been performed to help determine the genetic risk associated with certain single nucleotide polymorphisms (SNPs) and susceptibility to AAA and the likelihood of rupture.[30] When assessing the conclusions of genetic association studies, several editorial comments have suggested the following issues to be considered:[31]

- adequate sample size
- replication
- functional data
- confirmation by experimentation

It is important to understand the biology and potential impact of a polymorphism on gene function. TABLE 4 provides a list of inflammatory gene polymorphisms studied in various AAA populations and the outcomes of these studies. Because of the variability in the patient populations and the size of the population studied, it is difficult to draw any conclusions regarding the role these polymorphisms play in AAA.[31,32] As with atherosclerosis, the genetic background may play only a minor role when compared to the role of risk factors, particularly smoking, hypertension, and hypercholesterolemia in the pathogenesis of AAAs.

## FEATURES OF AUTOIMMUNITY IN AAA

In his opening remarks at the 2004 International Congress on Autoimmunity in Budapest, Hungary, Yehuda Shoenfeld said roughly 80 autoimmune diseases have been described today, affecting approximately one in five individuals. Autoimmune diseases range from those that fit a classical definition of autoimmunity such as rheumatoid arthritis (RA) and systemic lupus erythematosus (SLE), to diseases that may have an autoimmune basis such as autism, epilepsy, and cardiovascular diseases.[33]

## MOLECULAR MIMICRY AND BYSTANDER ACTIVATION

In 1996 Gregory et al. described autoimmune features of AAA.[34] They extracted immunoglobulin G (IgG) from AAA tissues and detected immunohistochemical reactivity to fixed sections of normal aorta. They also found that AAA IgG reacted with a band of about 80 kDa in size from tissue extracts from both normal aorta and AAA using immunoblotting techniques. The following year Ozsvath et al. published a paper introducing the concept of molecular mimicry as a possible mechanism for the features of autoimmunity previously described in AAA.[36] Molecular mimicry occurs in susceptible individuals who are infected by pathogens expressing epitopes that are immunologically similar to host antigenic determinants, yet possess enough antigenic differences to induce an immune response. In such cases tolerance to self may be breached, thus directing a pathogen-specific response to self.[35] The partial sequencing of the potential autoantigen done by Ozsvath revealed homology to bovine aortic microfibril-associated glyprotein-36 kDa (MAGP-36). Sequencing also revealed homologies to two pathogenic microorganisms that had been associated with aneurysms; a bacterium known to cause venereal disease, Treponema

**TABLE 4. Published studies of inflammatory gene polymorphisms and AAA**

| Author, Year | Polymorphisms | Number of subjects | Controls | Population | Conclusions |
|---|---|---|---|---|---|
| Fatini,[47] 2005 | ACE I/D<br>AII receptors: AT1R<br>A1166C | 250 each AAA and Control | Age, gender-matched | Caucasian; Central and Southern Italians | ACE D/D more common in AAA |
| Hamano,[48] 1999 | ACE I/D | 125 AAA<br>153 Control | Matched: age, gender, DM, hyperlipidemia | Japanese | No ACE I/D association with AAA |
| Pola,[49] 2001 | ACE I/D | 124 AAA (55% HT, 45% non-HT)<br>112 Control (non-HT) | Age, gender, BMI-matched | Caucasian; Central and Southern Italians | ACE DD and ID associated with non-HT AAA |
| Bown,[50] 2002 | IL-1β +3953<br>IL-6 -174<br>IL-10 -1082<br>TNF-α -308 | 100 AAA | None | Caucasians from the United Kingdom, 80% male | Plasma cytokine levels did not correlate with AAA genotype |
| Bown,[51] 2003 | IL-1β +3953<br>IL-6 -174<br>IL-10 -1082<br>TNF-α -308 | 100 AAA<br>100 Control | Age, gender-matched | White Europeans | IL-10 -1082 A allele associated with AAA. |

*Continued.*

**TABLE 4. Continued**

| Author, Year | Polymorphisms | Number of subjects | Controls | Population | Conclusions |
|---|---|---|---|---|---|
| Bown,[51] 2004 | IL-1β +3953<br>IL-6 -174<br>IL-10 -1082<br>TNF-α -308 | 135 AAA | None | No ethnicity specified, 79% male | Postop cytokine levels related to AAA outcome, polymorphism associations unclear |
| Jones,[52] 2001 | IL-6 -174 | 466 small AAA | None | Majority male | AAA source of IL-6, weak association with -174 G allele and cardiovascular mortality |
| Ghilardi,[53] 2004 | Chemokine receptor CCR5 Δ32 deletion | 70 AAA<br>76 PAOD<br>62 Carotid<br>172 Control | Age, gender-matched | Not specified | CCR5 32 deletion more frequent in AAA and associated with rupture |

HT = hypertension; DM = diabetes mellitus; BMI = body mass index; PAOD = peripheral artery occlusive disease.

palidum (T pall) and the herpes simplex virus.[36] It is also plausible that features of autoimmunity in AAA may result from the exposure of sequestered antigens as a result of degradation of the matrix associated with the inflammatory response. This mechanism is called bystander activation. Ongoing inflammation of the aortic wall may lead to the release or exposure of sequestered, chemoattractive antigens, degraded elastin peptides, for example. Presentation of these newly exposed self-antigens by the host can prime naïve self-reactive lymphocytes, leading to their activation.[37]

## GENETIC FACTORS: MAJOR HISTOCOMPATIBILITY COMPLEX (MHC) AND HUMAN LEUKOCYTE ANTIGEN (HLA)

The MHC represents a set of genes on human chromosome 6 that code for cell-surface histocompatibility antigens. They are the principal determinants of tissue type and transplant compatibility. Many autoimmune diseases are associated with particular MHC haplotypes. The HLA system comprises a group of genes within the MHC that encode cell-surface antigens used in the recognition of self. Certain autoimmune diseases are known to associate with specific HLA gene profiles. For example, individuals with HLA-B8, -DR3 have a higher incidence of type I diabetes and lupus.[33] Rasmussen and colleagues published several papers reporting specific loci of the HLA class II genes that associated with inflammatory abdominal aortic aneurysms (IAAA) and AAA.[38–40] They found that IAAA risk was mapped to HLA-DR B1 and risk of AAA was associated with HLA-DR B1*02, -*04 alleles in Caucasian populations. Genetics of populations differ, and Hirose reported AAA risk associated with HLA-DR2(15),[41] while more recently Sugimoto found association with HLA-A2 and HLA-B61 in Japanese populations.[42] In a Spanish population with confirmed Spanish ancestors, Monux reported AAA associated with HLA-DR B1*0401.[43] Monux also noted that the HLA-DR B1*0401 subtype has been associated with a severe form of rheumatoid arthritis, a classic autoimmune disease. Although these HLA-AAA association studies do not identify the same HLA subtypes for all AAA populations (see the summary in TABLE 4), which would be unlikely due to the inherent genetic differences seen in other disease associations across populations, collectively they provide evidence that phenomena linked to autoimmunity play a role in aneurysm disease. HLA typing associations vary between AAA and IAAA, and suggest that the etiology of the two diseases may be distinct. Haug *et al.* reported an association between a group of IAAA patients and an increased incidence of autoimmune disease compared to a group of noninflammatory AAA patients.[44] However, in both AAA and IAAA, implications of autoimmunity may change diagnostic and risk assessment as well as provide a new set of therapeutic targets.

## AAA: AN AUTOIMMUNE DISEASE?

At this time most investigators hesitate to define AAA as an autoimmune disease and prefer to qualify the use of this term using phrases like aspects of autoimmunity, possible basis in autoimmunity, et cetera. This is for good reason. Many questions remain unanswered. Does the presence of chronic inflammation categorize a disease as autoimmune? If that were the case, many more diseases would be considered autoimmune. What about the presence of autoantibodies? Some of these are naturally occurring and function to eliminate debris from the body. A number of healthy individuals have circulating autoantibodies of the type that are typically found in SLE, but never show signs of the disease in their lifetimes. Aging is also a factor in immune response. Lacroix-Desmazes *et al.* reported data that showed a decreasing incidence and severity of autoimmune disease with aging, yet also observed increased autoantibodies in the serum of elderly patients, which did not correlate with overt autoimmune disease.[45] Tomer and Shoenfeld published a review on aging and autoantibodies finding an increase in the production of autoantibodies with age, yet an overall decreased immune responsiveness in general.[46] They concluded that these two opposing phenomena resulted from an alteration in immunoregulatory function, marked by an increased incidence of malignant, infectious, and nonclassical autoimmune diseases that accompany aging.

## COMMENT

Although we may not know the etiology of AAAs, a better understanding of the inflammatory process and its regulatory points will help develop new strategies for the treatment of AAA. In addition, one of the difficulties in understanding the pathogenesis of AAA is the lack of precise definition of the phenotype. Most studies on human AAA combine what may be more than one phenotype as a single disease process. For example, is a patient with multiple aneurysms the same as a patient with a single AAA or one with diffused arteriomegally? The nature of AAA disease is multifactorial; some aneurysms may have a stronger genetic component while environmental factors such as smoking play a greater role in others. Ultimately, the underlying process in AAA may be of an immunologic nature based on an abnormal inflammatory response to injury and not a single disease entity.

## REFERENCES

1. GROSS, J. & C.M. LAPIERE. 1962. Collagenolytic activity in amphibian tissue: a tissue culture assay. Proc. Natl. Acad. Sci. USA **48:** 1014–1022.

2. BRINCKERHOFF, C.E. & L.M. MATRISIAN. 2002. Matrix metalloproteinases: a tail of a frog that became a prince. Nat. Rev. Mol. Cell Biol. **3:** 207–214.

3. VAN DEN STEEN, P.E., B. DUBOIS, I. NELISSEN, et al. 2002. Biochemistry and molecular biology of gelatinase B or matrix metalloproteinase-9 (MMP-9). Crit. Rev. Biochem. Mol. Biol. **37:** 375–536.

4. KUZUYA, M. & A. IGUCHI. 2003. Role of matrix metalloproteinases in vascular remodeling. J. Atheroscler. Thromb. **10:** 275–282.

5. LEE, M.H. & G. MURPHY. 2004. Matrix metalloproteinases at a glance. J. Cell. Sci. **117:** 4015–4016.

6. STAMENKOVIC, I. 2003. Extracellular matrix remodelling: the role of matrix metalloproteinases. J. Pathol. **200:** 448–464.

7. SOMERVILLE, R.P., S.A. OBLANDER & S.S. APTE. 2003. Matrix metalloproteinases old dogs with new tricks. Genome Biol. **4:** 216.1–216.11.

8. SINHA, I., K.K. HANNAWA, J.L. ELIASON, et al. 2004. Early MT-1 MMP expression following elastase exposure is associated with increased cleaved MMP-2 activity in experimental rodent aortic aneurysms. Surgery **136:** 176–182.

9. MOTT, J.D. & Z. WERB. 2004. Regulation of matrix biology by matrix metalloproteinases. Cur. Opin. Cell. Biol. **16:** 558–564.

10. MANNELLO, F., F. LUCHETTI, E. FALCIERI, et al. 2005. Multiple roles of matrix metalloproteinases during apoptosis. Apoptosis **10:** 19–24.

11. VANWART, H.E. & H. BIRKEDAL-HANSEN. 1990. The cysteine switch: a principle of regulation of metalloproteinase activity with potential applicability to entire metalloproteinase gene family. Proc. Natl. Acad. Sci. USA **87:** 5578–5582.

12. MARTIGNETTI, J.A., A.A. AQEEL, W. AL SEWAIRI, et al. 2001. Mutation of the matrix metalloproteinases 2 gene (MMP2) causes a multicentric osteolysis and arthritis syndrome. Nat. Gen. **28:** 261–265.

13. NAKAHARA, H., L. HOWARD, E.W. THOMPSON, et al. 1997. Transmembrane/cytoplastmic domain-mediated membrane type 1-matrix metalloproteinase docking to invadopodia is required for cell invasion. Proceedings of the National Academy of Science of the United States of America. **94:** 7959–7964.

14. YE, S. 2000. Polymorphism in matrix metalloproteinase gene promoters: implication in regulation of gene expression and susceptibility of various diseases. Matrix Biol. **19:** 623–629.

15. BUSUTTIL, R.W., A.M. ABOU-ZAMZAM & H.I. MACHLEDER. 1980. Collagenase activity of the human aorta. A comparison of patients with and without abdominal aortic aneurysms. Arch. Surg. **115:** 1373–1378.

16. LONGO, G.M., S.J. BUDA, N. FIOTTA, et al. 2005. MMP-12 has a role in abdominal aortic aneurysms in mice. Surgery **137:** 457–462.

17. WASSEF, M., B.T. BAXTER, R.L. CHISHOLM, et al. 2001. Pathogenesis of abdominal aortic aneurysms: a multidisciplinary research program supported by the National Heart, Lung, and Blood Institute. J. Vasc. Surg. **34:** 730–738.

18. PYO, R., J.K. LEE, J.M. SHIPLEY, et al. 2000. Targeted gene disruption of matrix metalloproteinase-9 (gelatinase B) suppresses development of experimental abdominal aortic aneurysms. J. Clin. Invest. **105:** 1641–1649.

19. MAO, D., J.K. LEE, S.J. VANVICKLE, et al. 1999. Expression of collagenase-3 (MMP-13) in human abdominal aortic aneurysms and vascular smooth muscle cells in culture. Biochem. Biophys. Res. Com. **261:** 904–910.

20. LONGO, G.M., W. XIONG, T.C. GREINER, et al. 2002. Matrix metalloproteinases 2 and 9 work in concert to produce aortic aneurysms. J. Clin. Invest. **110(5):** 625–632.

21. FATINI, C., G. PRATESI, F. SOFI, *et al.* 2005. ACE DD genotype: a predisposing factor for abdominal aortic aneurysm. Eur. J. Vasc. Endovasc. Surg. **29:** 227–232.
22. HAMANO, K., I. OHISHI, M. UEDA, *et al.* 1999. Deletion polymorphism in gene for ACE is not a risk factor predisposing to abdominal aortic aneurysm. Eur. J. Vasc. Enodvasc. Surg. **18:** 158–161.
23. POLA, R., E. GAETANI, A. SANTOLIQUIDO, *et al.* 2001. Abdominal aortic aneurysm in normotensive patients: association with ACE gene polymorphism. Eur. J. Vasc. Endovasc. Surg. **21:** 445–449.
24. BOWN, M.J., T. HORSBURGH, M.L. NICHOLSON, *et al.* 2003. Cytokine gene polymorphisms and the inflammatory response to abdominal aortic aneurysm repair. Br. J. Surg. **90(9):** 1085–1092.
25. PARKS, W.C. 2002. A confederacy of proteinases. J. Clin. Invest. **110:** 613–614.
26. NEPTUNE, E.R., P.A. FRISCHMEYER, D.E. ARKING, *et al.* 2003. Dysregulation of TGF-β activation contributes to pathogenesis in Marfan syndrome. Nat. Gen. **33:** 407–411.
27. ELKINGTON, P.T.G., C.M. KANE & J.S. FRIEDLAND. 2005. The paradox of matrix metalloproteinases in infectious disease. Clin. Exper. Immunol. **142:** 12–20.
28. PARKS, W.C., C.L. WILSON & Y.S. LOPEZ-BOADO. 2004. Matrix metalloproteinases as modulators of inflammation and innate immunity. Nat. Rev. Immunol. **4:** 617–629.
29. NATHAN, C. 2002. Points of control in inflammation. Nature **420:** 846–852.
30. NENAN, S., E. BOICHOT, V. LAGENTE, *et al.* 2005. Macrophage elastase (MMP-12): a pro-inflammatory mediator? Mem. Inst. Oswaldo Cruz **100**(Suppl 1): 167–172.
31. MARIAN, A.J. 2001. On genetics, inflammation, and abdominal aortic aneurysm: can single nucleotide polymorphisms predict the outcome? Circulation **103:** 2222–2224.
32. MARIAN, A.J. & E. BOERWINKLE.2002. "Into Thin Air" and the genetics of complex traits. Circulation **106:** 768–769.
33. SHOENFELD, Y. & G. ZANDMAN-GODDARD. 2003. Autoimmune Diseases – The Enemy from Within. First edition. Bio-Rad Laboratories. USA.
34. GREGORY, A.K., N.X. YIN, J. CAPELLA, *et al.* 1996. Features of autoimmunity in the abdominal aortic aneurysm. Arch. Surg. **131:** 85–88.
35. LAHITA, R.G., N. CHIORAZZI & W.H. REEVES, Eds.: 2000. Textbook of the Autoimmune Diseases. Lippincott Williams & Wilkins. Philadelphia.
36. OZSVATH, K.J., H. HIROSE, S. XIA, *et al.* 1997. Molecular mimicry in human aortic aneurysmal diseases. Ann. N. Y. Acad. Sci. **800:** 288–293.
37. SARVETNICK, N. 2000. Etiology of autoimmunity. Immunol. Res. **21/2-3:** 357–362.
38. RASMUSSEN, T.E., J.W. HALLETT, R.L. MATHIEU METZGER, *et al.* 1997. Genetic risk factors in inflammatory abdominal aortic aneurysms: polymorphic residue 70 in the HLA-DR B1 gene as a key genetic element. J. Vasc. Surg. **25:** 356–364.
39. RASMUSSEN, T.E., J.W. HALLETT, S. SCHULTE, *et al.* 2001. Genetic similarity in inflammatory and degenerative abdominal aortic aneurysms: a study of human leukocyte antigen class II disease risk genes. J. Vasc. Surg. **34:** 84–89.
40. RASMUSSEN, T.E., J.W. HALLETT, H.D. TAZELAAR, *et al.* 2002. Human leukocyte antigen class II immune response genes, female gender, and cigarette smoking as risk and modulating factors in abdominal aortic aneurysms. J. Vasc. Surg. **35:** 988–993.

41. HIROSE, H., M. TAKAGI, N. MIYAGAWA, et al. 1998. Genetic risk factor for abdominal aortic aneurysm: HLA-DR2(15), a Japanese study. J. Vasc. Surg. **7:** 500–503.
42. SUGIMOTO, T., M. SADA & H. YAO. 2003. Genetic analysis on HLA loci in Japanese patients with abdominal aortic aneurysm. Eur. J. Vasc. Endovasc. Surg. **26:** 215–218.
43. MONUX, G., F.J. SERRANO, P. VIGIL & E.G. DE LA CONCHA. 2003. Role of HLA-DR in the pathogenesis of abdominal aortic aneurysm. Eur. J. Vasc. Endovasc. Surg. **26:** 211–214.
44. HAUG, E.S., J.F. SKOMSVOLL, G. JACOBSEN, et al. 2003. Inflammatory aortic aneurysm is associated with increased incidence of autoimmune disease. J. Vasc. Surg. **38:** 492–497.
45. LACROIX-DESMAZES, S., L. MOUTHON, S.V. KAVERI, et al. 1999. Stability of natural self-reactive antibody repertoires during aging. J. Clin. Immunol. **19:** 26–34.
46. TOMER, Y. & Y. SHOENFELD. 1998. Review: ageing and autoantibodies. Autoimmunity **1:** 141–149.
47. FATINI, C., G. PRATESI, F. SOFI, et al. 2005. ACE DD genotype: a predisposing factor for abdominal aortic aneurysm. Eur. J. Vasc. Endovasc. Surg. **29:** 227–232.
48. HAMANO, K., I. OHISHI, M. UEDA, et al. 1999. Deletion polymorphism in gene for angiotensin converting enzyme is not a risk factor predisposing to abdominal aortic aneurysm. Eur. J. Vasc. Endovasc. Surg. **18:** 158–161.
49. POLA, R., E. GAETANI, A. SANTOLIQUIDO, et al. 2001. Abdominal aortic aneurysm in normotensive patients: association with ACE gene polymorphism. Eur. J. Vasc. Endovasc. Surg. **21:** 445–449.
50. BOWN, M.J., P.R. BURTON, T. HORSBURGH, et al. 2003. The role of cytokine gene polymorphisms in the pathogenesis of abdominal aortic aneurysms: a case-control study. J. Vasc. Surg. **37:** 999–1005.
51. BOWN, M.J., T. HORSBURGH, M.L. NICHOLSON, et al. 2004. Cytokines, their genetic polymorphisms, and outcome after abdominal aortic aneurysm repair. Eur. J. Vasc. Endovasc. Surg. **28:** 274–280.
52. JONES, K.G., D.J. BRULL & L.C. BROWN. 2001. Interleukin-6 (IL-6) and the prognosis of abdominal aortic aneurysms. Circulation **103:** 2260–2265.
53. GHILARDI, G., M.L. BIONDI, L. BATTAGLIOLI, et al. 2004. Genetic risk factor characterizes abdominal aortic aneurysm from arterial occlusive disease in human beings: CCR5 Δ32 deletion. J. Vasc. Surg. **40:** 995–1000.

# The Intraluminal Thrombus as a Source of Proteolytic Activity

JESPER SWEDENBORG[a] AND PER ERIKSSON[b]

[a]Department of Vascular Surgery, Karolinska University Hospital and Institute, Stockholm, Sweden

[b]King Gustav Vth Research Institute, Department of Medicine, Karolinska University Hospital and Institute, Stockholm, Sweden

ABSTRACT: Most abdominal aortic aneurysms (AAAs) with a diameter indicating need for surgical repair contain intraluminal thrombus (ILT). The development of AAA is linked to degradation of elastin and collagen. These changes are more pronounced in the aneurysm wall covered by the ILT, which also shows more signs of inflammation and is thinner compared to the aneurysm wall exposed to flowing blood. The rate of increase in diameter of AAA correlates with increased thrombus growth and rupture. CT examinations of patients with rupture have demonstrated contrast appearing in the thrombus suggesting bleeding into it. Studies using gene array of human aneurysm specimens have shown that most matrix metalloproteinases (MMP) were upregulated in the thrombus-free wall. Analyses by zymography, however, demonstrate gelatinase activity in the interface between the thrombus and the underlying wall and in the media of the wall not covered by a thrombus. The thrombus contains large amounts of neutrophils. Neutrophil gelatinase associated lipocalin (NGAL) is involved in the regulation of MMP-9 activity and prevents its inactivation, thus augmenting the proteolytic effect. It has been identified in all layers of the ILT. The presence of NGAL/MMP-9 complexes throughout the thrombus and in the thrombus-covered wall may contribute to the increased proteolytic degradation seen in this wall segment. In conclusion, the presence, growth, and thickness of the ILT have been shown to be associated with growth and risk of rupture. The wall underlying the thrombus is thinner and shows more signs of proteolytic degradation. Increased proteolytic activity by MMP-9 may be mediated by binding to NGAL.

KEYWORDS: abdominal aortic aneurysm; thrombus; lipocalin; rupture

Abdominal aortic aneurysm (AAA) is a disease associated with aging. The prevalence is low before the age of 55 years and then increases and reaches a

Address for correspondence: Jesper Swedenborg, Department of Vascular Surgery N1:06, Karolinska University Hospital, 17176, Stockholm, Sweden. Voice: +46-8-51772348; fax: +46-8-51776642.
e-mail: jesper.swedenborg@ki.se

Ann. N.Y. Acad. Sci. 1085: 133–138 (2006). © 2006 New York Academy of Sciences.
doi: 10.1196/annals.1383.044

plateau at age 75 years.[1] It is more common in men than in women with a ratio of 4–6:1. The development of AAA is linked to loss of structural integrity of the major ground substances elastin and collagen. It has been suggested that the loss of elastin leads to dilatation, whereas loss of collagen predisposes for rupture.[2] Loss of elastin primarily causes a decrease in longitudinal strength leading to elongation and tortuosity of the major arteries including the abdominal aorta. The curvatures of the aorta cause asymmetric and turbulent flow profiles and abnormal wall stress leading to endothelial injury.[3] If the normal nonthrombogenic properties of endothelial cell lining are damaged, prerequisites for thrombus formation in areas with turbulent flow increases. Patients with AAA have atherosclerotic disease and atheroma of the wall of the AAA is regularly observed. The presence of atherosclerosis may further increase the risk for thrombus formation within the aneurysm.

The rate of increase in diameter of AAA correlates with increased thrombus growth.[4] Consequently, most patients with large AAA (>5 cm diameter) have an intraluminal thrombus (ILT). In most cases, the ILT is located eccentrically leaving some areas of the aneurysm wall covered by thrombus and some exposed to the flowing blood. The thrombus volume has been reported to be larger in patients with rupture, but the ratio between diameter and thrombus volume is the same in patients with and without rupture of their AAA.[5] In a follow-up study of patients undergoing serial CT scans, it has been concluded that the growth of the thrombus is a stronger predictor of rupture and impending rupture than growth of the AAA. In the reported patient material, there were a few patients without ILT; none of them experienced rupture or threatening rupture.[6]

Comparisons between wall segments covered by thrombus and not covered by thrombus from patients undergoing elective aneurysm repair have demonstrated that elastic degradation and signs of inflammation are greatly increased in the AAA wall covered by thrombus. The wall segment under the thrombus also shows a decrease in number of smooth muscle cells (SMC), many of which have undergone apoptosis. The number of T cells, both helper and cytotoxic cells, are increased in the wall covered by thrombus.[7] No differentiation between Th1 and Th2 cells were made in this study. In a study using human blood lymphocytes from patients with arterial disease, elastin degradation products (EDP) were shown to cause an orientation toward differentiation to Th1 cells. This causes the Th1 cytokines interferon-γ and IL-2 to be enhanced by EDP.[8] On the other hand, reports examining wall segments of AAA state that Th2 cells predominate, but the study reporting this finding did not differentiate between wall segments covered and not covered by thrombus.[9] The wall covered by ILT is thinner[7] and less resistant to wall stress.[10] Various findings regarding the protective effect of the ILT for the underlying wall have been reported. Some authors suggest that the ILT reduces and redistributes the stress in the wall[11] and that the thrombus lowers pressure in the aneurysm sac.[12] The latter argument has been used for the introduction of endovascular aneurysm repair

(EVAR), where the thrombus is left inside the aneurysm and thus possibly could contribute to decreased wall tension.

A possible reduction of the wall tension by the ILT, however, requires that it is intact and prevents blood from reaching the underlying wall. Association between rupture and thrombus as stated above is further supported by Satta et al. who also stated that the thickness of the thrombus correlates with the risk of rupture.[13] The question is if and how the blood reaches the weakened wall covered by the thrombus. In patients with ruptured AAA stable enough to undergo CT, the so-called crescent sign has been demonstrated. This implies contrast enhancement in the thrombus due to blood leaking into it.[14,15] Consequently, theoretical prerequisites exist for rupture occurring through the thrombus covered wall by blood entering the thrombus. Similar findings have also been found using ultrasonography.[16]

What is the cause of the increased degradation of the wall under the ILT? Is its proteolytic activity derived from constituents of the wall or the thrombus itself including the interphase fluid often observed between the ILT and the underlying wall? In most cases, the thrombus consists of distinct layers. The inner layer is a red thrombus, which is rather thin and toward the abluminal side where one or two layers of impacted fibrin are found. In many cases, there is also an interstitial fluid phase between the most abluminal layer and the wall. The ILT has been reported to contain high amounts of predominantly metalloproteinases (MMP)-9 with higher amounts in the luminal part of the thrombus.[17] The presence of MMP-9 in the luminal part of the ILT has also been demonstrated by Fontaine et al.,[18] who also demonstrated that spontaneous clotting of whole blood induces release of pro-MMP-9 into the serum, a process which is further accentuated by fibrinolysis. It is likely that cellular penetration occurs predominantly from the luminal layer of the ILT, but the structure of the thrombus with large canaliculi could also enable macromolecular penetrations into the deeper layers of the thrombus.[19] Signs of collagenolytic activity based on hydroxyproline derived from collagen degradation products have also been shown to be present in the ILT.[20]

In experimental models of AAA induced by elastase or calcium chloride no major thrombus formation is observed.[21] Xenografting of the aorta, however, leads to aneurysm formation with a thrombus. By definition plasminogen is present in the thrombus because it is bound to fibrin. When activated into plasmin it participates in the activation of several MMPs. Plasminogen itself does not cause AAA development in experimental animals but inhibitors of both plasminogen and MMP-9 (PAI-1 and TIMP-1) attenuate aneurysm development and rupture in xenograft models of AAA.[22]

Even though the wall underlying the thrombus in human aneurysm tissue obtained at surgery shows increased signs of proteolysis, mRNA expression of MMP 1, 7, 9, and 12 was upregulated in the wall not covered by ILT, but so were the inhibitors PAI-1 and TIMP-1. To examine functional activity, gelatinolysis was studied by in situ zymography. Gelatinolytic activity was detected in both the media of the wall not covered by ILT and in the interphase between the ILT and the wall. The activity could be inhibited by the MMP inhibitor 10-phenantroline.[23] The findings of proteolytic activity in the interphase fluid are supported by Fontaine et al.[18]

Activation of c-Jun-N-terminal-kinase (JNK), which is involved in cellular stress responses, has been shown to be an important signaling molecule in the pathogenesis of AAA.[24] JNK causes upregulation of both MMP-9 and lipocalin. Neutrophil gelatinase associated lipocalin (NGAL) binds to MMP and prevents its degradation.[25] This mechanism combined with the presence of leucocytes in the thrombus led us to hypothesize that NGAL could be of importance for the destruction of the underlying wall. In the ILT and particularly in the interphase between it and the underlying wall, it could be demonstrated that NGAL was colocalized with MMP-9. NGAL was, however, also present in the wall segments without ILT, but only in the media. NGAL expression colocalized with areas of CD-66b expressing neutrophils, but was also found in the tissue without association with cells indicating secretion of NGAL. Further analyses by immunoprecipitation and Western blot indicated that complexes of various sizes including NGAL and MMP-9 were present, suggesting binding of various molecular amounts of MMP-9 to one molecule of NGAL (own unpublished observations). In an experimental elastase-induced model of AAA, neutrophil depletion was shown to attenuate the development of AAA. This effect was, however, shown to be independent of neutrophil collagenase (MMP-8).[26] The absence of NGAL after could provide an explanation for the inhibition of AAA development caused by neutrophil depletion.

## CONCLUSION

The ILT and its growth are associated with growth and rupture of AAA. The wall underlying ILT is thinner and shows more signs of inflammation and proteolytic degradation than the wall exposed to flowing blood. The ILT and the interphase region between it and the AAA wall contain proteolytic activity which explains the degradation of the underlying wall. Consequently there is evidence that the ILT plays an important role in the pathogenesis of aneurysm growth and rupture. This relationship needs to be further studied. In the meantime, it is important that studies using human material from AAA are defined based on whether or not the specimens are taken from walls covered by ILT.

## REFERENCES

1. VARDULAKI, K.A. et al. 1998. Growth rates and risk of rupture of abdominal aortic aneurysms. Br. J. Surg. **85:** 1674–1680.

2. DOBRIN, P.B. & R. MRKVICKA. 1994. Failure of elastin or collagen as possible critical connective tissue alterations underlying aneurysmal dilatation. Cardiovasc. Surg. **2**: 484–488.

3. NICHOLS, W.W. & M.F. O'ROURKE. 2005. McDonald's blood flow in arteries. Hodder Arnold. London.

4. WOLF, Y.G. *et al.* 1994. Computed tomography scanning findings associated with rapid expansion of abdominal aortic aneurysms. J. Vasc. Surg. **20**: 529–535; Discussion 535–538.

5. HANS, S.S. *et al.* 2005. Size and location of thrombus in intact and ruptured abdominal aortic aneurysms. J. Vasc. Surg. **41**: 584–588.

6. STENBAEK, J., B. KALIN & J. SWEDENBORG. 2000. Growth of thrombus is a better predictor for rupture than diameter in patients with abdominal aortic aneurysms. Eur. J. Vasc. Endovasc. Surg. **20**: 466–469.

7. KAZI, M. *et al.* 2003. Influence of intraluminal thrombus on structural and cellular composition of abdominal aortic aneurysm wall. J. Vasc. Surg. **38**: 1283–1292.

8. DEBRET, R. *et al.* 2005. Elastin-derived peptides induce a T-helper type 1 polarization of human blood lymphocytes. Arterioscler. Thromb. Vasc. Biol. **25**: 1353–1358.

9. SCHONBECK, U. *et al.* 1997. Regulation of matrix metalloproteinase expression in human vascular smooth muscle cells by T lymphocytes: a role for CD40 signaling in plaque rupture? Circ. Res. **81**: 448–454.

10. VORP, D.A. *et al.* 2001. Association of intraluminal thrombus in abdominal aortic aneurysm with local hypoxia and wall weakening. J. Vasc. Surg. **34**: 291–299.

11. DI MARTINO, E. *et al.* 1998. Biomechanics of abdominal aortic aneurysm in the presence of endoluminal thrombus: experimental characterisation and structural static computational analysis. Eur. J. Vasc. Endovasc. Surg. **15**: 290–299.

12. HINNEN, J.W., M.J. VISSER & J.H. VAN BOCKEL. 2005. Aneurysm sac pressure monitoring: effect of technique on interpretation of measurements. Eur. J. Vasc. Endovasc. Surg. **29**: 233–238.

13. SATTA, J., E. LAARA & T. JUVONEN. 1996. Intraluminal thrombus predicts rupture of an abdominal aortic aneurysm. J. Vasc. Surg. **23**: 737–739.

14. ARITA, T. *et al.* 1997. Abdominal aortic aneurysm: rupture associated with the high-attenuating crescent sign. Radiology **204**: 765–768.

15. MEHARD, W.B., J.P. HEIKEN & G.A. SICARD. 1994. High-attenuating crescent in abdominal aortic aneurysm wall at CT: a sign of acute or impending rupture. Radiology **192**: 359–362.

16. CATALANO, O. & A. SIANI. 2005. Ruptured abdominal aortic aneurysm: categorization of sonographic findings and report of 3 new signs. J. Ultrasound Med. **24**: 1077–1083.

17. SAKALIHASAN, N. *et al.* 1996. Activated forms of MMP2 and MMP9 in abdominal aortic aneurysms. J. Vasc. Surg. **24**: 127–133.

18. FONTAINE, V. *et al.* 2002. Involvement of the mural thrombus as a site of protease release and activation in human aortic aneurysms. Am. J. Pathol. **161**: 1701–1710.

19. ADOLPH, R. *et al.* 1997. Cellular content and permeability of intraluminal thrombus in abdominal aortic aneurysm. J. Vasc. Surg. **25**: 916–926.

20. PANEK, B., M. GACKO & J. PALKA. 2004. Metalloproteinases, insulin-like growth factor-I and its binding proteins in aortic aneurysm. Int. J. Exp. Pathol. **85**: 159–164.

21. DAUGHERTY, A. & L.A. CASSIS. 2004. Mouse models of abdominal aortic aneurysms. Arterioscler. Thromb. Vasc. Biol. **24:** 429–434.
22. ALLAIRE, E. *et al*. 1998. Prevention of aneurysm development and rupture by local overexpression of plasminogen activator inhibitor-1. Circulation **98:** 249–255.
23. KAZI, M. *et al*. 2005. Difference in matrix-degrading protease expression and activity between thrombus-free and thrombus-covered wall of abdominal aortic aneurysm. Arterioscler. Thromb. Vasc. Biol. **25:** 1341–1346.
24. YOSHIMURA, K. *et al*. 2005. Regression of abdominal aortic aneurysm by inhibition of c-Jun N-terminal kinase. Nat. Med. **11:** 1330–1338.
25. YAN, L. *et al*. 2001. The high molecular weight urinary matrix metalloproteinase (MMP) activity is a complex of gelatinase B/MMP-9 and neutrophil gelatinase-associated lipocalin (NGAL). Modulation of MMP-9 activity by NGAL. J. Biol. Chem. **276:** 37258–37265.
26. ELIASON, J.L. *et al*. 2005. Neutrophil depletion inhibits experimental abdominal aortic aneurysm formation. Circulation **112:** 232–240.

# Activators of Plasminogen and the Progression of Small Abdominal Aortic Aneurysms

JES S. LINDHOLT

ABSTRACT: The aim of this study was to examine the role of activating pathways of plasminogen in the natural history of abdominal aortic aneurysms (AAA). To fulfill this objective 70 male patients with small AAA (> 3 cm) were interviewed and examined. Their blood samples were taken at diagnosis. The patients were scanned annually for a minimum period of 1 year and a maximum of 5 years (mean 2.5 years), and referred for surgery if the AAA exceeded 5 cm in diameter. Plasma levels of urokinase-like plasminogen activator (uPA), tissue-type plasminogen activator (tPA), plasminogen-activator-inhibitor-1 (PAI-1), macrophage-inhibiting factor (MIF), transforming-growth-factor-$\beta 1$ (TGF-$\beta 1$), homocysteine, and serum levels of IgA-antibodies against *Chlamydia pneumoniae* (IgA-CP) and cotinine (a nicotine metabolite) were measured. The annual expansion rate correlated positively with tPA, IgA-CP, and S-cotinine; rho = 0.37 ($P = 0.004$), 0.28 ($P = 0.01$), and 0.24 ($P = 0.04$), while PAI-1, uPA, TGF-$\beta 1$, homocysteine, and MIF did not. S-cotinine and PAI-1 also correlated positively with tPA, rho = 0.24 ($P = 0.04$), and 0.33 ($P = 0.005$). IgA-CP did not correlate with tPA. By receiver operating characteristics (ROC) curve analysis, tPA showed to be predictive of cases expanding to above 5 cm within the first 5 years with an optimal sensitivity and specificity of 0.73 and 0.71, respectively ($P = 0.015$). The aortic matrix degradation in AAA may be partly caused by an activation of plasminogen by tPA, but not by uPA, which usually dominates matrix degradation. Smoking seems to be an important factor for this pathway, while the pathway of IgA-CP seems different.

KEYWORDS: abdominal aortic aneurysm; tissue-like plasminogen activator; cytokines; plasmin; hyperhomocysteinemia; smoking; surveillance; expansion; growth; progression

## BACKGROUND

There are at least three good reasons for developing tools for predicting aneurysmal progression. First, if we can predict which small abdominal aortic

Address for correspondence: Jes S. Lindholt, M.D., Ph.D., Vascular Research Unit, Department of Vascular Surgery, Viborg Hospital, Denmark. Voice: 0114589272447 or 01145353977; fax: 0114589273580.
e-mail: Jes.S.Lindholt@sygehusviborg.dk

Ann. N.Y. Acad. Sci. 1085: 139–150 (2006). © 2006 New York Academy of Sciences.
doi: 10.1196/annals.1383.023

aneurysms (AAAs) will require treatment later, treatment could be offered earlier, with decreased morbidity and mortality because age is one of the major risk factors,[1] and impairment in quality of life due to surveillance of small AAA could be reduced.[2,3] Second, only half of the patients with AAAs operated upon would have experienced ruptured AAA if they were left untreated. The growth rate reflects the magnitude of the degenerative process of the wall and thus becomes a surrogate marker of rupture. Consequently, biomarkers of growth could give us a more nuanced indication for surgery. The degradation products of the aortic matrix breakdown, elastin peptides, have been shown to correlate with AAA growth rate ($r = 0.40$ (0.20–0.57)), and be predictive of later rupture.[4,5] Finally, markers of aneurysm progression could be used for monitoring endovascularly excluded AAA for evidence of endoleaks. At present, a very consuming surveillance program is used.

At least three proteolytic systems seem to be involved in the degradation of aorta causing AAA.

1. *The serine-dependent proteases:* The levels of elastase are elevated in the circulation and in aneurysmal walls compared with aortic walls of occlusive atherosclerosis.[6] Furthermore, systemic levels are predictive of aneurysm expansion (rho $= 0.30$, $P < 0.001$) and cases expanding to sizes demanding operation.[7]

2. *The cysteine-dependent proteases:* Circulating levels of cystatin C—the major inhibitor of cysteine proteases—have been reported to be decreased in aneurysmal cases compared with controls,[8] correlate negatively to aneurysmal expansion rate ($r = -0.24$ (−0.75–0.05)), and are predictive for cases expanding to sizes demanding operation.[9]

3. *The metallodependent matrix proteases:* Levels of various metallodependent matrix proteases, especially matrix metalloproteinases (MMP)-2 and MMP-9, are elevated in aneurysmal aortic walls compared with aortic walls of occlusive atherosclerosis.[10] The plasma level of MMP-9 has also been correlated with the expansion of small AAAs ($r = 0.33$ (0.01–0.53)).[11]

Besides its fibrinolytic function in plasma, plasmin also plays a central role in tissue degenerative processes and is a common activator of the mentioned proteases.[12–14] Plasmin-antiplasmin-complexes correlate with aneurysmal expansion ($r = 0.39$ (0.16–0.56)) and are predictive for cases expanding to sizes requiring an operation, indicating a key role in AAA progression.[15] Consequently, this study was performed to study the pathways of plasmin activation during AAA development.[16]

As potential activators of tPA or uPA, smoking (expressed as cotinine—a nicotine metabolite), homocysteine, IgA against *Chlamydia pneumoniae* (IgA-CP), macrophage-inhibiting factor (MIF), and transforming-growth-factor-β1 (TGF-β1) were also studied.[13,14]

## MATERIALS AND METHODS

In 1994 half (4,404) of all 65- to 73-year-old males in Viborg County, Denmark, were invited to B-mode ultrasonographic screening for AAA at their regional hospital. Men having an AAA diagnosed were informed, interviewed, and examined, including a rescan, by the trial physician. An AAA was defined as an infrarenal aortic diameter of 30 mm or more. Patients with AAAs > 50 mm were referred for surgery, while those with AAAs 30–49 mm were offered yearly follow-up examinations to check for expansion.[17]

Strong efforts were made to limit the observer variation, by standardization of measurement, and using only one scanner and two observers for the first 7 years of the study. Consequently, a quite low interobserver variation (2SD) of 1.4 mm was achieved.[18] Those offered annual control had blood samples taken at base line. Plasma samples were stabilized with EDTA and serum samples were left at 18°C in 45 min for coagulation. The samples were subsequently stored in multiple aliquots until analysis.

Plasminogen-activator-inhibitor-1 (PAI-1) was measured with the ELISA (Imulyse PAI-1,Biopool Int., Umeå, Sweden). The within and between-assay CV is 5% and 9%, respectively.[19] Similarly, tPA was measured with the ELISA (Imulyse tPA, Biopool Int., Umeå, Sweden).The within and between assay coefficient of variation is 8% and 10%, respectively.[20] UPA was measured with ELISA (Imulyse uPA, Biopool Int., Umeå). The within and between assay co efficient of variation is 5% and 9%, respectively.[21] MIF were measured with a routine MIF-specific sandwich ELISA (in-house) using recombinant human MIF as standard. The coefficient of variation was 18.5%.[22] TGF-β1 levels were determined using a commercial ELISA Kit (BioSource International, Camarillo, CA, USA). The coefficient of variation was 28%. Homocysteine was analyzed using gas chromatography mass spectrometry after reduction with dithiothreitole. The inter- and intra-assay coefficient of variation was 5% and 3%.[23] Creatinine was analyzed using the Vitros CREA slide on the Vitros 950 Chemistry System (Ortho-Clinical Diagnostics, Rochester, NY, USA). The creatinine clearance was estimated by the Cockroft-Gault formula: $((140\text{-age})^*\text{weight(kg)})/(0.825^*\text{s-creatinine}(\mu\text{mol/L}))$.[9] IgA antibodies against *C. pneumoniae* were measured by means of microimmunoflourescence tests. S-cotinine levels were determined by a commercial radioimmunoassay (Diagnostic Products Corp., LA, USA) modified as suggested by Perkins *et al.*[24] The analytical coefficient of variation was 5.4%. The trial was approved by the local scientific ethics committee and reported to the data protection authorities.

### *Statistical Tests*

The mean annual expansion rate was calculated based upon 5 years of observation using a linear model of expansion calculated as the change in the anteriorposterior (AP) diameter during the whole observation period, transformed to annual units. Spearmann's correlation analyses were used to correlate the parameters with uPA, tPA, and mean annual expansion rate. Logarithmic transformation of S-cotinine was performed to carry out a multiple regression analysis concerning tPA and expansion rate adjusting for smoking. Wilcoxon's Rank Sum test for unpaired data was used to compare cases expanding above and below 2 mm annually. Finally, receiver operating characteristics (ROC) curve analysis of tPA in predicting cases of small AAAs expanding to operation recommendable sizes (>5 cm) within the first 5 years of observation was performed.

## RESULTS

Of the 4,404 men invited to screening, 3,344 (76%) attended and AAA was diagnosed in 141 of these (4.2%). Nineteen AAAs were more than 5 cm in diameter and these patients were referred for surgery. The remaining 122 cases were offered annual control scans and referred for surgery if the AAA expanded to more than 5 cm in diameter. Ten cases were lost to follow-up due to death or severe illness during the first year, and the rest have been followed for 1 to 5 years, in average 2.5 years. A random sample of 70 men attending follow-up was used for this study. The selected cases had a mean age of 68.8 ± 2.67 years. The AAA sizes were 34.2 ± 5.1 mm on average with a mean expansion rate of 2.69 ± 2.05 mm/year.

The results of bivariate correlation analyses are listed in TABLE 1. Briefly, the annual expansion rate correlated positively with tPA (rho = 0.37, $P$ = 0.004, FIG. 1), but not with uPA (rho = 0.001, $P$ = 0.993, FIG. 1). PAI-1 correlated with tPA (rho = 0.328, $P$ = 0.006), but not with expansion rate (rho = 0.015, $P$ = 0.871). S-cotinine correlated with expansion rate (rho = 0.234, $P$ = 0.038) and tPA (rho = 0.238, $P$ = 0.049). Not unexpected, IgA-CP correlated with expansion rate (rho = 0.28, $P$ = 0.01), but interestingly no significant correlation with tPA was noticed (rho = 0.135, $P$ = 0.252).

MIF, TGF-β1, and homocysteine did not correlate with AAA growth rate, but homocysteine correlated with creatinine clearance (rho = 0.30, $P$ = 0.003, FIG. 2). In addition, cases were classified as AAA expanding above or less than 2 mm annually according to the interobserver variation of the measurements. Again, tPA and IgA-CP were significantly associated with expansion rates above 2 mm, persisting after correction for chance findings, while S-cotinine failed to show significance.

Logarithmic transformation of S-cotinine and tPA normalized their distributions. In multiple linear regression analyses adjusting for S-cotinine, the correlation between tPA and expansion rate remained significantly correlated, while S-cotinine failed to reach significance and *vice versa* if the sequence of independent variables was reversed.

**TABLE 1. Nonparametric correlation matrix between activators and inhibitors of plasminogen, and progression of small AAAs**

|  | tPA | uPA | PAI-1 | MIF | TGF-$\beta$1 | Homocysteine | Cotinine | IgA-CP |
|---|---|---|---|---|---|---|---|---|
| Expansion rate (mm/year) | 0.368* | 0.001 | 0.015 | 0.224 | 0.000 | 0.063 | 0.234* | 0.290* |
|  | (0.002) | (0.993) | (0.871) | (0.061) | (0.999) | (0.535) | (0.038) | (0.006) |
| tPA (ng/mL) |  | 0.125 | 0.328* | −0.046 | −0.002 | 0.091 | 0.238* | 0.135 |
|  |  | (0.308) | (0.006) | (0.703) | (0.984) | (0.414) | (0.049) | (0.252) |
| uPA (ng/mL) |  |  | 0.005 | 0.119 | −0.082 | 0.048 | −0.345* | −0.053 |
|  |  |  | (0.966) | (0.419) | (0.570) | (0.691) | (0.006) | (0.690) |

Spearmann's correlation coefficients. *P* values in parentheses.

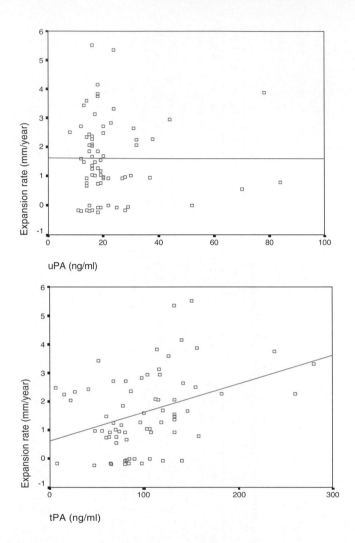

**FIGURE 1.** Scatter plots of the correlation of the mean annual expansion rate of small AAAs and P-uPA (rho = 0.001, $P$ = 0.993) and tPA (rho = 0.37, $P$ = 0.002), respectively.

Finally, by ROC curve analysis, the level of tPA was predictive of cases expanding to operation recommendable sizes (> 5 cm), within the first 5 years of observation with an optimal sensitivity and specificity as high as 0.73 and 0.71, respectively ($P$ = 0.015, FIG. 3).

## DISCUSSION

The study showed significant correlations between aneurysmal progression rate, tPA, and S-cotinine, but not with uPA, which usually dominates

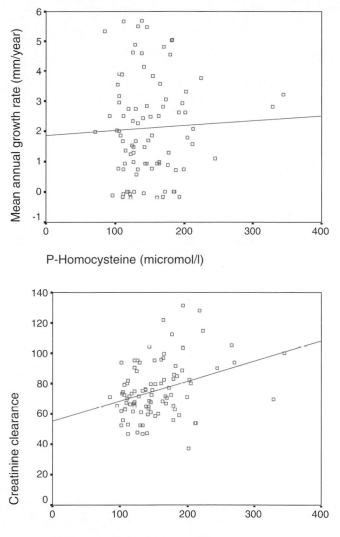

**FIGURE 2.** Scatter plots of the correlation between P-homocysteine and the mean annual expansion rate of small AAAs (rho = 0.063, $P$ = 0.535) and creatinine clearance (rho = 0.30, $P$ = 0.003).

plasmin-mediated matrix degradation. The latter may be due to the binding of uPA to their specific receptors on the membrane of the cells, which is stable and long lasting. It may prevent inactivation, but may also affect relevant systemic detection. However, Reilly *et al.*[25,26] reported elevated fibrinolytic activity in AAA compared with normal and atherosclerotic aortas. This was mainly caused by free tPA, as uPA concentrations did not differ from

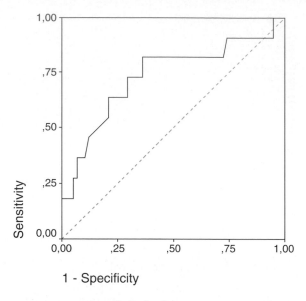

**Area Under the Curve**

Test Result Variable(s): TPA

| Area | Std. Error[a] | Asymptotic Sig.[b] | Asymptotic 95% Confidence Interval | |
|---|---|---|---|---|
| | | | Lower Bound | Upper Bound |
| ,733 | ,094 | ,015 | ,549 | ,916 |

a. Under the nonparametric assumption

b. Null hypothesis: true area = 0.5

**FIGURE 3.** ROC curve concerning the predictive value of the level of P-tPA C in predicting cases of small AAAs expanding to sizes recommended for operation (> 5 cm) within the first 5 years.

controls. They also reported that tPA in normal aortas are only present in the intima, while tPA is diffusely present in the intima and media of AAA walls. In contrast, uPA was only present in the infiltrative monocellular cells in the adventitia.

The positive correlations between S-cotinine, tPA, and expansion rate suggest smoking is participating in this pathway as smoking has been associated with AAA development and aneurysm progression.[27–30] This is in accordance with the findings in the multiple linear regression analyses where the correlation between tPA and expansion rate remained significant, while S-cotinine failed to reach significance. If the sequence of independent variables was reversed, the opposite was true. This indicates that this association is not due to confounding factors, but likely an overadjustment suggesting that smoking and tPA are located on the same line of causality. Genetic polymorphisms in PAI-1 have been associated with familial AAAs,[31] and PAI-1 correlated positively with tPA in this study. However, PAI-1 did not correlate with the expansion rate suggesting a minor, if any role, in the progression of AAA.

Not surprisingly, antibodies against *C. pneumoniae* correlated positively with expansion rate. We have earlier reported this in another sample from the present cohort and in a British cohort.[32–34] However, no significant correlation with tPA was noticed suggesting that the antibodies have a different pathway. However, antibiotic trials have been disappointing,[35,36] and today the presence of CP in AAA and plaques is questioned.[36,37] It is puzzling as to what these antibodies actually express as we have shown earlier that such antibodies purified from AAA patients cross-react with elements in the AAA wall. Perhaps early infections in life trigger an immune response, which is reactivated later in life by vessel lesions triggering an autoimmune reaction.

Hyperhomocysteinemia has also been associated with intense remodeling of the extracellular matrix in arterial walls, particularly elastolysis involving metalloproteinases, which are known to take part in the aneurysmal degradation.[38,39] In theory, homocysteine could activate uPA or tPA as levels of homocysteine are increased in AAA cases.[40,41] However, no significant correlation with aneurysm growth was documented. A significant correlation between homocysteine and creatinine clearance has been documented.[42] As AAA patients in general have impaired renal function due to coexisting atherosclerosis and hypertension compared to the general population, confounders may explain the current findings.

Finally, TGF-β1 and MIF did not correlate with tPA or AAA expansion rate. However, MIF levels tended, but insignificantly, to correlate to expansion rate (rho $= 0.224$, $P = 0.061$). We were recently able to show a positive correlation with aneurysm expansion with a larger sample size.[22] TGF-β1 is suspected to activate tPA and PAI-1.[13,14] However, we were not able to demonstrate any associations. The relatively high coefficient of variation of the measurements of TGF-β1 and aortic size combined with the pollution of TGF-β1 originating from nonaortic locations could hide a weak correlation.

## CONCLUSION

The aortic matrix degradation in AAA may be partly caused by an activation of plasminogen by tPA, and not by uPA, which usually dominates matrix degradation. Smoking seems to be an important factor for this pathway, while lack of association with IgA-CP suggests other proteolytic pathways are involved in the wall degradation in AAA.

### REFERENCES

1. IRVINE, C.D., E. SHAW, K.R. POSKITT, *et al.* 2000. A comparison of the mortality rate after elective repair of aortic aneurysms detected either by screening or incidentally. Eur. J. Vasc. Endovasc. Surg. **20:** 374–378.

2. LINDHOLT, J.S., S. VAMMEN, H. FASTING & E.W. HENNEBERG. 2000. Psychological consequences of screening for abdominal aortic aneurysm and conservative treatment of small abdominal aortic aneurysms. Eur. J. Vasc. Endovasc. Surg.**20:** 79–83.

3. UK SMALL ANEURYSM TRIAL MANAGEMENT COMMITTEE. 1998. Health service costs and quality of life for early elective surgery or ultrasonographic surveillance for small abdominal aortic aneurysms. Lancet **352:** 1656–1660.

4. LINDHOLT, J.S., L. HEICKENDORFF, E.W. HENNEBERG & H. FASTING. 1997. Serum-elastin-peptides as a predictor of expansion of small abdominal aortic aneurysms. Eur. J. Vasc. Endovasc. Surg. **14:** 12–16.

5. LINDHOLT, J.S., H.A. ASHTON, L. HEICKENDORFF & R.A. SCOTT. 2001. Serum elastin peptides in the preoperative evaluation of abdominal aortic aneurysms. Eur. J. Vasc. Endovasc Surg. **22:** 546–50.

6. DUBICK, M.A., G.C. HUNTER, E. PEREZ-LIZANO, G. MAR & M.C. GEOKAS. 1988. Assessment of the role of pancreatic proteases in human abdominal aortic aneurysms and occlusive disease. Clin. Chim. Acta **177:** 1–10.

7. LINDHOLT, J.S., B. JORGENSEN, N.A. KLITGAARD & E.W. HENNEBERG. 2003. Systemic levels of cotinine and elastase, but not pulmonary function, are associated with the progression of small abdominal aortic aneurysms. Eur. J. Vasc. Endovasc. Surg. **26:** 418–422.

8. SHI, G.P., G.K. SUKHOVA, A. GRUBB, *et al.* 1999. Cystatin C deficiency in human atherosclerosis and aortic aneurysms. J. Clin. Invest. **104:** 1191–1197.

9. LINDHOLT, J.S., E.J. ERLANDSEN & E.W. HENNEBERG. 2001. Cystatin C deficiency is associated with the progression of small abdominal aortic aneurysms. Br. J. Surg. **88:** 1472–1475.

10. THOMPSON, R.W. & W.C. PARKS. 1996. Role of matrix metalloproteinases in abdominal aortic aneurysms. Ann. N. Y. Acad. Sci. **800:** 157–174.

11. LINDHOLT, J.S., S. VAMMEN, H. FASTING, *et al.* 2000. The plasma level of matrix metalloproteinase 9 may predict the natural history of small abdominal aortic aneurysms. A preliminary study. Eur. J. Vasc. Endovasc. Surg. **20:** 281–285.

12. JEAN-CLAUDE, J., K.M. NEWMAN, H. LI, *et al.* 1994. Possible key role for plasmin in the pathogenesis of abdominal aortic aneurysms. Surgery **116:** 472–478.

13. MAYER, M. 1990. Biomedical and biological aspects of the plasminogen activation system. Clin. Biomed. **23:** 197–211.

14. SAKSELA, O. & D.B. RIFKIN. 1988. Cell associated plasminogen activation: regulation and physiological functions. Ann. Rev. Cell. Biol. **4:** 93–126.

15. LINDHOLT, J.S., B. JORGENSEN, H. FASTING & E.W. HENNEBERG. 2001. Plasma levels of plasmin-antiplasmin-complexes are predictive for small abdominal aortic aneurysms expanding to operation-recommendable sizes. J. Vasc. Surg. **34:** 611–615.

16. LINDHOLT, J.S., B. JORGENSEN, G.P. SHI & E.W. HENNEBERG. 2003. Relationships between activators and inhibitors of plasminogen, and the progression of small abdominal aortic aneurysms. Eur. J. Vasc. Endovasc. Surg. **25:** 546–551.

17. LINDHOLT, J.S., S. JUUL, H. FASTING & E.W. HENNEBERG. 2005. Screening for abdominal aortic aneurysms: single centre randomised controlled trial. BMJ **330:** 750–754.

18. LINDHOLT, J.S., S. VAMMEN, S. JUUL, *et al.* 1999. The validity of ultrasonographic scanning as screening method for abdominal aortic aneurysm. Eur. J. Vasc. Endovasc. Surg. **17:** 472–475.

19. DECLERCK, P.J., M.C. ALESSI, M. VERSTREKEN, *et al.* 1988. Measurement of plasminogen activator inhibitor 1 in biologic fluids with a murine monoclonal antibody-based enzyme-linked immunosorbent assay. Blood **71:** 220–225.

20. RANBY M., G. NGUYEN, P.Y. SCARABIN & M. SAMAMA. 1989. Immunoreactivity of tissue plasminogen activator and of its inhibitor complexes. Biochemical and multicenter validation of a two site immunosorbent assay. Thromb. Haemost. **61:** 409–414.

21. GARCIA FRADE, L.J., A. SUREDA, M.C. TORRADO & A. GARCIA AVELLO. 1992. High plasma urokinase-type plasminogen activator levels are present in patients with acute nonlymphoblastic leukemia. Acta Haematol. **88:** 7–10.

22. PAN, J.H., J.S. LINDHOLT, G.K. SUKHOVA, *et al.* 2003. Macrophage migration inhibitory factor is associated with aneurysmal expansion. J. Vasc. Surg. **37:** 628–635.

23. MØLLER, J., K. RASMUSSEN & L. CHRISTENSEN. 1999. External quality assessment of methylmalonic acid and total homocysteine. Clin. Chem. **45:** 1536–1542.

24. PERKINS, L., J.F. LIVESEY, E.A. ESCARES, *et al.* 1991. High performance liquidchromatographic method compared with a modified radioimmunoassay of Cotinine in plasma. Clin. Chem. **37:** 1989–1993.

25. REILLY, J.M., G.A. SICARD & C.L. LUCORE. 1994. Abnormal expression of plasminogen activators in aortic aneurysmal and occlusive disease. J. Vasc. Surg. **19:** 865–872.

26. REILLY, J.M. 1996. Plasminogen activators in abdominal aortic aneurysmal disease. Ann. N. Y. Acad. Sci. **800:** 151–156.

27. THE UK SMALL ANEURYSM TRIAL PARTICIPANTS. 2000. Smoking, lung function and the prognosis of abdominal aortic aneurysm. Eur. J. Vasc. Endovasc. Surg. **19:** 636–642.

28. BRADY, A.R., S.G. THOMPSON, F.G. FOWKES, *et al.* 2004. Abdominal aortic aneurysm expansion: risk factors and time intervals for surveillance. Circulation **110:** 16–21.

29. CRONENWETT, J.L. 1996. Variables that affect the expansion rate and rupture of abdominal aortic aneurysms. Ann. N. Y. Acad. Sci. **800:** 56–67.

30. MACSWEENEY, S.T., M. ELLIS, P.C. WORRELL, *et al.* 1994. Smoking and growth rate of small abdominal aortic aneurysms. Lancet **344:** 651–652.

31. ROSSAAK, J.I., A.M. VAN RIJ, G.T. JONES & E.L. HARRIS. 2000. Association of the 4G/5G polymorphism in the promoter region of plasminogen activator inhibitor-1 with abdominal aortic aneurysms. J. Vasc. Surg. **31:** 1026–1032.

32. LINDHOLT, J.S., S. JUUL, S. VAMMEN, *et al.* 1999. Immunoglobulin A antibodies against Chlamydia pneumoniae are associated with expansion of abdominal aortic aneurysm. Br. J. Surg. **86:** 634–638.

33. LINDHOLT, J.S., H.A. ASHTON & R.A. SCOTT. 2001. Indicators of infection with Chlamydia pneumoniae are associated with expansion of abdominal aortic aneurysms. J. Vasc. Surg. **34:** 212–215.

34. VAMMEN, S., J.S. LINDHOLT, P.L. ANDERSEN, *et al.* 2001. Antibodies against Chlamydia pneumoniae predict the need for elective surgical intervention on small abdominal aortic aneurysms. Eur. J. Vasc. Endovasc. Surg. **22:** 165–168.

35. VAMMEN, S., J.S. LINDHOLT, L. OSTERGAARD, *et al.* 2001. Randomized double-blind controlled trial of roxithromycin for prevention of abdominal aortic aneurysm expansion. Br. J. Surg. **88:** 1066–1072.

36. LINDHOLT, J.S., J. STOVRING, P.L. ANDERSEN, et al. 2003. Review of macrolide treatment of atherosclerosis and abdominal aortic aneurysms. Curr. Drug Targets Infect. Disord. **3:** 55–63.
37. LINDHOLT, J.S., H. FASTING, E.W. HENNEBERG & L. OSTERGAARD. 1999. A review on atherosclerosis and Chlamydia pneumoniae. Eur. J. Vasc. Endovasc. Surg. **17:** 283–289.
38. BESCOND, A., T. AUGIER, C. CHAREYRE, et al. 1999. Influence of homocysteine on matrix metalloproteinase2: activation and activity. Biochem. Biophys. Res. Commun. **263:** 498–503.
39. GIUSTI, B., R. MARCUCCI, I. LAPINI, et al. 2004. Role of hyperhomocysteinemia in aortic disease. Cell. Mol. Biol. (Noisy-le-grand) **50:** 945–952.
40. BRUNELLI, T., D. PRISCO, S. FEDI, et al. 2000. High prevalence of mild hyperhomocysteinemia in patients with abdominal aortic aneurysm. J. Vasc. Surg. **32:** 531–536.
41. SOFI, F., R. MARCUCCI, B. GIUSTI, et al. 2005. High levels of homocysteine, lipoprotein (a) and plasminogen activator inhibitor-1 are present in patients with abdominal aortic aneurysm. Thromb. Haemost. **94:** 1094–1098.
42. LINDHOLT, J.S., J. MOLLER & E.W. HENNEBERG. 2002. Mild hyperhomocysteinaemia is correlated with impaired renal function but not with the progression of small abdominal aortic aneurysms. Int. J. Angio. **11:** 95–98.

# Is There a Role for the Macrophage 5-Lipoxygenase Pathway in Aortic Aneurysm Development in Apolipoprotein E–Deficient Mice?

COLIN D. FUNK,[a] RICHARD YANG CAO,[a] LEI ZHAO,[b]
AND ANDREAS J.R. HABENICHT[c]

[a]Departments of Physiology and Biochemistry, Queen's University, Kingston, ON K7L 3N6 Canada

[b]Cordis Corp., Warren, NJ, 07059, USA

[c]Institute for Vascular Medicine, Friedrich-Schiller-University of Jena, Bachstr. 18, 07743 Jena, Germany

ABSTRACT: Activation of the 5-lipoxygenase (5-LO) pathway leads to the biosynthesis of proinflammatory leukotriene (LT) lipid mediators in macrophages, mast cells, and other inflammatory cell types. A recent surge in interest in this pathway within the cardiovascular system has arisen from a variety of exciting findings using genetic, pathological specimen, and biochemical approaches in humans and mice. We found that a subset of CD68-positive macrophages, localized within the adventitial layer of apolipoprotein E (apo E)-deficient mice, expressed 5-LO and that these cells represented a significant cellular component of aortic aneurysms induced by an atherogenic diet containing cholate. Surprisingly, almost no 5-LO-expressing cells were observed in atherosclerotic lesions in the same mice. Correspondingly, lesion size in the fat-fed mice did not depend on 5-LO gene expression but aneurysm incidence was reduced in the absence of the 5-LO pathway. We are currently exploring the potential mechanisms for 5-LO/LT involvement in aneurysm pathogenesis and if this pathway might come into play in other models such as induction by angiotensin II.

KEYWORDS: lipoxygenase; macrophage; aneurysm; leukotriene; chemokine; atherosclerosis; inflammation; arachidonic acid

Address for correspondence: Colin D. Funk, Ph.D., Department of Physiology, Botterell Hall, Room no. 433, Stuart Street, Queen's University, Kingston, ON K7L 3N6 Canada. Voice: 613-533-3242; fax: 613-533-6880.
e-mail: funkc@post.queensu.ca

Ann. N.Y. Acad. Sci. 1085: 151–160 (2006). © 2006 New York Academy of Sciences.
doi: 10.1196/annals.1383.012

# BACKGROUND

The 5-lipoxygenase (5-LO) pathway metabolizes arachidonic acid, released by cytosolic phospholipase $A_2$ from membrane phospholipids in inflammatory cells, to a family of leukotriene (LT) molecules (LTA$_4$, B$_4$, C$_4$, D$_4$, E$_4$).[1–3] LTs are secreted extracellularly by means of specific transporters and can bind to G-protein-coupled receptors (GPCRs) of which there are four, referred to as B-LT1, B-LT2, Cys-LT1, and CysLT2 (FIG. 1).[1–3] LTs possess a broad array of biological activities ranging from neutrophil/T lymphocyte subset chemotactic activity and enhancement of endothelial cell integrin expression (LTB$_4$) to modulation of endothelial cell permeability and sustained smooth muscle constriction (LTC$_4$, LTD$_4$).[1–3] Emerging data implicate 5-LO in cardiovascular disease (CVD).

## Brief History of Cardiovascular-Related Biological Activities of LTs (1980–2000)

Shortly after the structural elucidation of the various members in the LT family, researchers intensified efforts to unravel biological activities of these arachidonate metabolites. From 1980–1982 LTs were demonstrated to promote plasma leakage and leukocyte adhesion in postcapillary venules and in separate studies to induce a systemic arterial hypotensive effect.[4–6] LTD$_4$ elicited a potent coronary artery vasoconstrictor response associated with impaired ventricular contraction.[7] Subsequently, a number of studies indicated various vasoactive actions in different vascular beds in a species-specific manner that influenced cardiovascular hemodynamic properties.[8,9] At the molecular level, Cys-LTs induced P-selectin expression, vonWillebrand factor secretion, and platelet-activating factor synthesis,[10–12] while LTB$_4$ enhanced CD11b/CD18 endothelial cell expression,[13] all events of importance in leukocyte activation and subsequent emigration into sites of inflammation.

LTs were detected in atherosclerotic lesions and human coronary vessels with disease and were found to be hypersensitive to CysLT action.[14,15] However, many investigators shied away from the potential connection of the 5-LO pathway with atherogenesis and perhaps in general to CVD throughout the 1990s since the enzyme did not appear to be detected in macrophages/foam cells within the human vessel wall as detected by the *in situ* hybridization technique.[16]

## 5-LO Pathway and CVD (2000–Present)

A significant turn of events happened when investigators[17] compiled a large and diverse set of human coronary and carotid artery disease specimens and found evidence for 5-LO expression in atherosclerotic lesions. Moreover, the various components in the complete LT biosynthetic cascade were also

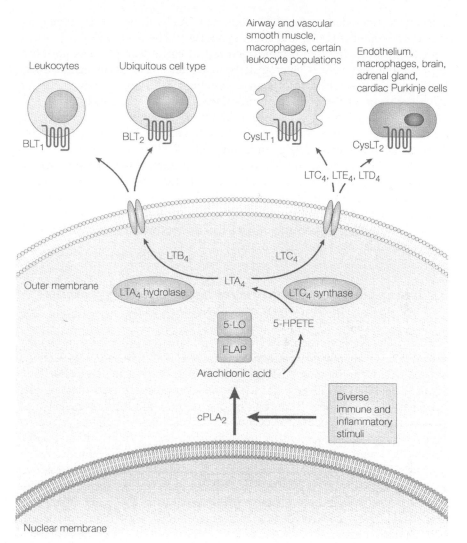

**FIGURE 1.** LT biosynthetic cascade. Various stimuli induce release of arachidonic acid from the sn-2 position of membrane phospholipids by the action of cytosolic phospholipase $A_2$, allowing metabolism by 5-LO. FLAP facilitates the transfer of substrate to the enzyme by unknown mechanisms. A complex of 5-LO, FLAP, LTC$_4$ synthase, and possibly LTA$_4$ hydrolase forms at the nuclear envelope with only the synthase and FLAP integrally associated in the membrane. Tissue specificity of expression yields either LTB$_4$ or the cysteinyl LT, LTC$_4$, or both products. Specific proteins facilitate transport of these molecules outside the cell where metabolism to LTD$_4$ and LTE$_4$ occurs and activation of GPCRs takes place. (Reproduced with permission from Funk)[3]

found, which included the four LT receptors, $LTA_4$ hydrolase, 5-lipoxygenase-activating protein (FLAP), and $LTC_4$ synthase.[17] The reason why 5-LO was detected in these diseased samples and not in earlier samples has not been resolved, but may reflect heterogeneity in expression patterns and/or assay conditions. Noteworthy, recent human genetic studies revealed evidence for polymorphisms in the 5-LO gene promoter linked to a surrogate marker of atherosclerosis (carotid intima-media thickness)[18] and certain haplotypes in the FLAP gene (known as *ALOX5AP*) were linked to CVD susceptibility, including risk of myocardial infarction and stroke.[19,20]

While the human studies on 5-LO expression in relation to CVD were emerging, mouse genetic studies were in progress and a locus on mouse chromosome 6 in which the 5-LO gene resides was found to be a "hot spot" for determination of lesion size in atherosclerotic-resistant strains of mice.[21] Since 2001 several studies have implicated one arm of the LT pathway, toward $LTB_4$ synthesis, in early atherosclerotic lesion development.[22–25]

### Is the 5-LO Pathway Involved in the Inflammatory Component of Atherosclerosis and Aortic Aneurysms?

Atherosclerosis is considered a chronic inflammatory process that is characterized by macrophage infiltration into the vessel wall in response to retained and modified lipoproteins with subsequent foam cell generation and fatty streak formation.[26,27] Over time, the streaks progress to large plaques that are occasionally unstable leading to plaque rupture and the subsequent triggering of thrombotic occlusive events. Aortic aneurysm is characterized by medial degeneration and involves multiple processes including inflammation, immunologic cell infiltration, and proteolysis. Adventitial infiltrations (periarteritis), immune reactions (attraction of T cells), and neoangiogenesis are associated with advanced atherosclerotic plaques as well as aneurysm pathogenesis,[28,29] although mouse aneurysms, in contrast to those in humans, are almost exclusively associated with atherosclerotic lesions in mouse models of hypercholesterolemia.[30]

The different genetic determinants for susceptibility to aneurysm development and plaque formation[31] necessitate identification of critical pathways involved in these cardiovascular events and we have turned our attention to the 5-LO/LT pathway as one such potential determinant. Since the mouse studies implicating the 5-LO pathway in atherogenesis were striking,[22,23] we set out to confirm and expand upon these data. Using 5-LO-deficient mice crossbred to apolipoprotein E (apoE) or low-density lipoprotein receptor (LDL-R)-deficient mice fed either a normal mouse chow diet or a Western-type high-fat diet, respectively, surprisingly we were unable to detect a difference in atherosclerotic lesion development between 5-LO-expressing and 5-LO-deficient mice.[32]

To understand the reason for the lack of effect on lesion development we determined the expression of 5-LO in the arterial wall of apoE$^{-/-}$ mice.[32] 5-LO was scarcely detectable in apoE$^{-/-}$ foam cells in intimal lesions at various ages. In contrast, adventitial macrophages were strongly 5-LO positive. Greater than 95% of all 5-LO-expressing cells in 8-month or 1-year-old mice were present in the adventitial layer, with a few positive cells in the intima, and almost none in the medial layer. Expression of 5-LO in the adventitial macrophages was accompanied by a significant increase of adventitial T lymphocytes, lacking 5-LO as the mice became older.[33]

Since the 5-LO expression pattern within atherosclerotic lesions differed significantly from that reported previously in LDL-R-deficient mice,[23] we undertook a study[32] on the same atherogenic diet (colloquially known as the "Paigen" diet; named for the investigator who developed a suitable diet for inducing lesion formation in atherosclerotic-resistant mice).[34] While this diet is not recommended in atherosclerotic-susceptible strains because of its potent proinflammatory gene-inducing effects and potential to cause cholelithiasis due to the presence of cholic acid,[35,36] it was necessary to determine if this diet via specific interactions with the 5-LO pathway affects atherogenesis.

The high-fat, cholate-containing diet is known to induce aortic aneurysms in apoE$^{-/-}$ mice.[37] To explore the participation of 5-LO in aneurysm formation, we examined 5-LO expression in aneurysms induced by feeding this diet to apoE$^{-/-}$ mice. We observed a significant subpopulation of 5-LO-expressing macrophages among CD68-positive cells in adventitial granulomas that had formed around aneurysmal arteries. Interestingly, aneurysmal granuloma macrophages, unlike adventitial macrophages of mice on standard mouse chow, accumulated lipid.[32] Aneurysmal granulomas contained an extensive *vasa vasorum* and the 5-LO-expressing macrophages accumulated preferentially in proximity to these blood vessels. These data indicate that macrophages containing 5-LO are a major cellular constituent of aneurysmal granuloma tissue and that the macrophages may enter the adventitia through *vasa vasorum*.

The incidence of aneurysm in apoE$^{-/-}$/5-LO$^{-/-}$ mice was significantly less than in apoE$^{-/-}$ mice (2/17 vs. 16/34 mice, aneurysm positive) after 8 weeks feeding of the Paigen diet.[32] Moreover, the two aneurysms in the double knockout mice were smaller and less severe than those in apoE$^{-/-}$ mice. In this hyperlipidemic/cholate diet-induced model, the aneurysms were present most often at the abdominal/thoracic diaphragmatic border. Histological analysis revealed complete disruption of media and elastin fibers in apoE$^{-/-}$ mice, while it was apparent that the extent of media disruption was reduced in apoE$^{-/-}$/5-LO $^{/-}$ mice. In parallel studies with mice deficient for another LO, known as 12/15-LO, the incidence and severity of aneurysm development were the same as for 5-LO-positive mice, thus ruling out 12/15-LO involvement in aneurysm pathogenesis (FIG. 2).

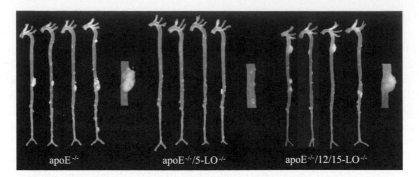

**FIGURE 2.** 5-LO, but not 12/15-LO deficiency, reduces hyperlipidemic diet-induced aortic aneurysm formation. Four representative aortas in each of apoE$^{-/-}$, apoE$^{-/-}$/5-LO$^{-/-}$, and apoE$^{-/-}$/12/15-LO groups of mice are shown.

To explore potential mechanisms for the 5-LO pathway to mediate aneurysm pathogenesis, we sought to understand the molecular events. One of the CysLTs, LTD$_4$, induced expression of distinct subsets of genes in endothelial cells and monocyte/macrophages.[32,38] Two chemokine genes in particular, macrophage inflammatory protein 1-alpha (MIP-1$\alpha$, also known as CCL3) and MIP-2, were potently induced in the respective cell types. Coordinated changes in chemokines and cytokines can mediate inflammatory responses in the vasculature. MIP-1$\alpha$ was increased in hyperlipidemic mice and 5-LO deficiency induced a gene dose-dependent reduction in plasma levels of this chemokine.[32] The LTD$_4$ action on MIP-1$\alpha$ gene expression was mediated via the CysLT$_1$ receptor subtype.[32,38] MIP-1$\alpha$ possesses the ability to induce T lymphocyte chemotaxis; these cells are a prominent component of adventitial inflammation in mice.

The extracellular matrix-degrading metalloproteinases (MMP)-2 and MMP-9 participate in aneurysm development.[39,40] 5-LO deficiency attenuated aortic activities of these enzymes in apoE$^{-/-}$ mice, however, only the decrease of MMP-2 was significant.[32] The data suggest that 5-LO may indirectly affect these enzymes and participate in aneurysm development via proinflammatory LTs as one potential pathway in pathogenesis.

## CONCLUDING REMARKS

Based on our studies whereby disruption of the 5-LO gene reduces both incidence and extent of aortic aneurysm development, a finding consistent with 5-LO expression in the adventitial layer, we created a model to evaluate further how 5-LO significantly contributes to atherosclerotic diet-induced aortic aneurysm formation in apoE$^{-/-}$ mice. 5-LO links hyperlipidemia and systemic inflammatory chemokine production and may alter adaptive immune responses via the biosynthesis of LTs (FIG. 3).

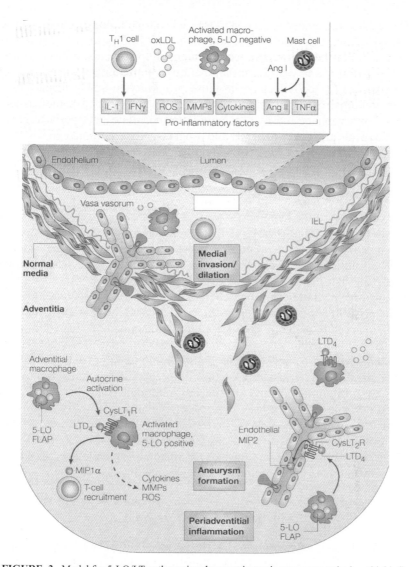

**FIGURE 3.** Model for 5-LO/LT pathway involvement in aortic aneurysm and adventitial inflammation pathogenesis. Adventitial macrophages express 5-LO and FLAP, and generate LTs, which set in motion a number of proinflammatory events. One of the LTs, $LTD_4$, causes autocrine activation of macrophages through binding to $CysLT_1$ receptors. Increased LT formation also promotes the recruitment of monocytes, the precursors of tissue macrophages, in addition to T lymphocytes. Specifically, $LTD_4$ binds to $CysLT_2$ receptors on endothelial cells of the many microvessels present in the adventitia and media (*vasa vasorum*), resulting in increased endothelial release of MIP-2 and leukocyte extravasation. Activated macrophages also release MIP-1$\alpha$, which may further promote T cell recruitment. Independent of the 5-LO pathway, activated macrophages generate other proinflammatory factors, including MMPs that weaken the media. Atherosclerosis in the intima may act synergistically with adventitial inflammation. Intimal macrophages, $T_H1$ cells, and mast cells secrete many proinflammatory factors, including IFN-$\gamma$, IL-1, MMPs, and TNF-$\alpha$. Hypercholesterolemia is an essential factor of both adventitial and intimal inflammation. (Reproduced with permission from Funk)[3]

Several lines of evidence related to arterial wall pathology, cellular composition of inflammatory infiltrates, and the action of LTs *in vivo* and *in vitro* establish similarities between mice and men, and mechanistic links between the 5-LO pathway and vascular inflammation in both humans and mice, begin to emerge: 5-LO$^+$ cells localize in close proximity to newly formed blood vessels in human CVD adventitia, intima, and aneurysmal granulomas as in mice;[17,32] macrophage and T cell accumulation correlate in the periarteritic tissues of patients afflicted with CVD and progressively accumulate in adventitia of apoE$^{-/-}$ mice;[17,32,33] the CC-chemokine MIP-1α/CCL3 is upregulated in macrophages in response to LTD$_4$, through activation of the CysLT$_1$ receptor in murine and human myeloid cells, and MIP-1α/CCL3 levels are attenuated in 5-LO-deficient mice.[32]

Our data support the hypothesis that LTs produced by macrophages, in addition to targeting their own CysLT$_1$ receptor in an autocrine fashion, may target T cells and endothelial cells in a paracrine manner (FIG. 3), resulting in the recruitment of inflammatory cells in human-diseased tissue through mechanisms that involve CC- and CXC-type chemokines. These 5-LO-rich inflammatory infiltrates in which chemokines and their receptors are found may conceivably promote pathophysiological levels of matrix-degrading proteases. However, the relation between eicosanoid action and chemokines merits close attention as they suggest previously unrecognized links between the arachidonic acid cascade generating potent lipid mediators and the powerful peptide chemokines. Thus, strong amplifying signals are generated to initiate cycles of inflammation and arterial wall remodeling in which 5-LO plays a regulatory role. 5-LO pathway pharmacologic antagonism may represent a potential therapeutic target site for intervention in aortic aneurysm development. In ongoing studies, we are currently exploring 5-LO/LT involvement in aneurysm pathogenesis in other aortic aneurysm models such as the one induced by angiotensin II minipump infusion over the course of 4 weeks.[30]

## ACKNOWLEDGMENTS

This work was supported by CIHR grant MOP-67146 and NIH grant HL53558 to C.D. Funk, by grants supported by the Deutsche Forschungsgemeinschaft (Ha 1083/13-1/13-2/13-3/13-4/12-5/12-6), the European Union research network (QLG1-CT-2001-01521), and the Interdisziplinäre Zentrum für Klinische Forschung Jena to A.J.R. Habenicht. CDF holds a Tier I Canada Research Chair in Molecular, Cellular, and Physiological Medicine and is a Career Investigator of the Heart and Stroke Foundation of Canada.

## REFERENCES

1. FUNK, C.D. 2001. Prostaglandins and leukotrienes: advances in eicosanoid biology. Science **294:** 1871–1875.

2. LOTZER, K., C.D. FUNK & A.J. HABENICHT. 2005. The 5-lipoxygenase pathway in arterial wall biology and atherosclerosis. Biochim. Biophys. Acta **1736:** 30–37.
3. FUNK, C.D. 2005. Leukotriene modifiers as potential therapeutics for cardiovascular disease. Nat. Rev. Drug Discov. **4:** 664–672.
4. DAHLEN, S.E. *et al.* 1981. Leukotrienes promote plasma leakage and leukocyte adhesion in postcapillary venules: *in vivo* effects with relevance to the acute inflammatory response. Proc. Natl. Acad. Sci. USA **78:** 3887–3891.
5. DRAZEN, J.M. *et al.* 1980. Comparative airway and vascular activities of leukotrienes C-1 and D *in vivo* and in vitro. Proc. Natl. Acad. Sci. USA **77:** 4354–4358.
6. SMEDEGARD, G. *et al.* 1982. Leukotriene C4 affects pulmonary and cardiovascular dynamics in monkey. Nature **295:** 327–329.
7. MICHELASSI, F. *et al.* 1982. Leukotriene D4: a potent coronary artery vasoconstrictor associated with impaired ventricular contraction. Science **217:** 841–843.
8. LETTS, L.G. 1987. Leukotrienes: role in cardiovascular physiology. Cardiovasc. Clin. **18:** 101–113.
9. FEUERSTEIN, G. 1984. Leukotrienes and the cardiovascular system. Prostaglandins **27:** 781–802.
10. DATTA, Y.H. *et al.* 1995. Peptido-leukotrienes are potent agonists of von Willebrand factor secretion and P-selectin surface expression in human umbilical vein endothelial cells. Circulation **92:** 3304–3311.
11. MCINTYRE, T.M., G.A. ZIMMERMAN & S.M. PRESCOTT. 1986. Leukotrienes C4 and D4 stimulate human endothelial cells to synthesize platelet-activating factor and bind neutrophils. Proc. Natl. Acad. Sci. USA **83:** 2204–2208.
12. PEDERSEN, K.E., B.S. BOCHNER & B.J. UNDEM. 1997. Cysteinyl leukotrienes induce P-selectin expression in human endothelial cells via a non-CysLT1 receptor-mediated mechanism. J. Pharmacol. Exp. Ther. **281:** 655–662.
13. ARFORS, K.E. *et al.* 1987. A monoclonal antibody to the membrane glycoprotein complex CD18 inhibits polymorphonuclear leukocyte accumulation and plasma leakage *in vivo*. Blood **69:** 338–340.
14. DE CATERINA, R. *et al.* 1988. Leukotriene B$_4$ production in human atherosclerotic plaques. Biomed. Biochim. Acta **47:** S182–S185.
15. ALLEN, S. *et al.* 1998. Differential leukotriene constrictor responses in human atherosclerotic coronary arteries. Circulation **97:** 2406–2413.
16. YLA-HERTTUALA, S. *et al.* 1991. Gene expression in macrophage-rich human atherosclerotic lesions. 15-lipoxygenase and acetyl low density lipoprotein receptor messenger RNA colocalize with oxidation specific lipid-protein adducts. J. Clin. Invest. **87:** 1146–1152.
17. SPANBROEK, R. *et al.* 2003. Expanding expression of the 5-lipoxygenase pathway within the arterial wall during human atherogenesis. Proc. Natl. Acad. Sci. USA **100:** 1238–1243.
18. DWYER, J.H. *et al.* 2004. Arachidonate 5-lipoxygenase promoter genotype, dietary arachidonic acid, and atherosclerosis. N. Engl. J. Med. **350:** 29–37.
19. HELGADOTTIR, A. *et al.* 2004. The gene encoding 5-lipoxygenase activating protein confers risk of myocardial infarction and stroke. Nat. Genet. **36:** 233–239.
20. HELGADOTTIR, A. *et al.* 2005. Association between the gene encoding 5-lipoxygenase-activating protein and stroke replicated in a Scottish population. Am. J. Hum. Genet. **76:** 505–509.
21. MEHRABIAN, M. *et al.* 2001. Genetic locus in mice that blocks development of atherosclerosis despite extreme hyperlipidemia. Circ. Res. **89:** 125–130.

22. AIELLO, R.J. *et al*. 2002. Leukotriene $B_4$ receptor antagonism reduces monocytic foam cells in mice. Arterioscler. Thromb. Vasc. Biol. **22:** 443–449.
23. MEHRABIAN, M. *et al*. 2002. Identification of 5-lipoxygenase as a major gene contributing to atherosclerosis susceptibility in mice. Circ. Res. **91:** 120–126.
24. SUBBARAO, K. *et al*. 2004. Role of leukotriene $B_4$ receptors in the development of atherosclerosis: potential mechanisms. Arterioscler. Thromb. Vasc. Biol. **24:** 369–375.
25. HELLER, E.A. *et al*. 2005. Inhibition of atherogenesis in BLT1-deficient mice reveals a role for LTB4 and BLT1 in smooth muscle cell recruitment. Circulation **112:** 578–586.
26. ROSS, R. 1999. Atherosclerosis-an inflammatory disease. N. Engl. J. Med. **340:** 115–126.
27. STEINBERG, D. 2002. Atherogenesis in perspective: hypercholesterolemia and inflammation as partners in crime. Nat. Med. **8:** 1211–1217.
28. HOUTKAMP, M.A. *et al*. 1995. Adventitial infiltrates associated with advanced atherosclerotic plaques: structural organization suggests generation of local humoral immune responses. J. Pathol. **193:** 263–269.
29. KUMAMOTO, M., Y. NAKASHIMA & K. SUEISHI. 1995. Intimal neovascularization in human coronary atherosclerosis: its origin and pathophysiological significance. Hum. Pathol. **26:** 450–456.
30. DAUGHERTY, A. & L.A. CASSIS. 2004. Mouse models of abdominal aortic aneurysms. Arterioscler. Thromb. Vasc. Biol. **24:** 429–434.
31. SHI, W. *et al*. 2003. Genetic backgrounds but not sizes of atherosclerotic lesions determine medial destruction in the aortic root of apolipoprotein E-deficient mice. Arterioscler. Thromb. Vasc. Biol. **23:** 1901–1906.
32. ZHAO, L. *et al*. 2004. The 5-lipoxygenase pathway promotes pathogenesis of hyperlipidemia-dependent aortic aneurysm. Nat. Med. **10:** 966–973.
33. MOOS, M.P. *et al*. 2005. The lamina adventitia is the major site of immune cell accumulation in standard chow-fed apolipoprotein E-deficient mice. Arterioscler. Thromb. Vasc. Biol. **25:** 2386–2391.
34. PAIGEN, B. *et al*. 1985. Variation in susceptibility to atherosclerosis among inbred strains of mice. Atherosclerosis **57:** 65–73.
35. VERGNES, L. *et al*. 2003. Cholesterol and cholate components of an atherogenic diet induce distinct stages of hepatic inflammatory gene expression. J. Biol. Chem. **278:** 42774–42784.
36. KHANUJA, B. *et al*. 1995. Lith1, a major gene affecting cholesterol gallstone formation among inbred strains of mice. Proc. Natl. Acad. Sci. USA **92:** 7729–7733.
37. SILENCE, J. *et al*. 2001. Persistence of atherosclerotic plaque but reduced aneurysm formation in mice with stromelysin-1 (MMP-3) gene inactivation. Arterioscler. Thromb. Vasc. Biol. **21:** 1440–1445.
38. UZONYI, B. *et al*. 2006. Cysteinyl leukotriene 2 receptor and protease-activated receptor 1 activate strongly correlated gene signatures in endothelial cells. Proc. Natl. Acad. Sci. USA **103:** 6326–6331.
39. BRUEMMER, D. *et al*. 2003. Angiotensin II-accelerated atherosclerosis and aneurysm formation is attenuated in osteopontin-deficient mice. J. Clin. Invest. **112:** 1318–1331.
40. LONGO, G.M. *et al*. 2002. Matrix metalloproteinases 2 and 9 work in concert to produce aortic aneurysms. J. Clin. Invest. **110:** 625–632.

# Do Cathepsins Play a Role in Abdominal Aortic Aneurysm Pathogenesis?

GALINA K. SUKHOVA AND GUO-PING SHI

*Division of Cardiovascular Medicine, Brigham and Women's Hospital and Harvard Medical School, Boston, MA, USA*

ABSTRACT: Between 1998 and 1999 we suggested a role for cysteine proteases, particularly cathepsins S and K, in atherosclerosis and abdominal aortic aneurysm (AAA) formation. We also demonstrated the presence and activity of cathepsins S, K, and L in atherosclerotic and aneurysmal lesions in humans. Features unique to this family of extracellular enzymes indicate its likely participation in these vascular diseases. As very potent elastolytic enzymes, cathepsins are strong candidates as key participants in aneurysm development. Importantly, cathepsins express very high elastolytic activity in AAA due to reciprocal correlation with cystatin C, their most abundant endogenous inhibitor. Two opposite processes coexist in aneurysmal tissue: overexpression of elastolytic cathepsins, and severe suppression of cystatin C, probably due to differentially regulated expression and secretion of cathepsins and their inhibitors in response to inflammatory cytokines. Involvement of cathepsins in microvessel formation, a pathophysiological marker of human AAA, and programmed cell death (apoptosis), increases the likelihood of cathepsin participation in AAA formation and growth. We also summarize here results obtained in our and other laboratories that demonstrated reduced atherosclerosis and AAA in *in vivo* models using mice lacking different cathepsins. Deficiency of cysteine protease inhibitor cystatin C in atherosclerosis-prone ApoE-null mice leads to the development of specific features of AAA such as thinning of the tunica media and aortic dilatation. Taken together, such findings in humans *in vitro* with different cell types and *in vivo* in genetically altered mice demonstrate the importance of cysteine protease/protease inhibitor balance in dysregulated arterial integrity and remodeling during atherosclerosis and aortic aneurysm formation.

KEYWORDS: abdominal aortic aneurysm; cysteine proteases; cathepsins; elastase; collagenase

Address for correspondence: Galina K. Sukhova, Ph.D., Division of Cardiovascular Medicine, Brigham and Women's Hospital and Harvard Medical School, 77 Avenue Louis Pasteur, NRB-7, Room 730J, Boston, MA 02115. Voice: 617-525-4354; fax: 617-525-4380.
e-mail: gsukhova@rics.bwh.harvard.edu

Ann. N.Y. Acad. Sci. 1085: 161–169 (2006). © 2006 New York Academy of Sciences.
doi: 10.1196/annals.1383.028

# INTRODUCTION

The structural integrity and function of the vascular wall depend on extracellular matrix (ECM), especially elastin and collagen, and ECM remodeling contributes importantly to the pathogenesis of cardiovascular diseases such as atherosclerosis and abdominal aortic aneurysms (AAA).[1,2] In 1998, we suggested a role for cysteine proteases, particularly cathepsins S and K, in atherosclerosis and AAA formation.[3] Previously, unique features of this family of extracellular enzymes indicating their likely participation in atherogenesis and AAA formation were underestimated. First, cysteine proteases are expressed and stored in cells inside lysosomes, thus explaining why their enzymatic role had been limited to merely a housekeeping function, that is, terminal digestion of endocytozed proteins entering lysosomes.[4] Actually, several cell types undergoing activation can express, synthesize, and release cathepsins. Human macrophages release active cathepsins that function not only exclusively within acidic lysosomes, but also extracellularly, at or near cell surface.[5–7] In addition, we demonstrated that stimulated human smooth muscle cells (SMC) also express cathepsins-dependent elastolytic activity *in vitro*.[3] Another feature that limited interest in cathepsins was that optimal pH~5.5 required for cathepsins activity was nonphysiological and acidic. Some cathepsins such as cathepsins S and K, however, are active at neutral pH 7.2–7.4, although cathepsin K is stable at this pH for only a few hours.[8–10] More recently, findings regarding the generation of an acidic microenvironment at the interface between monocyte-derived macrophages and elastin indicate that macrophage-rich areas in atherosclerotic plaques or AAA lesions provide an optimal environment for cysteine protease function.[6]

# CYSTEINE PROTEASES ARE POTENT ELASTOLYTIC AND COLLAGENOLYTIC ENZYMES

Among the most common, constant, and defined features of AAA, high elastolytic activity in aneurysmal arteries that leads to massive degradation, fragmentation, and, in a worst-case scenario, complete loss of the elastic layer is a key event. As very potent elastolytic enzymes, cathepsins are strong candidates as key participants in aneurysm development. Cathepsin K is the most potent elastolytic enzyme known.[10] Cathepsins K, L, and S express collagenolytic enzyme activity against triple helical type I collagen at 37°C,[11] a function previously exclusively assigned to the matrix metalloprotease subfamily of collagenases. Interestingly, cathepsin L shares levels of elastolytic activity with cathepsin S and high collagenolytic capacity with cathepsin K, recognized as a central participant in bone resorption.[10,11]

## PRESENCE AND ACTIVITY OF CATHEPSINS IN HUMAN AAA

We demonstrated the presence of cathepsins S, K, and L in atherosclerotic and aneurysmal lesions in humans and localized them to all major cell types including SMC, macrophages, and endothelial cells (EC).[3,12,13] Representative immunohistochemical staining for cathepsin L shows increased expression of this enzyme in macrophage-rich areas and also in SMC of aneurysmal lesions compared to normal aortae (FIG. 1).

Even more importantly, cathepsins express very high elastolytic activity in AAA due to reciprocal correlation with cystatin C, their most abundant endogenous inhibitor.[12,14] Cystatin C is expressed in virtually all organs, it competitively inhibits cysteine proteases, and normally masks their activity. Interestingly, inflammatory processes reduce cystatin C levels and alter the enzyme/inhibitor balance.[15,16] Although Western blot analysis of tissue extracts from normal aortae showed very low expression of all three cathepsins tested (cathepsins S, K, and L) in extracts from normal tissue samples (FIG. 2),

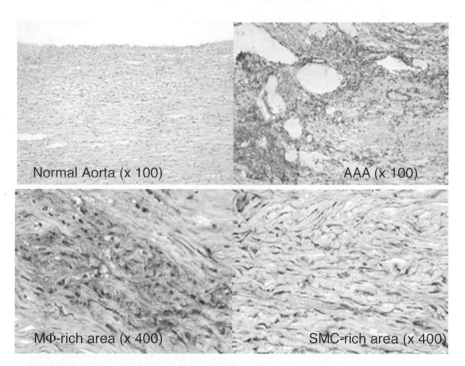

**FIGURE 1.** Increased expression of cathepsin L in human AAA compared to normal aortae. Immunohistochemistry performed on frozen sections using rabbit anti-human cathepsin L antibody. High power images (*bottom*) show cathepsin L- positive macrophages (*left*) and SMC (*right*). Original magnification is indicated.

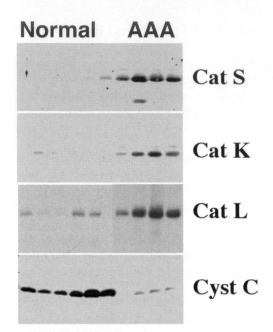

**FIGURE 2.** In human AAA cysteine protease/protease inhibitor balance is disturbed and shifted in favor of protease activity. Western blot analysis for tissue extracts from human AAA ($n = 4$) and control normal aortae ($n = 6$) showed high levels of cathepsins S, K, and L, but dramatically suppressed cystatin C levels in AAA compared to normal aortae.

cystatin C levels are high in all normal aortae tissue samples. Thus, cystatin C expression prevailed over cathepsins in normal aortae. Two opposite processes coexist in aneurysmal tissue: overexpression of elastolytic cathepsins, and severe suppression of cystatin C (FIG. 2). A group from Poland also demonstrated increased levels of cathepsin B, D, and L protein and activity in the wall of human aortic aneurysm, but decreased activity and concentration of cystatin C in AAA compared to control normal aortae in accordance with our findings.[14,17] A shift in protease/protease inhibitor balance in diseased arteries is likely due to differentially regulated expression and secretion of cysteine proteases and their inhibitors in response to inflammatory cytokines.[12,18] Indeed, although interferon (IFN)-γ boosted cathepsin S mRNA and protein expression, it did not affect cystatin C. On the other hand, transforming growth factor (TGF)-β did not change cathepsin S production or cystatin C mRNA levels, but significantly increased cystatin C protein expression and release. TGF-β (5 nM) completely blocked insoluble elastin degradation by IFN-γ-induced cultured SMC.[12]

Cystatin C deficiency in the serum of patients is associated with AAA progression and expansion rate. Cystatin C can influence AAA development and growth by disbalance of cysteine proteases/cysteine protease inhibitor both locally, in the wall of AAA, and systemically, in the blood of AAA patients. We found lower serum cystatin C levels ($0.516 \pm 0.2$ μg/mL) in patients with dilated aortae compared to patients with normal aortae ($1.3 \pm 1.1$ μg/mL) as well as inverse correlation between increased abdominal aortic diameter and decreased serum cystatin C levels.[12] In accord with our findings, Lindholt et al.[19] showed in a cohort of 142 men with small aneurysms followed for 3 years (mean) with annual ultrasonographic assessment and serum sampling that cystatin C deficiency is associated with the progression of small AAA (increased aneurysm size and expansion rate). In patients with lower blood serum concentrations of cystatin C, higher vulnerability to AAA formation resulted from a polymorphism in the signal peptide of the cystatin C gene likely due to lack of inhibition of cysteine proteases.[20,21]

## ROLE OF CYSTEINE PROTEASES IN NEOVASCULARIZATION

Microvessel formation is one of the pathophysiological features of human AAA;[1,22] interestingly, the ongoing process of angiogenesis also occurs in the mature aortic aneurysm.[23] Neovessel formation and growth require enzymatic degradation of the vascular basement membrane and the interstitial ECM. We demonstrated that cysteine protease (cathepsin S) contributes to angiogenesis in mice.[24] Cathepsin S-deficient EC demonstrated decreased elastolytic and collagenolytic activities, decreased matrigel and type I collagen gel invasion, and reduced capillary-like tube formation in vitro. Interestingly, the addition of recombinant cystatin C to wild-type EC dose-dependently inhibits microtube formation. Using a mouse model of skin wound healing-associated neovascularization as an in vivo model of angiogenesis, we observed a decreased number of microvessels (80%) in wound-healing areas of cathepsin S-null mice as shown by immunostaining with monoclonal antibody specific for mouse EC. These data supported the involvement of cysteine proteases in angiogenesis, thus implying an essential role for cathepsin S in ECM degradation.[24]

Several studies have shown that expression of cathepsins B, H, K, and L in the vasculature of human tumors is associated with increased angiogenesis and tumor growth.[25–27] Urbich et al. demonstrated a crucial role for cathepsin L in a model of postnatal neovascularization induced by infusion of endothelial progenitor cells using cathepsin L-deficient ischemic mice.[28] Inhibition of cathepsin activity by a broad-spectrum cysteine protease inhibitor also reduces neovascularization (vascular branching) in a model of pancreatic islet tumorigenesis.[29]

## ROLE OF CYSTEINE PROTEASES IN APOPTOSIS

Medial SMC undergo apoptosis during aneurysmal lesions formation.[30,31] Accumulating evidence supports a potential role of cysteine proteases in programmed cell death in AAA. Under physiological conditions cathepsins localize in cells in the lysosomes, but they could be released into the cytoplasm in response to proinflammatory mediators, triggering apoptotic cell death.[32] The protective effect of cathepsins B and L inhibitors on oxysterol-induced mononuclear cell death[33] as well as selective inhibition of cathepsin S and a null mutation (Cat S$^{-/-}$) on apoptosis induced by IFN-$\gamma$ in a murine pulmonary emphysema model suggest that cathepsins might mediate apoptosis.[34] Cathepsin L and to a lesser extent cathepsin S can promote caspase-dependent apoptosis,[32,35] and also by activating caspases indirectly via proteolytic cleavage of the proapoptotic Bcl-2 homolog Bid. This caspase-independent pathway was shown *in vitro* in various cellular models.[36]

## *IN VIVO* DIRECT EVIDENCE OF CYSTEINE PROTEASE INVOLVEMENT IN ATHEROSCLEROSIS AND AAA

We recently showed direct evidence that cysteine proteases participate in atherosclerosis and AAA formation *in vivo*. Interestingly, both low-density lipoprotein receptor (LDLr)- and apolipoprotein E (ApoE)-deficient mice develop atherosclerotic lesions that retain many features of human atheroma. All tested cathepsins showed higher expression in atherosclerotic lesions of both LDLr$^{-/-}$ and ApoE$^{-/-}$ mice compared to nonatherosclerotic control mice, but only cathepsin S was strongly positive in the tunica media.[37,38] Importantly, we co-localized cathepsin S-positive medial SMC with breaks in the elastic laminae similar to those shown previously for human atheroma.[3]

Very few laboratories use gene-targeting strategy to study the influence of different cathepsins in these vascular diseases. Our laboratory and a group from the Netherlands demonstrated that deficiency of both cathepsin S (Cat S$^{-/-}$LDLr$^{-/-}$) and cathepsin K (Cat K$^{-/-}$ ApoE$^{-/-}$) significantly reduced the size and severity of atherosclerotic lesions ($\sim$50% and 42%, respectively) as well as elastin degradation in the tunica media.[37,39] Additionally, new, exciting results showed reduced aortic dilatation (55%) in cathepsin S-deficient mice in a murine model of elastase-induced AAA (Shi G-P, Thompson RW unpublished data), clearly supporting the functional importance of cathepsin S and its necessity for the development of aneurysmal degeneration.

Systemic cystatin C deficiency in Cyst C$^{-/-}$Apo E$^{-/-}$ mice recapitulated many features of human athersclerotic aortic aneurysms including severe medial elastic laminae degradation, thinning of the tunica media, and aortic ectasia.[40] Atherosclerotic lesions in cystatin C-deficient mice augmented elastic laminae degradation due to increased elastolytic activity (shown by *in situ* zymography with DQ-elastin as a substrate). Interestingly, this enhanced elastolytic activity in CystC$^{-/-}$ApoE$^{-/-}$ intimal lesions resulted from amplified activity of cathepsins B, S, and L (shown by an active site labeling of cysteine proteases), but not matrix metalloproteinases (shown by gelatin zymography).

Although intimal lesion size did not change significantly in the aortic arch, the tunica media thinned in the aortic arch of cystatin C-null mice ($P < 0.005$), establishing that cystatin C maintains medial elastica integrity in the vessel wall.

Thus, findings in humans in different cell types *in vitro* and in genetically altered mice *in vivo* demonstrate the importance of maintaining a balance between cysteine protease and protease inhibitors. Disturbance of this balance plays an important role in dysregulated arterial integrity and remodeling during atherosclerosis and aortic aneurysm formation.

## ACKNOWLEDGMENTS

This work was supported by grants HL067249 (GKS) and HL60942 (GPS) from the National Institutes of Health.

## REFERENCES

1. THOMPSON, R.W. 1996. Basic science of abdominal aortic aneurysms: emerging therapeutic strategies for an unresolved clinical problem. Current Opin. Cardiol. **11:** 504–518.
2. LIBBY, P. 2003. Vascular biology of atherosclerosis: overview and state of art. Am. J. Cardiol. **91:** 3A–6A.
3. SUKHOVA, G.K., G-P. SHI, D.I. SIMON, *et al.* 1998. Expression of elastolytic cathepsins S and K in human atheroma and regulation of their production in smooth muscle cells. J. Clin. Invest. **102:** 576–583.
4. BARRETT, A.J. & H. KIRSCHKE. 1981. Cathepsin B, Cathepsin H, and Catepsin L. Methods Enzymol. **80:** 345–360.
5. REDDY, V.Y., Q.Y. ZHANG & S.J. WEISS. 1995. Pericellular mobilization of the tissue-destructive cysteine proteases, cathepsins B, L, and S, by human monocyte-derived macrophages. Proc. Natl. Acad. Sci. USA **92:** 3849–3853.
6. PUNTURIERI, A., S. FILIPPOV, E. ALLEN, *et al.* 2000. Regulation of elastolytic cysteine protease activity in normal and cathepsin K-deficient human macrophages. J. Exp. Med. **192:** 789–799.
7. HAKALA, J.K., R. OKSJOKI, P. LAINE, *et al.* 2003. Lysosomal enzymes are released from cultured human macrophages, hydrolyze LDL *in vitro*, and are present extracellularly in human atherosclerotic lesions. Arterioscler. Thromb. Vasc. Biol. **23:** 1430–1436.
8. XIN, X.-Q., B. GUNESEKERA & R.W. MASON. 1992. The specificity and elastinolytic activities of bovine cathepsins S and H. Arch. Biochem. Biophys. **299:** 334–339.
9. SHI, G.-P., J.S. MUNGER, J.P. MEARA, *et al.* 1992. Molecular cloning and expression of human alveolar cathepsin S, an elastolytic cysteine protease. J. Biol. Chem. **267:** 7258–7262.
10. CHAPMAN, H.A., R.J. RIESE & G-P. SHI. 1997. Emerging roles for cysteine proteases in human biology. Ann. Rev. Physiol. **59:** 63–88.
11. LI, Z., Y. YASUDA, W. LI, *et al.* 2004. Regulation of collagenase activity of human cathepsins by glycosaminoglycans. J. Biol. Chem. **279:** 5470–5479.

12. SHI, G.-P., G.K. SUKHOVA, A. GRUBB, et al. 1999. Cystatin C deficiency in human atherosclerosis and aortic aneurysms. J. Clin. Invest. **104:** 1191–1197.
13. LIU, J., G.K. SUKHOVA, J.S. SUN, et al. 2006. Cathepsin L expression and regulation in human abdominal aortic aneurysm, atherosclerosis, and vascular cells. Atherosclerosis **184:** 302–311.
14. GACKO, M., L. CHYCZEWSKI & L. CHROSTEK. 1999. Distribution, activity and concentration of cathepsin B and cystatin C in the wall of aortic aneurysm. Pol. J. Pathol. **50:** 83–86.
15. CHAPMAN, H.A., J.J. REILLY, R. YEE & A. GRUBB. 1990. Identification of cystatin C, a cysteine protease inhibitor, as a major secretory product of human alveolar macrophages in vitro. Am. Rev. Respir. Dis. **141:** 698–705.
16. WARFEL, A.H., D. ZUCKER-FRANKLIN, B. FRANGIONE & J. GHISO. 1987. Constitutive secretion of cystatin C (gamma-trace) by monocytes and macrophages and its down regulation after stimulation. J. Exp. Med. **166:** 1912–1917.
17. GACKO, M. & S. GLOWINSKI. 1999. Cathepsin D and cathepsin L activities in aortic aneurysm wall and parietal thrombus. Clin. Chem. Lab. Med. **36:** 449–452.
18. LIU, J., G.K. SUKHOVA, J.S. SUN, et al. 2004. Lysosomal cysteine proteases in atherosclerosis. Arterioscler. Thromb. Vasc. Biol. **24:** 1359–1366.
19. LINDHOLT, J.S., E.J. ERLANDSEN & E.W. HENNEBERG. 2001. Cystatin C deficiency is associated with the progression of small abdominal aortic aneurysms. Brit. J. Surg. **88:** 1472–1475.
20. ERIKSSON, P., H. DEGUCHI, A. SAMNEGARD, et al. 2004. Human evidence that the cystatin C gene is implicated in focal progression of coronary artery disease. Arterioscler. Thromb. Vasc. Biol. **24:** 1–7.
21. ERIKSSON, P., K.G. JONES, L.C. BROWN, et al. 2004. Genetic approach to the role of cysteine proteases in the expansion of abdominal aortic aneurysms. Brit. J. Surg. **91:** 86–89.
22. HOLMES, D.R., S. LIAO, W.C. PARKS & R.W. THOMPSON. 1995. Medial neovascularization in abdominal aortic aneurysms: a histopathologic marker of aneurysmal degeneration with pathophysiological implications. J. Vasc. Surg. **21:** 761–771.
23. PAIK, D.C., C. FU, J. BHATTACHARYA & M.D. TILSON. 2004. Ongoing angiogenesis in blood vessels of the abdominal aortic aneurysm. Exp. Mol. Med. **36:** 524–533.
24. SHI, G-P., G.K. SUKHOVA*, M. KUZUYA, et al. 2003. Deficiency of the cysteine protease cathepsin S impairs microvessel growth. Circ. Res. **92:** 493–500.
25. MIKKELSEN, T., P.S. YAN, K.L. HO, et al. 1995. Immunolocalization of cathepsin B in human glioma: implications for tumor invasion and angiogenesis. J. Neurosurg. **83:** 285–290.
26. KRUSZEWSKI, W.J., R. RZEPKO, J. WOJTACKI, et al. 2004. Overexpression of cathepsin B correlates with angiogenesis in colon adenocarcinoma. Neoplasma **51:** 38–43.
27. VAN HINSBERGH, V.W., M.A. ENGELSE & P.H. QUAX. 2006. Pericellular proteases in angiogenesis and vasculogenesis. Arterioscler. Thromb. Vasc. Biol. **26:** 716–728.
28. URBICH, C., C. HEESCHEN, A. AICHER, et al. 2005. Cathepsin L is required for endothelial progenitor cell-induced neovascularization. Nat. Med. **11:** 206–213.
29. GOCHEVA, V., W. ZENG, D. KE, et al. 2006. Distinct roles for cysteine cathepsin genes in multistage tumorigenesis. Genes. Dev. **20:** 543–556.
30. LOPEZ-CANDALES, A., D. HOLMES, S. LIAO, et al. 1997. Decreased vascular smooth muscle cell density in medial degeneration of human abdominal aortic aneurysms. Am. J. Path. **150:** 993–1007.

31. HENDERSON, E.L., Y.-J. GENG, G.K. SUKHOVA, *et al.* 1999. Death of smooth muscle cells and expression of mediators of apoptosis by T lymphocytes in human abdominal aortic aneurysms. Circulation **99:** 96–104.
32. CHWIERALSKI, C.E., T. WELTE & F. BUHLING. 2006. Cathepsin-regulated apoptosis. Apoptosis **11:** 143–149.
33. LI, W., H. DALEN, J.W. EATON & X-M. YUAN. 2001. Apoptotic death of inflammatory cells in human atheroma. Arterioscler. Thromb. Vasc. Biol. **21:** 1124–1130.
34. ZHENG, T., M.J. KANG, K. CROTHERS, *et al.* 2005. Role of cathepsin S-dependent epithelial cell apoptosis in IFN-gamma-induced alveolar remodeling and pulmonary emphysema. J. Immunol. **174:** 8106–8115.
35. ISHIKA, R., T. UTSUMI, T. KANNO, *et al.* 1999. Participation of a cathepsin L-type protease in the activation of caspase-3. Cell Struct. Funct. **24:** 465–470.
36. STOKA, V., B. TURK & V. TURK. 2005. Lysosomal cysteine proteases:structural features and their role in apoptosis. IUBMB Life **57:** 347–353.
37. SUKHOVA, G.K., Y. ZHANG, J-H. PAN, *et al.* 2003. Deficiency of cathepsin S reduces atherosclerosis in low-density lipoprotein receptor-deficient mice. J. Clin. Invest. **111:** 897–906.
38. JORMSJO, S., D.M. WUTTGE, A. SIRSJO, *et al.* 2002. Differential expression of cysteine and aspartic proteases during progression of atherosclerosis in apolipoprotein E-deficient mice. Am. J. Path. **161:** 939–945.
39. LUTGENS, E., S.P.M. LUTGENS, B.C.G. FABER, *et al.* 2006. Disruption of the cathepsin K gene reduces atherosclerosis progression and induces plaque fibrosis but accelerates macrophage foam cell formation. Circulation **113:** 98–107.
40. SUKHOVA, G.K., B. WANG, P. LIBBY, *et al.* 2005. Cystatin C deficiency increases elastin lamina degradation and aortic dilatation in apolipoprotein E-null mice. Circ. Res. **96:** 368–375.

# Matrix Metalloproteinase-2

## The Forgotten Enzyme in Aneurysm Pathogenesis

MATT THOMPSON AND GILLIAN COCKERILL

*St. George's Vascular Institute and Academic Department of Vascular Surgery, St. George's, University of London, UK*

ABSTRACT: The pathogenesis of abdominal aortic aneurysm (AAAs) involves progressive cycles of proteolysis and inflammation, the product of proteolysis driving subsequent inflammation. Little is yet known about the initiating events. We review the specific literature examining the possibility that MMP-2 may be the initial catalyst. Histologically, elastolysis is one of the earliest observable events in aneurysm genesis. Matrix metalloproteinase-2 (MMP-2), as the dominant gelatinase differentially expressed in aneurysmal tissue and cells derived from aneurysms, would be a good candidate. We report the results of *in vivo* and *in vitro* experiments, which lend support to the importance of MMP-2 as an aneurysmal initiator.

KEYWORDS: metalloproteinase; MMP-2; elastolysis

The biochemical and histopathological changes that characterize established abdominal aortic aneurysms (AAAs) have been extensively characterized. Aneurysms demonstrate arterial dilatation, wall thickening, and a reduction in the elastin/collagen ratio of the extracellular matrix. These structural changes are accompanied by a widespread inflammatory infiltrate, a rich cytokine milieu, and excessive local concentrations of a number of matrix metalloproteinases (MMP). These MMPs have been considered responsible for the widespread degradation and remodeling of the extracellular matrix that is demonstrated in established and expanding aneurysms.

Despite the breadth of knowledge that has accumulated regarding the expansion and rupture of AAA, relatively little attention has been directed toward the initiating events in aneurysm formation. The difficulty in investigating initiating events in AAA may be principally related to problems differentiating

Address for correspondence: Matt M. Thompson, Department of Vascular Surgery, St. George's Hospital, Blackshaw Road, Tooting, London, SW17 ORE, UK. Voice: 44-208-725-3205; fax: 44-208-725-3495.

e-mail: matt.thompson@stgeorges.nhs.uk

Ann. N.Y. Acad. Sci. 1085: 170–174 (2006). © 2006 New York Academy of Sciences.
doi: 10.1196/annals.1383.034

cause and effect of any biochemical/molecular changes in established end-stage aneurysmal tissue. To overcome these problems, alternative approaches are required that utilize animal models or interpretation of early changes in clinical samples.

The series of studies described in this abstract investigate the hypothesis that MMP-2 may play a pivotal role in early aneurysm genesis. Histologically, elastolysis is one of the earliest observable events in aneurysmal tissue. From a theoretical standpoint, fragmentation of elastin fibers within the aortic media may have the potential to drive the aneurysmal process. Degradation of elastin fibers in the aortic media would reduce the ability of the aortic tissue to withstand the tensile stresses of the circulation and cause collagen deposition. Fragmentation of elastin fibres would also generate elastin-derived peptides, small fragments which are powerfully chemotactic and might recruit inflammatory cells in to the aorta to further drive proteolysis and inflammation.

MMP-2 would be a good candidate to cause the initial elastolysis in tissue prone to aneurysmal degeneration. MMP-2 is constitutively expressed by vascular smooth muscle cells and fibroblasts, is activated by MT-MMP-1, and has substrate specificity for elastin and fibrillar collagen. Freestone et al.[1] demonstrated that MMP-2 was the dominant gelatinase in small aneurysms with the more researched MMP-9 only becoming important in the latter stages of aneurysm formation. Similarly, McMillan et al.[2] revealed that mesenchymal cells within the aortic wall expressed MMP-2 at high levels. In an interesting comparison, Davis et al.[3] reported that MMP-9 was expressed at comparable levels in aneurysmal and atherosclerotic tissue, whereas MMP-2 was differentially upregulated in aneurysmal aorta when compared to atherosclerotic or normal controls.

Circumstantial evidence therefore appears in the literature that MMP-2 may play a role in the early stages of aneurysm formation. These reports were strengthened by histological studies that demonstrated the presence of all components of the MMP-2 proteolytic system (MMP-2, MT-MMP, and TIMP-2) within normal and aneurysmal aortic media, localizing to smooth muscle cells.[4]

## STUDIES USING CULTURED VASCULAR SMOOTH MUSCLE CELLS

In an attempt to dissect the early events in aneurysm genesis, our group studied vascular smooth muscle cells cultured from aneurysmal and age-matched atherosclerotic aortic tissue.[5] Cultured cells were utilized in an attempt to remove these cells from the cytokine-rich environment of AAAs. Studies demonstrated that cells isolated from aneurysms secreted higher levels of MMP-2 than cells derived from atherosclerotic tissue (758 ng/mL compared to 262 ng/mL), and that aneurismal-derived cell lines exhibited higher MMP-2/TIMP-2 ratios (38.3 vs. 14.4). Both cell lines secreted equivalent quantities of MMP-1, MMP-3, and MMP-9. Expression studies demonstrated that the higher levels of MMP-2 secreted by the aneurysm-derived cell lines was due to higher levels of MMP-2 mRNA. Interestingly, dermal fibroblast cultures from the same patients demonstrated no differences in MMP expression suggesting that the phenotypic changes in aortic-derived smooth muscle cells were not part of a systemic mesenchymal cell process.

These data confirmed the findings of others that suggested elevated expression of MMP-2 in cells derived from the aneurysmal aorta. Although suggestive of a role for MMP-2 in early aneurysm formation, the results cannot be interpreted as causal because of the potential paracrine effects within the aortic tissue and because of the difficulty in interpreting results from cells at the end stage of a pathological process. An alternative approach was clearly required.

## STUDIES USING REMOTE VASCULAR TISSUE

One of the interesting aspects of patients with AAA is that they may exhibit a systemic dilating diathesis with manifestations of the aneurysmal process in sites remote from the aorta. This process was first described by Ward[6] who revealed that the mean diameters of all peripheral arteries were increased in patients with aneurysms. Similarly, Loftus et al.[7] reported that 40% of infrainguinal vein grafts performed for popliteal aneurysms suffered aneurysmal degeneration as compared to just 2% of grafts performed for atherosclerotic ischemic disease. One explanation for these phenomena was postulated by Baxter et al.[8] who demonstrated a reduction in the elastin/collagen ratio throughout the arterial vasculature of patients with AAA.

These observations led to the possibility of examining phenotypic changes in macroscopically normal tissue from patients with AAA. Our group performed a series of investigations using the inferior mesenteric vein harvested from patients with AAA and a series of controls.[9–11] The working hypothesis of these investigations was that tissue remote from the aorta was essentially preaneurysmal in that it might exhibit the molecular changes of a developing aneurysm without the degenerative changes of end-stage aneurysmal tissue.

Histological and biomechanical studies confirmed the promise of this approach. Histologic examination of the inferior mesenteric vein from patients with aneurysms revealed fragmentation of the elastic fibers in the media and a reduction in elastin concentration from 27% to 19%. There was no increase in inflammatory cells. Mechanical testing demonstrated a significant reduction in tensile strength (1.4 MPa vs. 2.9 MPa) and stiffness of the vessel. Remote venous tissue from patients with AAA therefore revealed changes comparable with arterial aneurysms.

Most significantly, tissue homogenates and isolated vascular smooth muscle cells from the inferior mesenteric veins of patients with AAA demonstrated elevated MMP-2 protein levels with no difference in TIMP-2 or MT1–MMP concentrations. Molecular studies confirmed elevated MMP-2 expression in these samples. *In situ* zymography confirmed that the MMP-2 activity in intact venous segments was localized to the fragmented elastin fibers in the media. At a functional level, the isolated vascular smooth muscle cells from patients with AAA demonstrated enhanced invasive properties associated with elevated MMP-2 production.

The data from these experiments suggested that overexpression of the MMP-2 gene may be responsible for the elastin fragmentation seen in early aneurysm formation.

## MMP-2 AND ANIMAL MODELS

Longo *et al.*[12] examined the role of MMP-2 and -9 in aneurysm formation in an experimental model. Using mice deficient in the expression of MMP-2 and MMP-9, this group demonstrated that mice deficient in either of these proteases were resistant to aneurysm formation. Infusion of competent macrophages into the deficient mice resulted in reconstitution of an aneurysm in the MMP-9-deficient, but not the MMP-2-deficient mice. These findings were interpreted to suggest that MMP-2 was required to facilitate MMP-9 aneurysm-driven expansion. It was suggested that both MMP-2 and MMP-9 were required to initiate aneurysm expansion in this model and that MMP-2 may be the primary driver of the disease.

## MMP-2 AS A CANDIDATE GENE FOR AAA

The data described above reviews a small proportion of the literature that suggests MMP-2 may play an important role in initiating aneurysm expansion. Recent important studies have defined a relationship between c-Jun N-terminal kinases (JNK) expression, activation of transforming growth factor (TGF)-β, and MMP-2 activity, which have strengthened the possibility of MMP-2 driving aneurysmal degeneration. Given the familial tendency to AAA formation, one obvious question is the potential of MMP-2 as a candidate gene for aneurysmal disease. At first inspection, MMP-2 does not appear to be a good candidate. MMP-2 is constitutively expressed by many cell types and its expression is not readily modulated. The promoter region of the MMP-2 gene lacks a TATA box and the AP-1 transcriptional factor binding motif common to other MMPs. However, MMP-2 has been observed to be differentially regulated in different tissue beds and recently several functional single nucleotide polymorphism (SNPs) have been described. Several of these promoter polymorphisms have been associated with disease states including coronary artery atherosclerosis and several cancers. Clearly, a study investigating the role of MMP-2 promoter polymorphisms in aneurysm formation is required.

## REFERENCES

1. FREESTONE, T., R.J. TURNER, A. COADY, *et al.* 1995. Inflammation and matrix metalloproteinases in the enlarging abdominal aortic aneurysm. Arterioscler. Thromb. Vasc. Biol. **15:** 1145–1151.
2. MCMILLAN, W.D., B.K. PATTERSON, R.R. KEEN & W.H. PEARCE. 1995. *In situ* localization and quantification of seventy-two-kilodalton type IV collagenase in aneurysmal, occlusive, and normal aorta. J. Vasc. Surg. **22:** 295–305.
3. DAVIS, V., L. BACA-REGEN, Y. ITOH, *et al.* 1998. Matrix metalloproteinase-2 production and its binding to the matrix are increased in abdominal aortic aneurysms. Arterioscler. Thromb. Vasc. Biol. **18:** 1625–1633.
4. CROWTHER, M., S. GOODALL, J.L. JONES, *et al.* 2000. Localization of matrix metalloproteinase 2 within the aneurysmal and normal aortic wall. Br. J. Surg. **87:** 1391–1400.
5. CROWTHER, M., S. GOODALL, J.L. JONES, *et al.* 2000. Increased matrix metalloproteinase 2 expression in vascular smooth muscle cells cultured from abdominal aortic aneurysms. J. Vasc. Surg. **32:** 575–583.
6. WARD, A.S. 1992. Aortic aneurysmal disease: a generalized dilating diathesis? Arch. Surg. **127:** 990–991.
7. LOFTUS, I.M., M.J. MCCARTHY, A. LLOYD, *et al.* 1999. Prevalence of true vein graft aneurysms: Implications for aneurysm pathogenesis. J. Vasc. Surg. **29:** 403–408.
8. BAXTER, B.T., V.A. DAVIS, D.J. MINION, *et al.* 1994. Abdominal aortic aneurysms are associated with altered matrix proteins of the nonaneurysmal aortic segments. J. Vasc. Surg. **19:** 797–803.
9. GOODALL, S., M. CROWTHER, D.M. HEMINGWAY, *et al.* 2001. Ubiquitous elevation of matrix metalloproteinase-2 expression in the vasculature of patients with abdominal aneurysms. Circulation **104:** 304–309.
10. GOODALL, S., M. CROWTHER, P.R. BELL & M.M. THOMPSON. 2002. The association between venous structural alterations and biomechanical weakness in patients with abdominal aortic aneurysms. J. Vasc. Surg. **35:** 937–942.
11. GOODALL, S., K.E. PORTER, P.R. BELL & M.M. THOMPSON. 2002. Enhanced invasive properties exhibited by smooth muscle cells are associated with elevated production of MMP-2 in patients with aortic aneurysms. Eur. J. Vasc. Endovasc. Surg. **24:** 72–80.
12. LONGO, G.M., W. XIONG, T.C. GREINER, *et al.* 2002. Matrix metalloproteinases 2 and 9 work in concert to produce aortic aneurysm. J. Clin. Invest. **110(5):** 625–632.

# Current Status of Endovascular Repair of Infrarenal Abdominal Aortic Aneurysms in the Context of 50 Years of Conventional Repair

NORMAN R. HERTZER

*Department of Vascular Surgery, The Cleveland Clinic Foundation, Cleveland, OH, USA*

ABSTRACT: The operative risk for conventional open repair of nonruptured infrarenal abdominal aortic aneurysms (AAAs) has steadily declined during the past several decades to the point that open procedures now can be done with a mortality rate of approximately 2% at tertiary referral centers. Nevertheless, population-based studies suggest that the mortality rate for open AAA repair remains nearly 7% in many communities, a finding that undoubtedly is influenced by a substantial risk for unfavorable outcomes in patients who represent less than ideal candidates for major abdominal operations on the basis of advanced age and the medical comorbidities that so often accompany it. Endovascular aneurysm repair (EVAR) is a landmark contribution to the management of such patients and has been associated with significant overall reductions in the operative mortality rate in statewide and national audits. This early advantage of EVAR comes at the price of a unique set of complications, secondary interventions, and related expenses, however, and randomized clinical trials of EVAR versus open repair have not yet demonstrated differences in survival or quality of life within 4 years of follow-up. Data from the Nationwide Inpatient Sample and other sources indicate that the mortality rate for open AAA repair appears to be less than 2% in patients who are 65 years of age or younger. This low operative risk may not justify exposure to whatever incidence of late complications the current generation of endografts may prove to have during the relatively long survival times that can be anticipated for these patients.

KEYWORDS: abdominal aortic aneurysm; open aortic aneurysm repair; endovascular aortic aneurysm repair

Address for correspondence: Norman R. Hertzer, M.D., F.A.C.S., Emeritus Office (EE-40), The Cleveland Clinic Foundation, 9500 Euclid Avenue, Cleveland, OH 44195. Voice: 216-444-5705; fax: 216-445-1521.
e-mail: hertzen@ccf.org

Ann. N.Y. Acad. Sci. 1085: 175–186 (2006). © 2006 New York Academy of Sciences.
doi: 10.1196/annals.1383.015

## INTRODUCTION

In the classic article published in the second volume of *Circulation* in 1950, Estes[1] described the clinical course of abdominal aortic aneurysms in a small but seminal series of 102 patients (mean age, 65 years) who were evaluated at the Mayo Clinic prior to 1948. Just two of these aneurysms were treated surgically, one by cellophane wrapping and the other by partial ligation because no other form of intervention yet existed. The cumulative 5-year survival rate for these 102 patients was only 19%, and ruptured aneurysms were responsible for 31 (63%) of the 49 deaths for which a cause was known. More than a half century has passed since Dubost *et al.*[2] then reported the first successful repair of an infrarenal abdominal aortic aneurysm (AAA) using an arterial homograft in 1952. Substantial improvements in graft materials, surgical and anesthetic management, perioperative care, and patient selection occurred during the next four decades, all of which enhanced the safety and durability of open AAA operations to the extent that they eventually became commonplace throughout much of the world.

The landscape of AAA repair again was altered dramatically in 1991 when Parodi *et al.*[3] introduced the concept of catheter-based transfemoral endograft replacement for patients who were poor candidates for conventional repair, generally because of advanced age, medical comorbidities, and/or multiple previous abdominal operations. The technology of endovascular aneurysm repair (EVAR) has matured rapidly since that time, revolutionizing the treatment of abdominal and thoracic aortic aneurysms and energizing the field of vascular surgery. The extraordinary level of interest in EVAR is clearly reflected by the number of publications that currently are devoted to it. In 2005 for instance, a total of 204 full-length original clinical articles appeared in the *Journal of Vascular Surgery*, 48 (24%) of which were on the topic of aortic aneurysms. Thirty-one (65%) of these 48 articles specifically addressed EVAR while only 7 (15%) were related in some way to open procedures.

Most technical aspects of open AAA repair have been standardized for many years. In comparison, those related to EVAR remain under evolution in order to resolve ongoing problems that potentially could lead to aneurysm rupture such as endoleaks (i.e., continued blood flow into the excluded aneurysm sac) and endograft migration. A large amount of data regarding EVAR has been generated by individual investigators, by device trials sponsored by industry and/or the Food and Drug Administration, and by the European collaborators on Stent/graft Techniques for aortic Aneurysm Repair (EUROSTAR) Registry, a voluntary archive of endograft results that now contains information from more than 17,000 cases that have been performed at 135 centers in 18 countries since 1996. The scope of the present report allows only an overview of this material. However, the contemporary evidence base for open AAA repair and EVAR is extensively tabulated in a recent American College of Cardiology/American

Heart Association guidelines document, the full text of which is available on the Internet.[4]

## OPERATIVE MORTALITY

The mortality rate of elective open repair has declined steadily to the point that it has been performed with an average early risk of approximately 2% at tertiary referral centers during the last decade. This is illustrated in FIGURE 1 using data reported by De Bakey,[5] Szilagyi,[6] Thompson,[7] Crawford,[8] and their associates for study periods prior to 1980 and 10 case series from other experienced sources since that time.[9–18] However, several statewide audits of open AAA procedures in New York,[19,20] Michigan,[21] California,[22] Maryland,[23] and Florida[24] have documented that their composite operative mortality rate of almost 7% does not conform to the exemplary results that have been reported from selected centers of excellence. Other population-based studies now reveal that EVAR currently is being employed in more than just high-risk cases, a trend that undoubtedly is being driven by patient preference in a competitive medical marketplace as well as by an effort to improve mortality rates. As one example, EVAR was used for only 9.6% of all AAA repairs in the state of New York during the year 2000, compared to 40% in 2001 and 53% in 2002.[25] As shown in FIGURE 2, wider deployment of EVAR has been associated with significantly lower overall operative mortality rates than open repair in New York as well as in Illinois.[25,26]

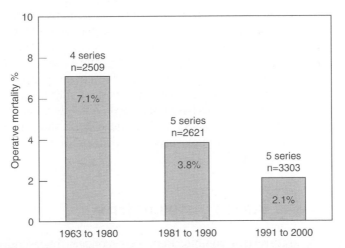

**FIGURE 1.** The declining operative mortality rate for open repair of nonruptured infrarenal abdominal aortic aneurysms at tertiary referral centers is illustrated by representative data for three consecutive study periods concluding in 1963 to 1980,[5–8] 1981 to 1990,[9–13] and 1991 to 2000.[14–18]

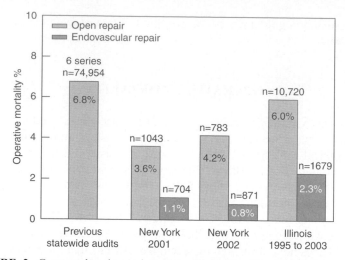

**FIGURE 2.** Compared to six previous statewide audits of open repair for nonruptured infrarenal abdominal aortic aneurysms,[19–24] endovascular repair has been associated with significantly lower overall operative mortality rates in New York (2001, $P = 0.0018$; 2002, $P < 0.0001$)[25] and Illinois ($P = 0.0003$).[26]

On the basis of a 5% random sample of inpatient claims, Dillavou et al.[27] have estimated that EVAR comprised 41% of the elective AAA procedures among Medicare patients in 2003 compared to 31% in 2001. There was a significant difference between the operative mortality rates for EVAR and open repair (1.9% vs. 5.2%, $P < 0.001$) on multivariable analysis. Age also had an independent influence on mortality rates, particularly among patients who were 85 years of age or older ($P = 0.02$). More than 60% of the Medicare patients in this age group underwent EVAR rather than open AAA repair in 2003 with a distinct advantage in their mortality rate (1.9% vs. 16%, $P < 0.001$). It seems likely that many of the deaths after open repair in such aged patients could have been linked in some way to underlying heart disease. In this regard, previous investigations have noted fewer hemodynamic alterations, less objective evidence of physiologic cardiac stress, and a lower incidence of elevated troponin levels indicating unsuspected myocardial injury after EVAR than after open AAA repair.[28,29]

## GRAFT COMPLICATIONS

The risk for graft-related complications or secondary interventions after open AAA repair is sufficiently low that it received little attention in the literature prior to the introduction of EVAR. In a report that frequently has been cited elsewhere, Hallett et al.[30] retrospectively reviewed 307 patients who underwent open repair from 1957 to 1990 at the Mayo Clinic or in the Minnesota community (Olmsted County) surrounding it. One hundred forty of these patients had follow-up imaging of their grafts with ultrasound scans or computed tomography. A total of 21 patients (6.8%) eventually were recognized to have late graft complications with a cumulative 10-year incidence of 3% for graft thrombosis, 4% for anastomotic pseudoaneurysm, and 5% for graft-enteric erosion and/or infection. In comparison, Cao et al.[31] described a prospective nonrandomized series in which abdominal ultrasound scans were obtained every 6 to 12 months during a mean follow-up interval of approximately 3 years after 585 open AAA operations and 534 endovascular procedures that were performed from 1997 to 2003. The 30-day mortality (0.9% vs. 4.1%, $P = 0.001$) and major morbidity (9.1% vs. 19%, $P < 0.0001$) rates were lower for EVAR than for open repair even though EVAR patients were slightly older and had a higher prevalence of cardiopulmonary disease. Nevertheless, EVAR was also associated with a significantly higher incidence of related reinterventions than open repair (16% vs. 2.9%, $P < 0.0001$). Fifty-seven (60%) of the 95 secondary interventions that were necessary after EVAR were done using catheter-based techniques, but 20 (24%) of the 84 patients who had any reintervention required conversion to open repair.

The early safety of EVAR comes at the price of a unique set of late complications that require life long surveillance with imaging studies and lead to follow-up expenses that exceed merely the high base cost (nearly $10,000 USD) of endograft devices.[32-34] Drury et al.[35] recently conducted a systematic review of 19,804 EVAR procedures and 9,255 open AAA operations from 61 reports that have been published since 2000. Some of the findings from this review are depicted in FIGURE 3. While EVAR had a significantly better 30-day mortality rate and a low incidence of AAA rupture or conversion to open repair, it also was associated with endoleaks and other problems for which secondary interventions were necessary in more than 15% of patients. Others have made similar observations regarding the expense of EVAR and have questioned whether it falls within an acceptable range of cost-effectiveness for emerging technology, especially in patients who have no medical contraindications to open AAA repair.[36,37]

# PATIENT SURVIVAL

## Randomized Trials

The comparative safety of EVAR often has been difficult to assess in published reports because it is not always possible to determine whether EVAR was performed only in high-risk surgical patients or in a blend of high-risk, average-risk, and low-risk patients. Like open AAA repair, survival rates after EVAR are influenced primarily by medical comorbidities and are lowest in

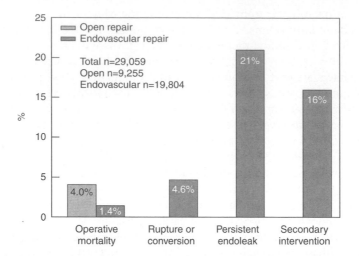

**FIGURE 3.** The early benefit in operative mortality ($P < 0.001$) and the long-term disadvantages of endovascular aortic aneurysm repair according to a systematic review of nearly 20,000 procedures reported in the literature from 2000 through 2004.[35]

series for which high surgical risk was a criterion for patient selection.[4] In an attempt to overcome such liabilities, at least three randomized clinical trials have been initiated to establish whether EVAR offers advantages over open repair in patients who are appropriate candidates for either procedure. Enrollment already has been completed for two trials involving 34 centers in the United Kingdom (EVAR trial 1)[38,39] and 28 centers in the Netherlands and Belgium (Dutch Randomized Endovascular Aneurysm Management [DREAM] Trial),[40,41] and recruitment is under way for another investigation by the Department of Veterans Affairs in the United States (Open Versus Endovascular Repair [OVER]Trial).[42]

TABLE 1 contains a summary of disclosures that presently are available from EVAR trial 1 and the DREAM Trial with respect to operative mortality and patient survival during 2 to 4 years of surveillance. Although EVAR had a lower operative mortality rate than open repair in each study, this difference was statistically significant only in the larger EVAR trial 1 and has not translated into any improvement in intermediate-term survival in either trial. All-cause mortality rates are similar for EVAR and for open repair in both trials, and a marginal difference in aneurysm-related mortality at 2 years of follow-up in the latest DREAM Trial report has been interpreted by its authors merely to reflect the lower operative mortality rate of EVAR.[41]

The additional analysis of secondary end points in these trials has produced findings in randomized cohorts that confirm previous observations from non-randomized series with respect to the intriguing advantages and disadvantages of EVAR. Although EVAR was associated with significant ($P < 0.001$)

**TABLE 1. Survival outcomes of two randomized clinical trials (EVAR trial 1[38,39] and the Dutch Randomized Endovascular Aneurysm Management [DREAM] Trial)[40,41] comparing open repair versus endovascular repair of nonruptured infrarenal abdominal aortic aneurysms**

| | EVAR trial 1 | | DREAM Trial | |
|---|---|---|---|---|
| | Open repair | Endovascular repair | Open repair | Endovascular repair |
| Randomized patients | 539 | 543 | 178 | 173 |
| Men | 489 | 494 | 161 | 161 |
| Women | 50 | 49 | 17 | 12 |
| Mean age (years ± SD) | 74.0 ± 6.1 | 74.2 ± 6.0 | 69.6 ± 6.8 | 70.7 ± 6.6 |
| Mean aneurysm diameter (cm ± SD) | 6.5 ± 1.0 | 6.5 ± 0.9 | 6.0 ± 0.8 | 6.1 ± 0.9 |
| Operative mortality rates in patients actually receiving treatment | | | | |
| 30-day | 4.7% (24/516) | 1.7% (9/531) P = 0.009 | 4.6%* (8/174) | 1.2%* (2/171) P = 0.10 |
| In-hospital | 6.2% (32/516) | 2.1% (11/531) P = 0.001 | | |
| Follow-up interval | 2.9 years (median) | 2.9 years (median) | 21 months (mean) | 22 months (mean) |
| All-cause mortality rates | | | | |
| Crude | 20% (109/539) | 18% (100/543) P = 0.46 | 10% (18/178) | 12%† (20/173) |
| Cumulative (Kaplan–Meier) | 29% (4 years) | 26% (4 years) P > 0.20 | 11% (2 years) | 11% (2 years) P = 0.86 |
| Aneurysm-related mortality rates | | | | |
| Crude | 6.3% (34/539) | 3.5% (19/543) P = 0.04 | 4.5% (8/178) | 1.2%† (2/173) |
| Cumulative (Kaplan–Meier) | 7% (4 years) | 4% (4 years) P > 0.20 | 5.7% (2 years) | 2.1% (2 years) P = 0.05 |

*Deaths within 30 days or during the same admission to the hospital, whichever was longer.
†Level of statistical significance not available in original report.

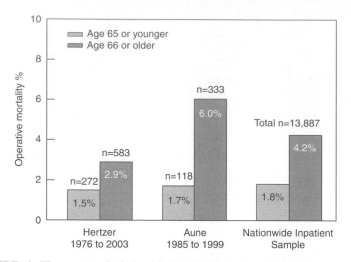

**FIGURE 4.** The suggested relationship ($P = \text{NS}$) between patient age and the mortality rate for open repair of nonruptured infrarenal abdominal aortic aneurysms in two personal series[16,44] is similar to the significant difference ($P < 0.001$) that has been demonstrated using data from the Nationwide Inpatient Sample in 1996 and 1997.[45]

reductions in operative time, blood loss, and transfusion requirements compared to open repair,[40] it also was associated with greater risk for reinterventions during the original hospital admission (9.8% vs. 5.8%, $P = 0.02$).[38] Furthermore, the cumulative 4-year incidence of graft-related complications (41% vs. 9%, $P < 0.0001$) and secondary interventions (20% vs. 6%, $P < 0.0001$) was significantly higher for EVAR than for open repair in EVAR trial 1,[39] and secondary procedures were especially common during the first 9 months after EVAR in the DREAM Trial (hazard ratio, 2.9; 95% confidence intervals, 1.1 to 6.2; $P = 0.03$).[41] There was an early advantage in quality of life immediately after EVAR, but this lasted for only 3 months.[39] Including follow-up costs, the mean expense of EVAR was 33% higher than open repair in EVAR trial 1.[39]

## Patient Age

Maher *et al.*[43] concluded from an evidence-based analysis of 22 studies prior to 2003 that it would be necessary to treat 57 patients by EVAR rather than by open procedures before one additional patient would be alive at 30 days postoperatively. Such estimates depend heavily on case mix, and patient age probably is the most important common denominator for many of the factors that determine it. As shown in FIGURE 4, data from two large personal series[16,44] and the significant findings reported by Dimick *et al.*[45] from an even larger data set in the Nationwide Inpatient Sample indicate that the operative mortality

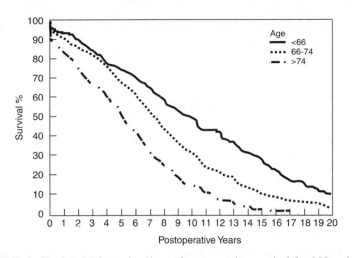

**FIGURE 5.** Kaplan–Meier estimations of postoperative survival for 855 patients who had elective open repair of infrarenal abdominal aortic aneurysms from 1976 through 2003. The survival rate for patients who were 65 years of age or younger ($n = 272$) was significantly better ($P < 0.001$) than for patients who were either 66 to 74 years of age ($n = 375$) or 75 years of age or older ($n = 208$) at the time of their operations.[44] (Reproduced with permission from the Society for Vascular Surgery.)

rate for conventional AAA repair generally is less than 2% in patients who are 65 years of age or younger. Moreover, as illustrated in FIGURE 5, long-term survival estimates after open repair in these patients (77% at 5 years, 52% at 10 years, and 29% at 15 years) are significantly higher ($P < 0.001$) than in any other age group.[44] An operative mortality rate of less than 2% for open operations may not warrant such prolonged exposure to whatever incidence of late complications eventually will be found to occur in the present generation of endografts.

## CONCLUSION

The appeal of EVAR is undeniable and justified. Many reports have established that it is associated with shorter operative times, less blood loss, reduced length of hospital stay, and more rapid return to full activity than open AAA repair.[4,35] Its low early mortality rate also makes it a landmark contribution to the care of high-risk patients for whom no good therapeutic alternative to open repair previously had been available. The wider use of EVAR understandably will be driven by patient preference for a less invasive procedure than open AAA repair, but this enthusiasm should be tempered by the present uncertainty regarding its long-term complications. Until endograft technology has improved to the point that this uncertainty no longer exists, it may not yet be appropriate to use EVAR in younger patients who predictably are at low risk for conventional open operations.

## REFERENCES

1. ESTES, J.E., JR. 1950. Abdominal aortic aneurysm: a study of one hundred and two cases. Circulation **2:** 258–264.
2. DUBOST, C.M., M. ALLARY & N. OECONOMOS. 1952. Resection of an aneurysm of the abdominal aorta: re-establishment of the continuity by a preserved human arterial graft, with result after five months. Arch. Surg. **64:** 405–408.
3. PARODI, J.C., J.C. PALMAZ & H.D. BARONE. 1991. Transfemoral intraluminal graft implantation for abdominal aortic aneurysms. Ann. Vasc. Surg. **5:** 491–499.
4. HIRSCH, A.T., Z.J. HASKAL, N.R. HERTZER, et al. ACC/AHA 2005 guidelines for the management of patients with peripheral arterial disease (lower extremity, renal, mesentereic, and abdominal aortic): a collaborative report from the American Association for Vascular Surgery/Society for Vascular Surgery, Society for Cardiovascular Angiography and Interventions, Society for Vascular Medicine and Biology, Society of Interventional Radiology, and the ACC/AHA Task Force on Practice Guidelines. Available at http://www.acc.org/clinical/guidelines/pad/index.pdf. Accessed January 24, 2006.
5. DE BAKEY, M.E., E.S. CRAWFORD, D.A. COOLEY, et al. 1964. Aneurysm of abdominal aorta. Analysis of results of graft replacement therapy one to eleven years after operation. Ann. Surg. **60:** 622–638.
6. SZILAGYI, D.E., R.F. SMITH, F.J. DeRUSSO, et al. 1966. Contribution of abdominal aortic aneurysmectomy to prolongation of life. Ann. Surg. **164:** 678–697.
7. THOMPSON, J.E., L.H. HOLLIER, R.D. PATMAN, et al. 1975. Surgical management of abdominal aortic aneurysms: factors influencing mortality and morbidity—a 20-year experience. Ann. Surg. **181:** 654–660.
8. CRAWFORD, E.S., S.A. SALEH, J.W. BABB, III, et al. 1981. Infrarenal abdominal aortic aneurysm: factors influencing survival after operation performed over a 25-year period. Ann. Surg. **193:** 699–709.
9. HERTZER, N.R., E.G. BEVEN, J.R. YOUNG, et al. 1984. Coronary artery disease in peripheral vascular patients. A classification of 1000 coronary angiograms and results of surgical management. Ann. Surg. **199:** 223–244.
10. REIGEL, M.M., L.H. HOLLIER, F.J. KAZMIER, et al. 1987. Late survival in abdominal aortic aneurysm patients: the role of selective myocardial revascularization on the basis of clinical symptoms. J. Vasc. Surg. **5:** 222–227.
11. GOLDEN, M.A., A.D. WHITTEMORE, M.C. DONALDSON, et al. 1990. Selective evaluation and management of coronary artery disease in patients undergoing repair of abdominal aortic aneurysms: a 16-year experience. Ann. Surg. **212:** 415–420.enlargethispage6pt
12. STARR, J.E., N.R. HERTZER, E.J. MASCHA, et al. 1996. Influence of gender on cardiac risk and survival in patients with infrarenal aortic aneurysms. J. Vasc. Surg. **23:** 870–880.
13. KOSKAS, F. & E. KIEFFER. 1997. Long-term survival after elective repair of infrarenal abdominal aortic aneurysm: results of a prospective multicentric study.

Association for Academic Research in Vascular Surgery (AURC). Ann. Vasc. Surg. **11:** 473–481.

14. SICARD, G.A., J.M. REILLY, B.G. RUBIN, *et al.* 1995. Transabdominal versus retroperitoneal incision for abdominal aortic surgery: report of prospective randomized trial. J. Vasc. Surg. **21:** 174–181.

15. LLOYD, W.E., P.S. PATY, R.C. DARLING, III, *et al.* 1996. Results of 1000 consecutive elective abdominal aortic aneurysm repairs. Cardiovasc. Surg. **4:** 724–726.

16. AUNE, S. 2001. Risk factors and operative results of patients aged less than 66 years operated on for asymptomatic abdominal aortic aneurysm. Eur. J. Vasc. Endovasc. Surg. **22:** 240–243.

17. HERTZER, N.R., E.J. MASCHA, M.T. KARAFA, *et al.* 2002. Open infrarenal abdominal aortic aneurysm repair: the Cleveland Clinic experience from 1989 to 1998. J. Vasc. Surg. **35:** 1145–1154.

18. MENARD, M.T., D.K.W. CHEW, R.K. CHAN, *et al.* 2003. Outcome in patients at high risk after open surgical repair of abdominal aortic aneurysm. J. Vasc. Surg. **37:** 285–292.

19. HANNAN, E.L., H. KILBURN, JR., J.F. O'DONNELL, *et al.* 1992. A longitudinal analysis of the relationship between in-hospital mortality in New York State and the volume of abdominal aortic aneurysm surgeries performed. Health Serv. Res. **27:** 517–542.

20. SOLLANO, J.A., A.C. GELIJNS, A.J. MOSKOWITZ, *et al.* 1999. Volume-outcome relationships in cardiovascular operations: New York State, 1990–1995. J. Thorac. Cardiovasc. Surg. **117:** 419–428.

21. KATZ, D.J., J.C. STANLEY & G.B. ZELENOCK. 1994. Operative mortality rates for intact and ruptured abdominal aortic aneurysms in Michigan: an eleven-year statewide experience. J. Vasc. Surg. **19:** 804–815.

22. MANHEIM, L.M., M.W. SOHN, J. FEINGLASS, *et al.* 1998. Hospital vascular surgery volume and procedure mortality rates in California, 1982–1994. J. Vasc. Surg. **28:** 45–56.

23. DARDIK, L., J.W. LIN, T.A. GORDON, *et al.* 1999. Results of elective abdominal aortic aneurysm repair in the 1990s: a population-based analysis of 2335 cases. J. Vasc. Surg. **30:** 985–995.

24. PEARCE, W.H., M.A. PARKER, J. FEINGLASS, *et al.* 1999. The importance of surgeon volume and training in outcomes for vascular surgical procedures. J. Vasc. Surg **29:** 768–776.

25. ANDERSON, P.L., R.R. ARONS, A.J. MOSKOWITZ, *et al.* 2004. A statewide experience with endovascular abdominal aortic aneurysm repair: rapid diffusion with excellent early results. J. Vasc. Surg. **39:** 10–19.

26. LEON, L.R., JR., N. LABROPOULOS, J. LAREDO, *et al.* 2005. To what extent has endovascular aneurysm repair influenced abdominal aortic aneurysm management in the state of Illinois? J. Vasc. Surg. **41:** 568–574.

27. DILLAVOU, E.D., S.C. MULUK & M.S. MAKAROUN. 2006. Improving aneurysm-related outcomes: nationwide benefits of endovascular repair. J. Vasc. Surg. **43:** 446–452.

28. CUYPERS, P.W.M., M. GARDIEN, J. BUTH, *et al.* 2001. Cardiac response and complications during endovascular repair of abdominal aortic aneurysms: a concurrent comparison with open surgery. J. Vasc. Surg. **33:** 353–360.

29. ABRAHAM, N., L. LEMECH, C. SANDROUSSI, *et al.* 2005. A prospective study of subclinical myocardial damage in endovascular versus open repair of infrarenal abdominal aortic aneurysms. J. Vasc. Surg. **41:** 377–381.

30. HALLETT, J.W., JR., D.M. MARSHALL, T.M. PETTERSON, *et al.* 1997. Graft-related complications after abdominal aortic aneurysm repair: reassurance from a 36-year population-based experience. J. Vasc. Surg. **25:** 277–286.

31. CAO, P., F. VERZINI, G. PARLANI, *et al.* 2004. Clinical effect of abdominal aortic aneurysm endografting: 7-year concurrent comparison with open repair. J. Vasc. Surg. **40:** 841–848.

32. VEITH, F.J., R.A. BAUM, T. OHKI, *et al.* 2002. Nature and significance of endoleaks and endotension: summary of opinions expressed at an international conference. J. Vasc. Surg. **35:** 1029–1035.

33. SAPIRSTEIN, W., P. CHANDEYSSON & C. WENTZ. 2001. The Food and Drug Administration approval of endovascular grafts for abdominal aortic aneurysm: an 18-month perspective. J. Vasc. Surg. **34:** 180–183.

34. LEE, W.A., J.W. CARTER, G. UPCHURCH, *et al.* 2004. Perioperative outcomes after open and endovascular repair of intact abdominal aortic aneurysms in the United States during 2001. J. Vasc. Surg. **39:** 491–496.

35. DRURY, D., J.A. MICHAELS, L. JONES, *et al.* 2005. Systematic review of recent evidence for the safety and efficacy of elective endovascular repair in the management of infrarenal abdominal aortic aneurysm. Br. J. Surg. **92:** 937–946.

36. HAYTER, C.L., S.R. BRADSHAW, R.J. ALLEN, *et al.* 2005. Follow-up costs increase the cost disparity between endovascular and open abdominal aortic aneurysm repair. J. Vasc. Surg. **42:** 912–918.

37. MICHAELS, J.A., D. DRURY & S.M. THOMAS. 2005. Cost-effectiveness of endovascular abdominal aortic aneurysm repair. Br. J. Surg. **92:** 960–967.

38. EVAR TRIAL PARTICIPANTS. 2004. Comparison of endovascular aneurysm repair with open repair in patients with abdominal aortic aneurysm (EVAR trial 1), 30-day operative mortality results: randomised controlled trial. Lancet **364:** 843–848.

39. EVAR TRIAL PARTICIPANTS. 2005. Endovascular aneurysm repair versus open repair in patients with abdominal aortic aneurysm (EVAR trial 1): randomised controlled trial. Lancet **365:** 2179–2186.

40. PRINSSEN, M., E.L.G. VERHOEVEN, J. BUTH, *et al.* 2004. A randomized trial comparing conventional and endovascular repair of abdominal aortic aneurysms. N. Engl. J. Med. **351:** 1607–1618.

41. BLANKENSTEIJN, J.D., S.E.C.A. DE JONG, M. PRINSSEN, *et al.* 2005. Two-year outcomes after conventional or endovascular repair of abdominal aortic aneurysms. N. Engl. J. Med. **352:** 2398–2405.

42. UNITED STATES DEPARTMENT OF VETERANS AFFAIRS. Standard open surgery versus endovascular repair of abdominal aortic aneurysm. Available at http://www.clinicaltrials.gov/ct/show/NCT00094575?order=1. Accessed October 20, 2004.

43. MAHER, M.M., A.M. MCNAMARA, P.M. MACENEANEY, *et al.* 2003. Abdominal aortic aneurysms: elective endovascular repair versus conventional surgery—evaluation with evidence-based medicine techniques. Radiology **228:** 647–658.

44. HERTZER, N.R. & E.J. MASCHA. 2005. A personal experience with factors influencing survival after elective open repair of infrarenal aortic aneurysms. J. Vasc. Surg. **42:** 898–905.

45. DIMICK, J.B., J.C. STANLEY, D.A. AXELROD, *et al.* 2002. Variation in death rate after abdominal aortic aneurysmectomy in the United States: impact of hospital volume, gender, and age. Ann. Surg. **235:** 579–585.

# Aortic Aneurysm, Thoracoabdominal Aneurysm, Juxtarenal Aneurysm, Fenestrated Endografts, Branched Endografts, and Endovascular Aneurysm Repair

ROY K. GREENBERG

*Department of Vascular Surgery, The Cleveland Clinic Foundation, Cleveland, Ohio, USA*

ABSTRACT: The development of endovascular devices to treat aneurysms that abut or involve the visceral vessels has occurred in an effort to reduce the significant procedural morbidity and mortality associated with conventional repair. To accomplish this, three systems have been trialed. The first technique was developed to treat juxtarenal aneurysms and involves the placement of customized fenestrations strategically placed within the fabric of the graft. These are aligned with the ostia of the visceral vessels incorporated by the repair and supplemented by the placement of a balloon expandable stent. In a similar fashion, aneurysms that involve the visceral vessels can be treated with a fenestrated graft where the fenestration is reinforced with a nitinol ring. This is then mated with a balloon-expandable stentgraft, allowing the devices to seal at the level of the nitinol ring. An alternative means of incorporating the visceral vessels is to use directional branches where one or more additional limbs (typically 8 mm) are anastomosed to the aortic graft, through which access into the visceral vessel is attained. Mating stentgrafts for the later design can be of a self-expanding or balloon expandable nature. The experience with fenestrated devices is mature and associated with a low perioperative mortality (<2%) without many long-term complications. The treatment of thoracoabdominal aneurysms with branches has provided us with optimism regarding the technique, but results are only short term in nature. Further device development is ongoing and dissemination of this technology is now occurring in Europe, Australia and Canada.

KEYWORDS: aortic aneurysm; thoracoabdominal aneurysm; juxtarenal aneurysm; fenestrated endografts; branched endografts; endovascular aneurysm repair

Address for correspondence: Roy K. Greenberg, M.D., Department of Vascular Surgery, The Cleveland Clinic Foundation, 9500 Euclid Avenue, Cleveland, OH 44195. Voice: 585-275-7741; fax: 216-445-6302.
e-mail: greenbr@ccf.org

Ann. N.Y. Acad. Sci. 1085: 187–196 (2006). © 2006 New York Academy of Sciences.
doi: 10.1196/annals.1383.038

# INTRODUCTION

Endovascular aneurysm repair is commonly utilized to treat infrarenal aneurysms with favorable anatomy. This technique has been shown to have a tenuous, but relevant aneurysm-related mortality benefit in healthy patients.[1–3] This observed risk reduction is significant despite the short-term nature of the benefit and the plethora of described failure modes associated with endovascular grafts.[4–12] However, the long-term benefit of such a repair remains to be proven. In fact, fears regarding the long-term instability of endovascular repairs has become a frequent subject of discussion.[6,7,13,14] Risks of device migration have approached 40% in some series.[13–15] Will this be the fate of all endografts, should the recipients live long enough, or only those with proximal neck degeneration? How can the stability of the minimally invasive repair be assessed before treatment? Are there ways to mitigate migration risk with the addition of fixation devices or modulation of the hemodynamic forces? These questions remain at the heart of the matter to maintain the success of endovascular treatments for a disease process that is poorly understood.

Yet infrarenal aneurysms represent the simplest form of aortic aneurysmal disease. Clearly, any mortality risk reduction benefit achieved with endovascular repair of both large and small infrarenal aortic aneurysms will pale in comparison to the potential for mortality risk reduction for aneurysms that are more proximal and involve the visceral segment. The mortality associated with conventional treatment of juxtarenal, suprarenal, and thoracoabdominal aneurysms ranges from 5% to 34%.[16–19] In addition, there is a significant incidence of major complications such as paraplegia, cardiopulmonary issues, and need for hemodialysis that approaches 8% in some series.[20] It is the application of endovascular technologies to this patient group that will change the face of aortic surgery. The acceptance of a technology to treat the complex aneurysms rests upon the spine of the perfection of technologies designed to treat simpler forms of the same disease. However, the simplicity of an infrarenal endoprosthesis is overshadowed by the intricacy of designing and implanting a device that will accommodate the renal, mesenteric, or brachiocephalic branches. Critical end organs will then be dependent upon flow through the prosthesis and thus, device-related complications that manifest following infrarenal aneurysm repair such as migration[13–15,21] or component separation[21,22] will likely be fatal if encountered following a repair that incorporates critical aortic branches.

# FENESTRATED ENDOGRAFTING

The use of devices incorporating fixation systems (uncovered bare stents with barbs) that extend across the ostia of the renal arteries has been suggested to improve device stability,[23–25] and does not appear to affect renal function.[24]

Although this fixation system as well as alternative mechanisms of fixation, have been proposed for suboptimal necks,[26,27] it is hard to consider the reported short- and intermediate-term results enthusiastically. Not only are such repairs tenuous with respect to the length of overlap with a sealing region, but the long-term health of the aorta in this region is also questionable. Such techniques are further limited to those aneurysms with some segment of infrarenal neck. Thus, the development of a device to treat aneurysms that abut or incorporate the visceral vessels was undertaken. Initially, devices with holes in the graft synchronized (based on preoperative imaging studies) to the visceral ostia, termed fenestrated grafts, allowed the incorporation of the renal arteries, and thus the endovascular treatment of juxtarenal aneurysms.[28–32] The technique has been previously reported. Fundamentally, a balloon expandable stent is placed through the customized fenestration aligned with the target visceral ostia. The balloon is inflated to the size of the target vessel and further flared with a larger balloon to rivet the stent against the graft and aortic wall. This is then repeated for the desired number of visceral vessels. Experience with this fenestrated stentgraft has now exceeded 1,000 cases worldwide. Data presented at the European Society for Vascular Surgery on 119 patients demonstrated both the feasibility and safety of the procedure. The long-term efficacy of this approach will require extended follow-up, but appears promising in the absence of any ruptures or conversions in this series.[33]

### Fundamental Fenestrated Concepts

The primary goal of treating an aneurysm with a fenestrated graft is to move the sealing and fixation region of the repair into healthy aorta. Although initially intended to treat patients with short proximal necks, the definition of such a neck requires detailed interrogation. Conical necks, atheroma depositions, and irregular-shaped necks all intimate disease. Whether an endovascular prosthesis can be placed in such a region and remain stable with respect to the native vasculature over time will likely depend upon how long the patient lives. It seems likely that such segments will ultimately dilate, subjecting the endograft to hemodynamic displacement forces without the stabilizing forces of the proximal neck resulting in migration. Therefore, the goal should be to place the sealing segment into healthy, parallel neck without wall defects. This type of approach will be more likely to provide the most stable, and therefore, durable exclusion of such aneurysms.

Despite adequate fixation within healthy aorta, the potential for displacement as a result of extreme hemodynamic forces remains significant. Migration of a device that incorporates the visceral vessels is potentially disastrous as the fenestrations and branched stents are not likely to confer added fixation and will therefore be sacrificed, along with their respective end organs should migration occur. It has been shown that the majority of the displacement forces affect the aortic bifurcation.[34] Therefore, the potential to decouple the aortic bifurcation segment from the portion of the device that incorporates the visceral branches should discourage migration of this critical segment. The two components would then be joined with a significant region of overlap, which as morphologic changes occur can serve as a stress relief mechanism. Thus, if 8 cm of overlap between the visceral and aortic bifurcation devices exists following implantation, up to 4 cm of overlap can be lost as the device morphology changes, before concern regarding complete component separation arises. This concept has the potential to provide truly long-term exclusion of complex aneurysms.

Based upon the aforementioned concepts, the planning for a fenestrated device begins with the decision of where the proximal sealing stent will reside. The intended location should be to place the stent in healthy aorta and preferably above marked aortic angulation. The length of this stent (approximately 20 mm) will dictate which vessels must be incorporated in the repair as fenestrations. The tubular component that transcends the desired portion of the visceral segment should be long such that the distal segment will provide a means to achieve excessive overlap with the bifurcated component. The iliac repair is not different than conventional infrarenal endovascular concepts.

## THORACOABDOMINAL ANEURYSMS

### Reinforced Fenestrated Graft

The addition of a ring supporting the circumference of the customized fenestration and substitution of the uncovered stent with a stentgraft represents the simplest form of branch vessel grafting. In this manner, aneurysms that involve the renal arteries or aneurysms involving all of the visceral vessels can be treated with an endovascular approach. Such a procedure is more challenging than a simple fenestrated procedure in that there exists a space between the fenestration and branch ostium, which can complicate cannulation. Furthermore, longer balloon-expandable stentgraft must be used to traverse this space, resulting in less flexible delivery systems that must be larger in size (7F) in contrast to uncovered stents. Additionally, it must be recognized that such a design depends upon the seal between the aortic component and branch that is dependent upon the joint between the mating stentgraft and the nitinol ring reinforcing the fenestration. Not only is this a relatively narrow region, but blood must also traverse a right angle to flow through the desired branch. This is not optimal from an engineering perspective but is currently necessary when working within a small lumen. The delivery system for such a device is identical with a fenestrated system (18–20F), but more frequently a greater number of visceral vessels must be incorporated into the repair. This creates a challenge with device design. The accurate design of a device with a single fenestration provides the user with a substantial margin of error. As more branches are added to the design, the greater the need for complete accuracy to properly align each ostium. Thus, optimally one would achieve proficiency with a fenestrated device prior to embarking on a reinforced fenestrated design to treat more proximal aneurysms.

### *Directional Branch Concepts*

The purpose of a directional branch is threefold. First, the branch provides a means to mate a small vessel stentgraft with the primary aortic device. Preferably the overlap should be long and allow the use of self-expanding stentgrafts rather than limit the armamentarium of small vessel devices to the relatively stiff balloon-expandable stentgrafts. Secondly, the branch should allow any angulation between the aorta and branch to be gently accommodated, avoiding the need to create steep angles that may inhibit blood flow and also detrimentally affect device durability. Importantly, the length of the seal between the aortic component and small vessel branch in a device with a directional branch is much longer than the joint within a reinforced fenestrated device where the entire sealing region consists of the nitinol ring surrounding the fenestration. Lastly, directional branches may be constructed in a manner to optimize the flow dynamics between the aorta and its branches. These branches are utilized in preference to a reinforced fenestrated design when there is a large aortic lumen or angulation of the aorta in the region of a critical branch.

Although directional branches are conceptually superior to reinforced fenestrations with respect to joint durability and flow direction, certain challenges remain with the implementation of such technology. The branches take up space within the aneurysm as well as the delivery system. Such devices are frequently bulky and may require introduction of 24F sheaths for delivery. The procedures, which require placement of an aortic device followed by one or more self-expanding stentgrafts into each of the visceral branch targets requires extensive fluoroscopy exposure, contrast dosing, and significant proficiency with catheter and wire techniques. Such branch devices may optimally be combined with other forms of visceral vessel accommodation (fenestrated or reinforced fenestrated designs) to create a device that will reside appropriately within the anatomy at hand. Lastly, the creation of such complex implants requires customization, which may result in delays for such repairs, challenges with respect to production, which will likely be sold for higher costs.

## RESULTS AND DISCUSSION

Following the initial descriptions of fenestrated cases,[28,29] larger series have been published[32,33,35] demonstrating the mid-term safety and efficacy of the repair. In the largest series from The Cleveland Clinic, 119 patients were treated with a perioperative (30 day) mortality of under 2%, and survival at 12, 24, and 36 months of 92%, 83%, and 79%, respectively. Aneurysm sac shrinkage was noted in 79% of the patients at 12 months, ensuring the concept that the natural history of the disease treated with this device was reversed. Endoleaks were uncommon and noted in 9% of the patients at 30 days (all type II), and 4%, 6%, and 3% at 12, 24, and 36 months respectively. A comprehensive analysis on renal dysfunction following fenestrated endovascular repair noted a parallel or lower incidence of renal function deterioration following endovascular repair[36] in contrast to open surgical repair of comparable aneurysms.[37] However, the technology is young, with only mid-term follow-up data available. The long-term stability of the repair remains suspect as does the ability to disseminate this technology. Yet, clear benefits over open procedures, the fact that a six-center U.S. trial with this device has been completed and is under review at the FDA, and the device is commercially available in Europe, Australia, and Canada, create an optimistic air about the future of fenestrated endovascular grafting.

Branched endografting to treat thoracoabdominal aneurysms is more complex and the results are less mature. Early case reports[38,39] provided an impetus to develop more versatile, durable designs. The first series of cases was presented at the Society for Vascular Surgery in 2005 and included 50 patients, of which 20 had suprarenal aneurysms and 9 had type II or type III thoracoabdominal aneurysms.[40] The patient population studied was considered to be at high risk for an open surgical procedure given the severity of the associated risk factors. Despite these issues, there was only one perioperative death as a result of a myocardial infarction in a patient that required an iliac conduit, iliac endarterectomy, and ilio-femoral bypass to address severe concomitant occlusive disease. There were two cases of spinal cord injury; both occurred in the setting internal iliac artery compromise combined with extensive aortic coverage (one type II and one type III aneurysm). The two neurologic events prompted concern with respect to the treatment of additional patients with baseline compromise of their internal iliac circulation who may have required long thoracoabdominal repairs in deference to open techniques where intercostal reimplantation is possible. However, despite these complications and other more minor complications, the majority of patients underwent the procedure with an abbreviated hospital stay without serious morbidity. Thus, the potential to treat such complex aneurysms has the potential to be a marked advance for aortic disease treatments.

In spite of the optimism associated with endovascular repair of thoracoabdominal aneurysms, concern remains for the longevity of the devices, particularly the most commonly utilized design (reinforced fenestrated). The joint in such a device consists of the balloon-expandable stentgraft and the nitinol ring surrounding the fenestration in the aortic device. Thus, the joint is quite thin and should it fail, the ensuing endoleak and sac repressurization result in rapid expansion and rupture. For this reason, and others, attention has been directed toward developing longer segments to establish a seal for the mating devices. Yet, the use of such branches is limited to patients with larger aortic lumens (to allow expansion of the aortic component and each branch) and without severe aortic angulation. Both reinforced fenestrated grafts and directional branched devices may take a long time to manufacture, given the patient specific requirements, requiring an uncomfortable wait from the time a patient decides to have the aneurysm addressed and device implantation. Regardless, when such techniques are contrasted with the surgical treatment of these aneurysms,[41] the importance of new advances in this field is underscored.

## CONCLUSIONS

It is quite clear that the entire aorta is within the domain of the aortic interventionalist. Today, there are no true contraindications to endovascular repair; instead it is the risk/benefit ratio of each possible treatment option that must be considered. Several roadblocks will slow the dissemination of this technology. Issues include the development of technical skills, conceptual understanding, and proficiency with image interpretation and manipulation techniques. Endovascular grafting of conventional infrarenal aorta, the treatment of renal and mesenteric occlusive disease, and attention to cross-sectional imaging techniques mandatorily precede training for more complex procedures. The devices are more complex to manufacture, they are more costly than infrarenal and thoracic counterparts, and each case requires additional small vessel stentgrafts that are still in various stages of development. Furthermore, following such a repair the patients still require close monitoring, most frequently in the intensive care unit, with length of stays considerably longer than less complex repairs. All of these factors will cause several financial issues regarding aneurysm repair that have not yet been addressed. However, the benefit of these technologies for this patient population is marked, and thus, as physicians, we should place great emphasis on the support of these technological developments and methods by which these skills can be disseminated.

## REFERENCES

1. GREENHALGH, R.M., L.C. BROWN , G.P. KWONG, et al. 2004. Comparison of endovascular aneurysm repair with open repair in patients with abdominal aortic aneurysm (EVAR trial 1), 30-day operative mortality results: randomised controlled trial. Lancet. **364:** 843–848.
2. EVAR trial participants. 2005. Endovascular aneurysm repair and outcome in patients unfit for open repair of abdominal aortic aneurysm (EVAR trial 2): randomised controlled trial. Lancet. **365:** 2187–2192.

3. EVAR trial participants. 2005. Endovascular aneurysm repair versus open repair in patients with abdominal aortic aneurysm (EVAR trial 1): randomised controlled trial. Lancet. **365:** 2179–2186.

4. ZARINS, C., R. WHITE & T. FOGARTY. 2000. Aneurysm rupture after endovascular repair using the AneuRx stent graft. J. Vasc. Surg. **31:** 960–970.

5. BUTH, J., P.L. HARRIS & M.C. VAN. 2002. Causes and outcomes of open conversion and aneurysm rupture after endovascular abdominal aortic aneurysm repair: can type II endoleaks be dangerous? [Review] [8 refs]. J. Am. Coll. Surg. **194:** S98–S102.

6. OHKI, T., F.J. VEITH, P. SHAW, et al. 2001. Increasing incidence of midterm and long-term complications after endovascular graft repair of abdominal aortic aneurysms: a note of caution based on a 9-year experience. Ann. Surg. **234:** 323–334.

7. BEEBE, H.G. 2003. Lessons learned from aortic aneurysm stent graft failure: observations from several perspectives. Semin. Vasc. Surg. **16:** 129–138.

8. BEEBE, H.G., J.L. CRONENWETT, B.T. KATZEN, et al. 2001. Results of an aortic endograft trial: impact of device failure beyond 12 months. J. Vasc. Surg. **33:** S55–S63.

9. RIEPE, G., P. HEILBERGER, T. UMSCHEID, et al. 1999. Frame dislocation of body middle rings in endovascular stent tube grafts. Eur. J. Vasc. Endovasc. Surg. **17:** 28–34.

10. BOHM, T., J. SOLDNER, A. ROTT, et al. 1999. Perigraft leak of an aortic stent graft due to material fatigue. AJR Am. J. Roentgenol. **172:** 1355–1357.

11. MALEUX, G., H. ROUSSEAU, P. OTAL, et al. 1998. Modular component separation and reperfusion of abdominal aortic aneurysm sac after endovascular repair of the abdominal aortic aneurysm: a case report. J. Vasc. Surg. **28:** 349–352.

12. JACOBS, T.S., J. WON, E.C. GRAVEREAUX, et al. 2003. Mechanical failure of prosthetic human implants: a 10-year experience with aortic stent graft devices. J. Vasc. Surg. **37:** 16–26.

13. CONNORS, M.I., W.I. STERNBERG, G. CARTER, et al. 2002. Endograft migration one to four years after endovascular abdominal aortic aneurysm repair with the AneuRx device: a cautionary note. J. Vasc. Surg. **36:** 476–484.

14. CAO, P., F. VERZINI, S. ZANNETTI, et al. 2002. Device migration after endoluminal abdominal aortic aneurysm repair: analysis of 113 cases with a minimum follow-up of 2 years. J. Vasc. Surg. **35:** 229–235.

15. LEE, J., J. LEE, I. AZIZ, et al. 2002. Stent-graft migration following endovascular repair of aneurysms with large proximal necks: anatomical risk factors and long-term sequelae. J. Endovasc. Ther. **9:** 652–654.

16. CAMBRIA, R.P., W.D. CLOUSE, J.K. DAVISON, et al. 2002. Thoracoabdominal aneurysm repair: results with 337 operations performed over a 15-year interval. Ann. Surg. **236:** 471–479.

17. COSELLI, J.S. 1994. Thoracoabdominal aortic aneurysms: experience with 372 patients. J. Card. Surg. **9:** 638–647.

18. HINES, G.L. & S. BUSUTIL. 1994. Thoraco-abdominal aneurysm resection. Determinants of survival in a community hospital. J. Cardiovasc. Surg. Torino. **35:** 243–246.

19. COX, G.S., P.J. O'HARA, N.R. HERTZER, et al. 1992. Thoracoabdominal aneurysm repair: a representative experience. J. Vasc. Surg. **15:** 780–787.

20. GODET, G., M.H. FLERON, E. VICAUT, *et al.* 1997. Risk factors for acute postoperative renal failure in thoracic or thoracoabdominal aortic surgery: a prospective study. Anesth. Analg. **85:** 1227–1232.
21. GREENBERG, R.K., A. TURC, S. HAULON, *et al.* 2004. Stent-graft migration: a reappraisal of analysis methods and proposed revised definition. J. Endovasc. Ther. **11:** 353–363.
22. OURIEL, K., D.G. CLAIR, R.K. GREENBERG, *et al.* 2003. Endovascular repair of abdominal aortic aneurysms: device-specific outcome. J. Vasc. Surg. **37:** 991–998.
23. GREENBERG, R.K., T.A. CHUTER, W.C. STERNBERGH III, *et al.* 2004. Zenith AAA endovascular graft: intermediate-term results of the US multicenter trial. J. Vasc. Surg. **39:** 1209–1218.
24. GREENBERG, R.K., T.A. CHUTER, M. LAWRENCE-BROWN, *et al.* 2004. Analysis of renal function after aneurysm repair with a device using suprarenal fixation (Zenith AAA Endovascular Graft) in contrast to open surgical repair. J. Vasc. Surg. **39:** 1219–1228.
25. LIFFMAN, K., M.M. LAWRENCE-BROWN, J.B. SEMMENS, *et al.* 2003. Suprarenal fixation: effect on blood flow of an endoluminal stent wire across an arterial orifice. J. Endovasc. Ther. **10:** 260–274.
26. GREENBERG, R.K., D. CLAIR, S. SRIVASTAVA, *et al.* 2003. Should patients with challenging anatomy be offered endovascular aneurysm repair? J. Vasc. Surg. **38:** 990–996.
27. GITLITZ, D., G. RAMASWAMI, D. KAPLAN, *et al.* 2001. Endovascular stent grafting in the presence of aortic neck filling defects: Early clinical experience. J. Vasc. Surg. **33:** 340–344.
28. BROWNE, T.F., D. HARTLEY, S. PURCHAS, *et al.* 1999. A fenestrated covered suprarenal aortic stent. Eur. J. Vasc. Endovasc. Surg. **18:** 445–449.
29. ANDERSON, J.L., M. BERCE, & D.E. HARTLEY. 2001. Endoluminal aortic grafting with renal and superior mesenteric artery incorporation by graft fenestration. J. Endovasc. Ther. **8:** 3–15.
30. STANLEY, B.M., J.B. SEMMENS, M.M. LAWRENCE-BROWN, *et al.* 2001. Fenestration in endovascular grafts for aortic aneurysm repair: new horizons for preserving blood flow in branch vessels. J. Endovasc. Ther. **8:** 16–24.
31. GREENBERG, R.K., S. HAULON, S.P. LYDEN, *et al.* 2004. Endovascular management of juxtarenal aneurysms with fenestrated endovascular grafting. J. Vasc. Surg. **39:** 279–287.
32. GREENBERG, R.K., S. HAULON, S. O'NEILL, *et al.* 2004. Primary endovascular repair of juxtarenal aneurysms with fenestrated endovascular grafting. Eur. J. Vasc. Endovasc. Surg. **27:** 484–491.
33. O'NEILL, S., R.K. GREENBERG, F. HADDAD, *et al.* 2006. A prospective analysis of fenestrated endovascular grafting: Intermediate-term outcomes. Eur. J. Vasc. Endovasc. Surg. **32(2):** 115–123.
34. LIFFMAN, K., M.M. LAWRENCE-BROWN, J.B. SEMMENS, *et al.* 2001. Analytical modeling and numerical simulation of forces in an endoluminal graft. J. Endovasc. Ther. **8:** 358–371.
35. VERHOEVEN, E.L., T.R. PRINS, I.F. TIELLIU, *et al.* 2004. Treatment of short-necked infrarenal aortic aneurysms with fenestrated stent-grafts: short-term results. Eur. J. Vasc. Endovasc. Surg. **27:** 477–483.
36. HADDAD, F., R.K. GREENBERG, E. WALKER, *et al.* 2005. Fenestrated endovascular grafting: the renal side of the story. J. Vasc. Surg. **41:** 181–190.

37. SARAC, T.P., D.G. CLAIR, N.R. HERTZER, *et al*. 2002. Contemporary results of juxtarenal aneurysm repair. J. Vasc. Surg. **36:** 1104–1111.
38. CHUTER, T.A., R.L. GORDON, L.M. REILLY, *et al*. 2001. Multi-branched stent-graft for type III thoracoabdominal aortic aneurysm. J. Vasc. Interv. Radiol. **12:** 391–392.
39. ANDERSON, J.L., D.J. ADAM, M. BERCE, *et al*. 2005. Repair of thoracoabdominal aortic aneurysms with fenestrated and branched endovascular stent grafts. J. Vasc. Surg. **42:** 600–607.
40. GREENBERG, R., K. WEST, J. FOSTER, *et al*. 2006. Beyond the aortic bifurcation: branched grafts for thoracoabdominal and aortoiliac aneurysms. J. Vasc. Surg. **43(5):** 879–886.
41. GRECO, G., N. EGOROVA, P.L. ANDERSON, *et al*. 2006. Outcomes of endovascular treatment of ruptured abdominal aortic aneurysms. J. Vasc. Surg. **43:** 453–459.

# Vibrometry

## A Novel Noninvasive Application of Ultrasonographic Physics to Estimate Wall Stress in Native Aneurysms

GAUTAM AGARWAL,[a] GEZA MOZES,[a] RANDALL R. KINNICK,[b]
PETER GLOVICZKI,[c] RUSSELL E. BRUHNKE,[d] MICHELE CARMO,[e]
TANYA L. HOSKIN,[f] KEVIN E. BENNETT,[d] AND JAMES L. GREENLEAF[g]

[a]Department of Vascular Surgery, Mayo Clinic, Rochester, Minnesota, USA

[b]Ultrasound Research Laboratory, Mayo Clinic, Rochester, Minnesota, USA

[c]Gonda Vascular Center, Mayo Clinic, Rochester, Minnesota, USA

[d]Division of Engineering, Mayo Clinic, Rochester, Minnesota, USA

[e]Tedd Rogers International Fellow, Mayo Clinic, Rochester, Minnesota, USA

[f]Division of Biostatistics, Mayo Clinic, Rochester, Minnesota, USA

[g]Department of Biophysics, Mayo Clinic, Rochester, Minnesota, USA

ABSTRACT: Our objective was to test vibrometry as a means to measure changes in aneurysm sac pressure in an *in vitro* aneurysm model. Explanted porcine abdominal aortas and nitrile rubber tubes were used to model an aneurysm sac. An ultrasound beam was used to vibrate the surface of the aneurysm model. The motion generated on the surface was detected either by reflected laser light or by a second ultrasound probe. This was recorded at different aneurysm pressures. The phase of the propagating wave was measured to assess changes in velocity and to see if there was a correlation with aneurysm pressure. The cumulative phase shift detected by laser or Doppler correlated well with increasing hydrostatic pressure in both the rubber and the porcine aorta model. The square of the mean pressure correlated well with the cumulative phase shift when dynamic pressure was generated by a pump. However, the pulse pressure was poorly correlated with the cumulative phase shift. Noninvasive measurement of changes in aortic aneurysm sac tension is feasible in an *in vitro* setting using the concept of vibrometry. This could potentially be used to noninvasively detect wall stress in native aneurysms and endotension after endovascular aneurysm repair (EVAR) and to predict the risk of rupture.

Address for correspondence: Peter Gloviczki, M.D., Chairman Gonda Vascular Center, Mayo Clinic, Rochester, MN 55905. Voice: 507-284-4652; fax: 507-266-7156.
e-mail: gloviczki.peter@mayo.edu

Ann. N.Y. Acad. Sci. 1085: 197–207 (2006). © 2006 New York Academy of Sciences.
doi: 10.1196/annals.1383.001

KEYWORDS: vibrometry; ultrasound; aneurysm

## BACKGROUND

The risk of rupture of an abdominal aortic aneurysm (AAA) is difficult to measure. This also applies to endovascular AAA repair (EVAR) as the risk of rupture is not completely eliminated.

AAA rupture relates primarily to the size of the aneurysm with a clear increase in risk over 5 cm.[1] Sequential imaging with either ultrasonography (US) or computed tomographic (CT) angiography is used conventionally to follow aneurysms. However, small aneurysms are also known to rupture. There is no true noninvasive technique that can measure the aneurysmal wall stress and predict aneurysm rupture.

EVAR also necessitates lifelong follow-up with imaging studies due to the potential for endoleak at attachment sites, structural failure of device, changes to arterial wall due to aging, and ongoing aneurysmal degeneration. The mainstay of current follow-up is CT angiography, supplemented selectively with US and catheter angiography, aiming at the detection of endoleaks, endograft deformation, migration, and enlargement of the aneurysm. Unfortunately, rupture after EVAR is reported in different series to occur at a 0.5–2% frequency over 3–5 years after repair.[2–4]

Significantly increasing or decreasing aneurysm size on follow-up images can suggest failure or success of the repair; however, in many patients, the size of the aneurysm remains unchanged. These patients, if no detectable endoleak is present, may have endotension and are exposed to an uncertain risk of aneurysm rupture.[5,6] Additionally, follow-up with CT angiography requires repeated exposure to ionizing radiation and to large volumes of nephrotoxic contrast dye.

Intuitively, the risk of rupture should be dependent on the pressure in the aneurysm sac. Current attempts at measuring pressure in the aneurysm sac require either invasive catheterization or the implantation of pressure sensors. No method is currently available for noninvasive monitoring of the aneurysm wall tension.

## OUR HYPOTHESIS

Our hypothesis in this study was that "vibrometry" is a suitable method to assess wall tension in an experimental *in vitro* aortic aneurysm model. Radiation pressure such as that generated by US can vibrate a surface from a distance without direct contact. The velocity ($v$) of the resulting waves within the surface depends on the tensile stress ($t$) of the vibrated surface and the material density ($d$): $v = (t/d)^{-2}$. By measuring the change in wave velocity, it is possible to detect the change in tensile stress and calculate the pressure through the vibrated surface. The aim of our study was to test this concept in an *in vitro* aneurysm model.

## MATERIALS AND METHODS

Explanted porcine aortas and elastic nitrile tubes (4.5 × 2.5 cm in diameter; 0.5 mm thick) were used to model the aneurysm sac (FIGS. 1 and 2). Segments (4.5 × 0.6–0.9 cm in diameter) of the infrarenal abdominal aorta of 40- to 45-kg Yorkshire pigs were harvested and prepared (side branches were ligated and periadventitial tissues were removed). Animal care and killing were in compliance with the corresponding institutional policies.

The aneurysm sac model was secured to 20- or 6-mm cannulas proximally and distally and connected to a hydrostatic (fluid column or pressure bag) or dynamic (Bio-Console Pump; Bio-Medicus, Minneapolis, MN, USA) pressure source with silicone rubber tubes and immersed in a water bath. The aneurysm sac was perfused with degassed water (nitrile tube) or a 0.9% sodium chloride solution (porcine aorta) at room temperature. Through a side connection of the distal cannula, a 7F angiocatheter was introduced into the lumen of

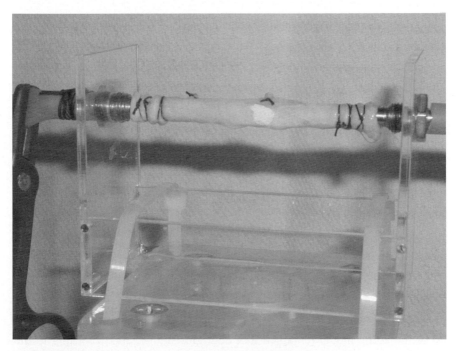

**FIGURE 1.** The porcine aorta aneurysm sac model.

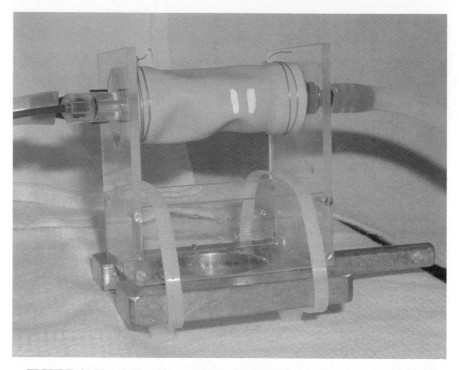

**FIGURE 2.** The nitrile rubber aneurysm sac model.

the aneurysm model and connected to a digital pressure monitor. A 45-mm-diameter 3 MHz drive transducer and a 5 MHz dual-element Doppler transducer were positioned near the axial center of the aneurysm with their focal points spaced 2.5 cm apart on the surface of the model. The focal lengths of the transducers were 10 and 8 cm, respectively. The surface of the aneurysm sac model was vibrated with a focused US beam with a center frequency of 3 MHz and amplitude modulated at 500 Hz. The resulting motion was detected either by a laser vibrometer (PSV-300; Polytec, Inc., Tustin, CA, USA) or by a Doppler transducer operating in continuous-wave mode (FIG. 3). The phase of the propagating wave was measured to assess changes in velocity with different pressures (e.g., at pressure 1 and 2 [P1 and P2, respectively]; FIG. 4). Phase measurements were taken in this manner at 10-mm Hg intervals over a range of 50 to 200 mm Hg. The lowest value of pressure used in this study was selected on the basis of visual observations of full inflation; this suggests that additional increases in pressure would have been associated with minimal changes in diameter. This setting allowed us to use pressure as a surrogate measure of wall tension because changes in the radius ($r$) and wall thickness ($t$) of the aortic model remained in a negligible range, and according to the law of Laplace ($\gamma = \Delta\, Pr/2t$), wall tension ($\gamma$) was primarily determined by

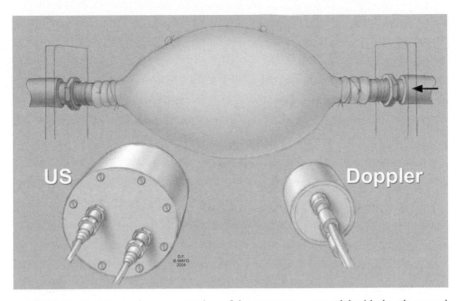

**FIGURE 3.** Schematic representation of the aneurysm sac model with the ultrasound and Doppler transducer.

pressure changes ($\Delta P$). The maximum pressure evaluated was determined by the capacity of the pressure sources and by the resistance of the experimental aneurysm model connections to leakage. Wall strain was not measured directly with a strain gauge because it would have required material properties to calculate tension. We did not have the appropriate scanner for measuring the diameter changes of the sac with pressure because the variation in diameter was a very small fraction of the baseline size of the aneurysm model.

A phase shift was calculated for each 10 mm Hg incremental increase in pressure. The wave phase at baseline (50 and 110 mm Hg mean pressure depending on the pressure source and 24 mm Hg pulse pressure) was normalized to 0°. The phase-shift values were sequentially added for each 10 mm Hg increase in pressure to obtain the cumulative phase-shift curve.

The relationship between cumulative phase shift and pressure was assessed visually, and linear regression models were used to describe the relationship between these two values for series measurements recorded across a range of pressures in a particular experiment. A simple linear regression model with only a pressure term was used when possible. However, when plots revealed curvature in the relationship, a quadratic term was included in the model. For each relationship assessed in this way, the strength of the association is reported as the coefficient of determination ($R^2$). In models that do not include the quadratic term, the square root of $R^2$ is equal to the correlation coefficient ($r$) between cumulative phase shift and pressure. In all cases, $R^2$ is interpreted as the percentage of variability in the response (cumulative phase shift) accounted

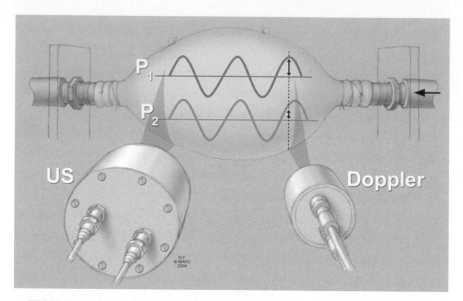

**FIGURE 4.** Phase shift measurement. The radiation force of an amplitude modulated ultrasound (US) beam vibrates the surface of the aneurysm. Continuous-wave (CW) Doppler detects the phase of the propagating wave at different pressures ($P_1$ and $P_2$). The difference between the phase of the wave at $P_1$ and $P_2$ pressures is the phase shift.

for by the model. In addition, overall $P$ values are reported for each model. Correlation coefficients are reported when a simple linear model is deemed appropriate. In experiments involving multiple animals, a separate correlation coefficient was calculated for each animal and an average correlation was calculated across animals. $P$ values $<0.05$ were considered statistically significant. Analyses were performed with JMP statistical software (version 5.1.2; SAS Institute, Inc., Cary, NC, USA).

## RESULTS

In the rubber aneurysm model (12 series of measurements), strong relationships were observed between cumulative phase shift and pressure. One experiment applied hydrostatic pressure by a static fluid column (50–110 mm Hg). Four series of cumulative phase-shift measurements were collected across this pressure range with 10 mm Hg incremental increases in pressure (FIG. 5). A quadratic regression model predicting cumulative phase shift using pressure and the square of pressure yielded $R^2 = 0.99$. The overall P value for this model was $<0.0001$, and both the linear and quadratic terms were highly significant ($P < 0.0001$). Similarly, four series of cumulative phase-shift measurements were collected for hydrostatic pressure applied by a pressure bag across

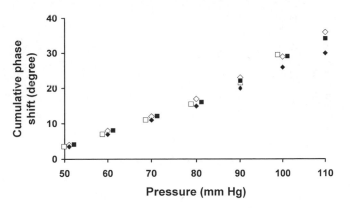

**FIGURE 5.** In the nitrile rubber aneurysm model the square of the hydrostatic pressure applied by a static fluid column (50–110 mm Hg) correlated well with the cumulative phase shift. (Different shapes [square, rhombus] of the plots label different sessions, while empty and dark plots with the same shape label different series within one session; $R^2 = 0.99$, $P < 0.0001$.)

pressures ranging from 110 to 200 mm Hg (FIG. 6). Again, a quadratic regression model using pressure and pressure squared explained nearly all of the variability in cumulative phase shift with $R^2 = 0.96$ and had a highly significant $P$ value for the entire model ($P < 0.0001$). Four series of measurements using a pump to generate dynamic pressure (110–200 mm Hg) in the same rubber aneurysm model resulted in $R^2 = 0.92$ ($P < 0.0001$) for the regression model using pressure and the square of pressure to predict the cumulative phase shift

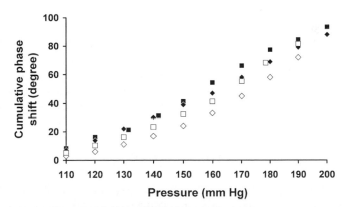

**FIGURE 6.** In the nitrile rubber aneurysm model the square of the hydrostatic pressure applied by a pressure bag (110–200 mm Hg) correlated well with the cumulative phase shift. (Different shapes [square, rhombus] of the plots label different sessions, while empty and dark plots with the same shape label different series within one session; $R^2 = 0.96$, $P < 0.0001$.)

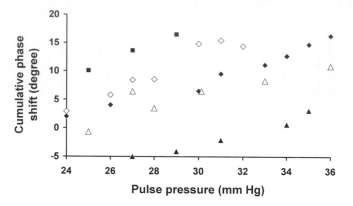

**FIGURE 7.** In the nitrile rubber aneurysm model cumulative phase shift correlated poorly with the pulse pressure. (Different shapes [square, rhombus, triangle] of the plots label different sessions, while empty and dark plots with the same shape label different series within one session $r = 0.38$, $P < 0.02$.)

detected by laser. In a new set of experiments, however, the cumulative phase shift showed only a weak correlation with the pulse pressure (24–36 mm Hg; FIG. 7). Specifically, the observed correlation coefficient between cumulative phase shift and pulse pressure was only 0.38 ($P= 0.02$).

In the porcine *in vitro* aortic sac model, 12 series of measurements were recorded by using aortas from five animals. In this model, the cumulative phase shift detected by laser showed a strong linear relationship with the dynamic pressure between 50 and 200 mm Hg. The correlation coefficients between the two measurements for each of the five animals were 0.99, 0.94, 0.98, 0.97, and 0.97 for an average correlation coefficient between cumulative phase shift and dynamic pressure across animals of 0.97 ($P < 0.0001$). In the same porcine model (six series of measurements in three animals), the cumulative phase shift detected by Doppler scan correlated well with the dynamic pressure between 50 and 200 mm Hg with an average correlation coefficient of 0.98 across the three animals; the three individual correlation coefficients between the measurements for these animals were 0.99, 0.96, and 0.98 (all $P < 0.0001$; FIG. 8).

## DISCUSSION

To identify patients noninvasively who are more likely to rupture would be "ideal." None of the currently available follow-up modalities, either alone or in combination, fulfill these requirements.

Aneurysms rupture when the material strength of the aortic wall is exceeded by the tangential wall tension. The current available methods do not estimate aortic wall tension directly. In fact, aneurysm diameter and pressure

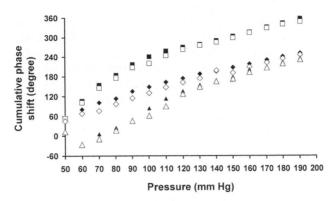

**FIGURE 8.** In the porcine model the cumulative phase shift detected by Doppler correlated well with the aneurysm pressure. (Different shapes [square, rhombus, triangle] of the plots label different sessions, while empty and dark plots with the same shape label different series within one session; $r = 0.96 - 0.99$.)

measurements are indirect indicators of wall tension and the risk of rupture. Vibrometry using Laplace's law ($\gamma = \Delta Pr/2t$, where $\gamma$ indicates wall tension, $\Delta P$ indicates pressure gradient, $r$ indicates radius, and $t$ indicates thickness of the wall) measures changes in aortic wall tension and may predict aneurysm rupture.[7]

Aneurysm sac shrinkage after EVAR occurs only in 39%, 60%, and 68% of cases at 1, 2, and 3 years, respectively. Sac enlargement is seen in 3.5% at 1 year, 11% at 2 years, and 21% at 3 years.[8] So aneurysm diameter, although the most established parameter predicting aneurysm rupture, may not be useful after EVAR. In spite of low rates of sac shrinkage, the incidence of aneurysm rupture after EVAR is low. Changes in the tangential wall tension of the excluded sac after EVAR can perhaps identify patients who are at increased risk of rupture.

Compartmentalization due to the presence of intrasac thrombus has been described after EVAR.[9] With any catheter-based technique or implanted pressure sensor, this could lead to erroneous intrasac pressure measurements. Recently, many centers have published their experience with the implantable pressure sensors.[9] Intrasac pressure measurement with implanted pressure sensors has the advantage of avoiding the need for repeat catheterization by using wireless charging and transducer techniques.[10,11] If sensors are implanted routinely at the time of repair, this method does not necessitate any secondary interventions; however, long-term implantation of the sensors may lead to compartmentalization. Moreover, these sensors are expensive and hence seldom used.

Our method directly measures changes in wall tension ($\gamma$) using vibrometry, whereas the previous methods measured variables on the left side of Laplace's equation (aneurysm size and intrasac pressure). The background of vibrometry in physics is that the velocity ($v$) of waves within a surface depends on the tensile stress ($t$) and the material density ($d$) of the vibrated surface[7]

$[v = (t/d)^{-2}]$. The general concept of using amplitude-modulated US and Doppler US for vibrometry has been described earlier by Fatemi and Greenleaf.[12] Our hypothesis in this study was that vibrometry is a suitable method to assess wall tension in an experimental *in vitro* aortic aneurysm model. We used the phase shift of the propagating wave instead of velocity because measuring velocity would have required more complex calibration without the addition of any information on the hypothesis tested. We had no other available method of measuring wall tension to serve as a control for vibrometry; therefore, we chose the experimental setting in a way that allowed us to use pressure for controlling wall tension. The aneurysm models were prestretched to a point at which additional changes in pressure were associated with minimal changes in diameter. Therefore, correlation between pressure and phase shift would represent well the correlation between wall tension and wave velocity or phase shift. In an *in vitro* aorta model, we found that the mean, but not the pulse, intrasac pressure correlated well with the phase shift of the propagating wave measured by vibrometry.

Our study has limitations that may be encountered when this technique is tested *in vivo*. First, even a prestretched *in vitro* aneurysm model is far from being an ideal spherical object, and, therefore, changes in the intrasac pressure will not perfectly reflect changes in wall tension. Second, in terms of clinical utility, a major concern is the need for calibration; during our study, we did not measure absolute values, but only changes in wall tension and in the corresponding intrasac pressure. There are two potential solutions for this problem: changes in wall tension can be evaluated before and after the exclusion during EVAR, or the surface of the nonaneurysmal aorta or the endograft can be used as an internal reference point. Material characteristics of an endograft can be measured before implantation. Therefore, if the tension of this surface is measured *in vivo* with vibrometry, the transmural pressure (transmural pressure = aortic pressure − intrasac pressure) can be calculated. Routine cuff blood pressure measurements can be used to approximate the aortic pressure in the absence of significant subclavian artery stenosis and the intrasac pressure can easily be calculated. The third limitation of our study may be technical: it is not known how changes in material density and elasticity or the presence of calcification will alter wave propagation and cause deterioration of the signal. Some of these problems may require complex electronic filtering of the wave signals detected to obtain appropriate sensitivity with vibrometry. The density of the aortic wall may vary among different patients; however, it is not expected to change significantly within the same aneurysm. Calcification may interfere with vibrometry and limit the evaluation to uncalcified areas of the aneurysm wall. Another limitation is that the experiment was set to examine pressure changes in a limited interval of 50 to 200 mm Hg, although we have no reason to think that vibrometry would not work at lower pressures as well.

Finally, *in vitro* application of vibrometry for noninvasive measurement of aortic aneurysm sac tension is feasible. The concept of vibrometry should be adopted to develop the technology to detect native aneurysm wall tension and endotension noninvasively or to assess aneurysm sac pressure associated with different endoleaks after endovascular repair.

## REFERENCES

1. THOMPSON, J.E., W.V. GARRETT, A.D. PATMAN, *et al*. 1982. Surgery for abdominal aortic aneurysms. *In* Aneurysms Diagnosis and Treatment. J. Bergan & J. Yao, Eds.: 287–299. Grune & Stratton. New York, NY.

2. OHKI, T., F.J. VEITH, P. SHAW, *et al*. 2001. Increasing incidence of midterm and long-term complications after endovascular graft repair of abdominal aortic aneurysms: a note of caution based on a 9-year experience. Ann. Surg. **234:** 323–334, discussion 334–335.

3. ZARINS, C.K., R.A. WHITE, F.L. MOLL, *et al*. 2001. The AneuRx stent graft: four-year results and worldwide experience 2000. J. Vasc. Surg. **33**(2 Suppl): S135–S145. [Erratum appears in J. Vasc. Surg. 2001;**33:** 1318].

4. HARRIS, P.L., S.R. VALLABHANENI, P. DESGRANGES, *et al*. 2000. Incidence and risk factors of late rupture, conversion, and death after endovascular repair of infrarenal aortic aneurysms: the EUROSTAR experience. European Collaborators on Stent/graft techniques for aortic aneurysm repair. J. Vasc. Surg. **32:** 739–749.

5. LIN, P.H., R.L. BUSH, J.B. KATZMAN, *et al*. 2003. Delayed aortic aneurysm enlargement due to endotension after endovascular abdominal aortic aneurysm repair. J. Vasc. Surg. **38:** 840–842.

6. SUROWIEC, S.M., M.G. DAVIES, A.J. FEGLEY, *et al*. 2004. Relationship of proximal fixation to postoperative renal dysfunction in patients with normal serum creatinine concentration. J. Vasc. Surg. **39:** 804–810.

7. SUMNER, D. 2000. Essential hemodynamic principles. *In* Vascular Surgery, 5th ed. R.B. Rutherford, Ed.: 73–120.WB Saunders. Philadelphia, PA.

8. OURIEL, K., D.G. CLAIR, R.K. GREENBERG, *et al*. 2003. Endovascular repair of abdominal aortic aneurysms: device-specific outcome. J. Vasc. Surg. **37:** 991–998.

9. SHARIF, H.E., A. CARROCCIO, R.A. LOOKSTEIN, *et al*. 2006. Abdominal aortic aneurysm sac shrinkage after endovascular aneurysm repair: correlation with chronic sac pressure measurement. J. Vasc. Surg. **43:** 2–7.

10. MILNER, R., H.J. VERHAGEN, M. PRINSSEN & J.D. BLANKENSTEIJN. 2004. Noninvasive intrasac pressure measurement and the influence of type 2 and type 3 endoleaks in an animal model of abdominal aortic aneurysm. Vascular **12:** 99–105.

11. ELLOZY, S.H., A. CARROCCIO, R.A. LOOKSTEIN, *et al*. 2004. First experience in human beings with a permanently implantable intrasac pressure transducer for monitoring endovascular repair of abdominal aortic aneurysms. J. Vasc. Surg. **40:** 405–412.

12. FATEMI, M. & J.F. GREENLEAF. 2000. Probing the dynamics of tissue at low frequencies with the radiation force of ultrasound. Phys. Med. Biol. **45:** 1449–1464.

# Combining Open and Endovascular Approaches to Complex Aneurysms

SCOTT A. LEMAIRE

*The Texas Heart Institute at St. Luke's Episcopal Hospital and The Division of Cardiothoracic Surgery, Michael E. DeBakey Department of Surgery, Baylor College of Medicine, Houston, TX, USA*

ABSTRACT: Patients with aortic aneurysms commonly present with anatomic issues that preclude them from receiving purely endovascular repairs. In these situations, open surgical procedures can be used to manage anatomic problems and facilitate endovascular aneurysm repair. This report focuses on combined approaches that enable repair of abdominal or thoracoabdominal aortic aneurysms that involve the mesenteric and/or renal circulation. Current experience with combined open/endovascular repairs is essentially anecdotal. The common feature among the open procedures is establishment of extra-anatomic perfusion of the visceral arteries to enable ligation and subsequent coverage of their ostia during endograft placement. The existing reports are notable for the marked variability in many factors including extent of aneurysm repair, surgical approach, mode of visceral revascularization, conduit for bypass, and type of endovascular device used. Overall, current reports demonstrate that patients with limited physiologic reserve and complex aortic anatomy can be treated successfully by combining open and endovascular repairs. As endograft design and endovascular techniques continue to improve, combined approaches are likely to play an increasingly important role in the treatment of extensive aortic disease.

KEYWORDS: aortic aneurysm; endovascular; surgery; hybrid procedures

Patients with aortic aneurysms commonly present with anatomic issues that preclude them from receiving purely endovascular repairs. In these situations, open surgical procedures can be used to manage anatomic problems and facilitate endovascular aneurysm repair. For example, open surgical approaches are commonly employed to enable device delivery through suboptimal peripheral arteries. Open operations can also be used to preserve the brachiocephalic circulation prior to placement of thoracic aortic endografts, or to preserve the internal iliac circulation prior to placing aortoiliac endografts.

Address for correspondence: Scott A. LeMaire, M.D., One Baylor Plaza, BCM 390, Houston, TX 77030, USA. Voice: 832-355-9910; fax: 832-355-9948.
e-mail: slemaire@bcm.tmc.edu

Ann. N.Y. Acad. Sci. 1085: 208–212 (2006). © 2006 New York Academy of Sciences.
doi: 10.1196/annals.1383.040

This report focuses on combined approaches that enable abdominal or thoracoabdominal aortic aneurysm repairs involving the mesenteric and/or renal circulation.

## RATIONALE FOR COMBINED APPROACHES

Two major factors that are considered when deciding between open and endovascular abdominal aortic aneurysm repairs are the patient's physiologic status and their vascular anatomy (TABLE 1).[1] The anatomic issues that preclude purely endovascular repairs generally involve landing zones that will not allow secure endograft fixation because of inadequate length, excessive angulation, extensive intraluminal thrombus, or severe vessel calcification. Open aortic aneurysm repairs are ideal for directly addressing complex anatomy but require considerable physiologic reserve. Endovascular repairs can reduce physiologic strain, but may not provide durable repairs in the setting of complex anatomy. Combining open and endovascular approaches capitalizes on the main advantages of both, thereby providing durable repairs in patients with problematic anatomy, while minimizing physiologic insult and postoperative morbidity and mortality. Therefore, combined approaches—commonly called "hybrid procedures"—seem particularly well suited for patients with limited physiologic reserve (precluding standard open repair) and complex aneurysm anatomy (precluding standard endovascular repair).

## CURRENT TECHNIQUES AND RESULTS

Compared to the vast experience that has accumulated for endovascular aortic repairs in general, experience with combined approaches remains essentially anecdotal. The existing literature is comprised primarily of single case reports and small case series.[2–14] The largest series was reported in 2005 by Fulton and colleagues[15]; they used combined approaches to repair juxtarenal, suprarenal, and thoracoabdominal aortic aneurysms in 10 patients, all of whom survived and remained well up to 13 months after operation.

The existing reports are notable for the marked variability in many factors including surgical approach (laparotomy vs. retroperitoneal exposure vs.

**TABLE 1. Treatment approaches based on the physiologic reserve of the patient and the anatomic complexity of the repair (Adapted from Greenberg et al.[1])**

| Physiologic risk | Anatomic complexity | Approach |
|---|---|---|
| Low | Low | Well served by open or endovascular repair |
| Low | High | Ideal for open repair |
| High | Low | Ideal for endovascular repair |
| High | High | Ideal for a combined approach |

thoracoabdominal incision), extent of repair, mode of revascularization (vessel translocation vs. ligation with bypass), conduit for bypass (reversed saphenous vein vs. prosthetic graft vs. transposed iliac artery), and type of endovascular device used. The timing of the open and endovascular repairs has also varied. While both procedures can be carried out in a single setting, they can also be staged, allowing a brief recovery period between the open procedure and the subsequent endovascular repair. Although patient ages have varied considerably (range 49–84 years, mean 68.7 ± 10.2 years), most patients presented with substantial comorbid conditions that precluded standard open repair. Solitary kidney was a common feature.

The extent of aortic coverage has varied widely ranging from short juxtarenal abdominal aortic aneurysm repairs to full thoracoabdominal aortic repairs. The most extreme examples have been reported by Flye and colleagues,[14] who described successful hybrid Crawford extent II thoracoabdominal aortic aneurysm repairs in three patients, and Svensson and colleagues,[13] who described endovascular completions of total aortic replacement in two patients who had previously undergone open aortic arch repairs using the elephant trunk technique.

The common feature among the open procedures is establishment of extra-anatomic perfusion of the mesenteric and/or renal arteries in order to enable ligation and subsequent coverage of their ostia during endograft placement. The sources of inflow for visceral bypass grafts have included the descending thoracic aorta, the infrarenal aorta, the common or external iliac arteries, pre-existing aortic or iliac grafts, and the hepatic artery. Alternative methods have included translocation of the celiac axis onto the superior mesenteric artery. Lawrence-Brown and colleagues[3] simply ligated a well-collateralized celiac trunk to optimize the distal landing zone during thoracoabdominal aortic repair; they also used the open approach to secure the distal end of the endograft using transaortic sutures and a periaortic Dacron wrap.

The lack of standardized reporting makes overall outcomes somewhat difficult to assess. It is clear, however, that most patients survived the procedures and were discharged from the hospital. Two early deaths have been reported, one due to ischemic pancreatitis and one due to multiple organ failure.[9,10] Reported early complications have included acute renal failure, bleeding from a ligated right renal stump, infected retroperitoneal hematoma, and transient cerebral ischemic attack.[2,3,6,14] One patient developed hepatic insufficiency that was attributed to kinking of the transposed iliac artery that had been used to revascularize the mesenteric circulation; the patient recovered well after revision of the conduit.[11] Paraplegia has not been reported despite coverage of a substantial proportion of the descending thoracic aorta during several of the procedures. Late deaths have been attributed to ruptured ascending aortic aneurysm (at 3 months) and cardiac disease (at 3 years).[3,10] Several reports[6,10,11,14,15] have documented survival of at least 1 year, and two reports[3,12] have documented 3-year survival.

Given their extensive disease and complex repairs, these patients should be followed with an aggressive postoperative surveillance imaging program; Greenberg and colleagues[1] obtain spiral computed tomography scans and four-view flat-plate radiographs before discharge, 1–3 months postprocedure, 6 months postprocedure, 12 months postprocedure, and annually thereafter. Type III endoleaks have been reported in two cases; one was successfully repaired with a bridging endovascular graft.[10,14]

## CONCLUSION

Several recent reports have demonstrated that patients with limited physiologic reserve and complex aortic anatomy can be treated successfully by combining open and endovascular repairs. As endograft design and endovascular techniques continue to improve, combined approaches are likely to play an increasingly important role in the treatment of extensive aortic disease.

## REFERENCES

1. GREENBERG, R.K., D. CLAIR, S. SRIVASTAVA, et al. 2003. Should patients with challenging anatomy be offered endovascular aneurysm repair? J. Vasc. Surg. **38:** 990–996.
2. QUINONES-BALDRICH, W.J., T.F. PANETTA, C.L. VESCERA & V.S. KASHYAP. 1999. Repair of type IV thoracoabdominal aneurysm with a combined endovascular and surgical approach. J. Vasc. Surg. **30:** 555–560.
3. LAWRENCE-BROWN, M., K. SIEUNARINE, G. VAN SCHIE, et al. 2000. Hybrid open-endoluminal technique for repair of thoracoabdominal aneurysm involving the celiac axis. J. Endovasc. Ther. **7:** 513–519.
4. YANO, O.J., P.L. FARIES, N. MORRISSEY, et al. 2001. Ancillary techniques to facilitate endovascular repair of aortic aneurysms. J. Vasc. Surg. **34:** 69–75.
5. AGOSTINELLI, A., S. SACCANI, A.M. BUDILLON, et al. 2002. Repair of coexistent infrarenal and thoracoabdominal aortic aneurysm: combined endovascular and open surgical procedure with visceral vessel relocation. J. Thorac. Cardiovasc. Surg. **124:** 184–185.
6. KHOURY, M. 2002. Endovascular repair of recurrent thoracoabdominal aortic aneurysm. J. Endovasc. Ther. **9:** II106–II111.
7. WATANABE, Y., S. ISHIMARU, S. KAWAGUCHI, et al. 2002. Successful endografting with simultaneous visceral artery bypass grafting for severely calcified thoracoabdominal aortic aneurysm. J. Vasc. Surg. **35:** 297–299.
8. OREND, K.H., T. KOTSIS, R. SCHARRER-PAMLER, et al. 2002. Endovascular repair of aortic rupture due to trauma and aneurysm. Eur. J. Vasc. Endovasc. Surg. **23:** 61–67.
9. OREND, K.H., R. SCHARRER-PAMLER, X. KAPFER, et al. 2003. Endovascular treatment in diseases of the descending thoracic aorta: 6-year results of a single center. J. Vasc. Surg. **37:** 91–99.

10. KOTSIS, T., R. SCHARRER-PAMLER, X. KAPFER, *et al.* 2003. Treatment of thoracoabdominal aortic aneurysms with a combined endovascular and surgical approach. Int. Angiol. **22:** 125–133.

11. IGURO, Y., G. YOTSUMOTO, N. ISHIZAKI, *et al.* 2003. Endovascular stent-graft repair for thoracoabdominal aneurysm after reconstruction of the superior mesenteric and celiac arteries. J. Thorac. Cardiovasc. Surg. **125:** 956–958.

12. LIN, P.H., K. MADSEN, R.L. BUSH & A.B. LUMSDEN. 2003. Iliorenal artery bypass grafting to facilitate endovascular abdominal aortic aneurysm repair. J. Vasc. Surg. **38:** 183–185.

13. SVENSSON, L.G., K.H. KIM, E.H. BLACKSTONE, *et al.* 2004. Elephant trunk procedure: newer indications and uses. Ann. Thorac. Surg. **78:** 109–116.

14. FLYE, M.W., E.T. CHOI, L.A. SANCHEZ, *et al.* 2004. Retrograde visceral vessel revascularization followed by endovascular aneurysm exclusion as an alternative to open surgical repair of thoracoabdominal aortic aneurysm. J. Vasc. Surg. **39:** 454–458.

15. FULTON, J.J., M.A. FARBER, W.A. MARSTON, *et al.* 2005. Endovascular stent-graft repair of pararenal and type IV thoracoabdominal aortic aneurysms with adjunctive visceral reconstruction. J. Vasc. Surg. **41:** 191–198.

# Engineering Improvements in Endovascular Devices

## Design and Validation

DAVID M. WILLIAMS

*Radiology Department, University of Michigan Hospitals, Ann Arbor, Michigan, USA*

ABSTRACT: Advances in endovascular treatment of vascular disease have focused on basic and translational research of vascular disease and endovascular devices. Clinical trials serve to establish the safety and efficacy of engineering advances that incorporate this research. Recent position statements by the Food and Drug Administration (FDA) emphasize that research into conducting these trials in a timely and cost-effective manner (critical path research) is as important to patient care as the engineering advances themselves. This article reviews the recent FDA documents discussing critical path research, highlighting those topics that the FDA emphasizes. Several directions of translational research in which engineering advances may contribute to enhanced device design and improved patient care are reviewed.

KEYWORDS: critical path research; endografts; Food and Drug Administration (FDA)

## INTRODUCTION

The endograft revolution is upon us. As we evaluate third and fourth generation devices for treating abdominal aortic aneurysms, wrestle with endoleaks, and debate how rigorously to follow device IFUs in treating the patient with marginal anatomy, it is tempting to think that engineering advances will solve our problems. However, when we are speaking of how to treat an aneurysm, our problems become our patients' problems. Several recent Food and Drug Administration (FDA) documents serve to remind us that the world of devices is more complicated than searching for engineering improvements. Basic science advances are a small part of adding a new device to the daily inventory of the interventionalist. While chemical engineering no doubt has much to

Address for correspondence: David M. Williams, M.D., Radiology Department, University of Michigan Hospitals, Ann Arbor, MI 48109-0030. Voice: 734-615-2890; fax: 734-615-1276.
e-mail: davidwms@med.umich.edu

Ann. N.Y. Acad. Sci. 1085: 213–223 (2006). © 2006 New York Academy of Sciences.
doi: 10.1196/annals.1383.021

contribute to endograft technology, a more pressing question is: What is the probability that a chemical (or other) engineering improvement will find its way into a new device on the shelf?

## CRITICAL PATH RESEARCH

The first of these FDA documents is a report from March 2004, Challenge and Opportunity on the Critical Path to New Medical Products.[1] According to the FDA, the applied sciences needed for product development have lagged advances in the basic sciences. Furthermore, there has not been "enough validated work towards showing how the safety and effectiveness of new products can be demonstrated faster, with more certainty, and at lower costs." Finally, the path of a device to market is "long, costly . . . inefficient," and, we may add, unsure. In support of these observations, the FDA presented evidence of steadily increasing financial outlays by the pharmaceutical R&D enterprises and the FDA (FIG. 1), and declining submissions of new molecular entities and biologics license applications (FIG. 2). Other data from the FDA web site show similar trends in submissions of original PMAs, IDEs, and HDEs (FIG. 3) and 510(k)s (FIG. 4).[2] While a comparable figure for device failure is not available, 75% of the cumulative research and development costs of new drugs are due to failure of the drug to meet safety or efficacy standards.[3] The

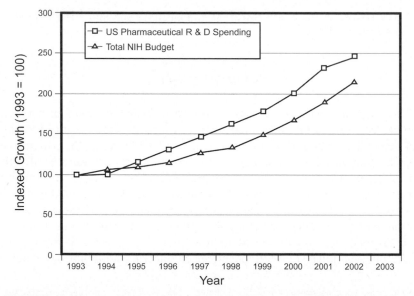

**FIGURE 1.** Graph showing increasing expenditure by pharmaceutical companies and the FDA for drug development (http://www.fda.gov/oc/initiatives/criticalpath/whitepaper.html).

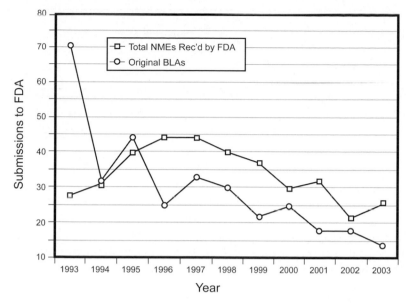

**FIGURE 2.** Graph showing declining submissions of new molecular entities and biologics license applications (http://www.fda.gov/oc/initiatives/criticalpath/whitepaper.html).

research model discussed in the FDA Critical Path report focuses separately on basic sciences research, translational research, and what the FDA calls "critical path research" (FIG. 4). The presentations in this symposium have been in the categories of basic sciences and translational research. Before taking up the charge of this presentation, namely surveying engineering advances that will improve endovascular treatment of aneurysms, which comprise another facet of translational research, it is worthwhile looking in greater detail at the FDA discussion of critical path research.

The FDA lists six areas of critical path research, four of which (TABLE 1) are pertinent to the medical and economical environment affecting development of current medical devices.[4] From a list of 66 specific topics within these four areas, 18 (27%) are pertinent to endovascular treatment of aneurysms (TABLES 2–5). The list is not exhaustive. Recent experience in conducting U.S. device trials has highlighted additional challenges and opportunities for improvement (TABLE 6). These challenges affected the Wallgraft trial for treatment of arterial pseudoaneurysms and numerous endograft trials for treatment of aortic aneurysm.

Recently, at the 2006 Centennial FDA Science Forum, a group of FDA staff, industry representatives, and university investigators met " . . . [to discuss] how emerging science and technology can be effectively applied in support of the FDA's public health mission, [and] . . . to revisit the investment in regulatory science and communicate not only the tangible results of that investment, but highlight the process by which that original commitment to high quality

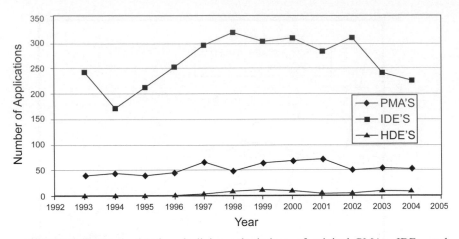

**FIGURE 3.** Graph showing declining submissions of original PMAs, IDEs, and HDEs adapted from web site (as of May 3, 2006) http://www.fda.gov/cdrh/annual/fy2004/ode/part3.html.

scientific achievement will translate into the future of science at [the] FDA."[5] From a list of 24 break-out sessions in this forum, eight (33%) discussed topics relevant to critical path research in medical device development (TABLE 7). To give the reader the flavor of the conference, some of these topics are listed in TABLE 8; for the sake of brevity, the presenter and parent institution have been omitted, but are available on the web site.

To summarize these recent discussions of critical path research, approximately one-third of the effort has been devoted to topics directly relevant to medical device development. Success in streamlining the path from device

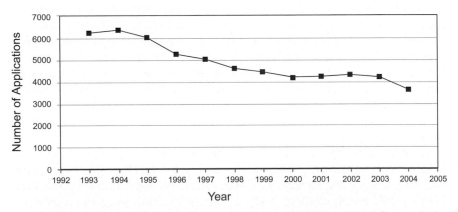

**FIGURE 4.** Graph showing declining submissions of 510(k)s adapted from web site (as of May 3, 2006) http://www.fda.gov/cdrh/annual/fy2004/ode/part3.html.[2]

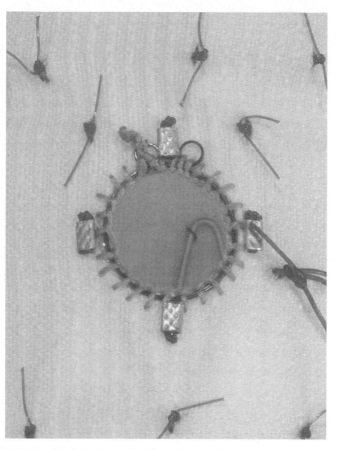

**FIGURE 5.** Detail of fenestrated endograft showing nitinol-reinforced fenestration, radio-opaque markers, and securing sutures in this hand-sewn device.

design to implantation is critical for economic, scientific, and medical reasons.


## ENGINEERING OPPORTUNITIES IN ENDOVASCULAR TREATMENT OF ANEURYSMS

Many speakers at this symposium have reported on exciting developments in understanding the biology, hemodynamics, and treatment of aneurysms. The remainder of this presentation is to illustrate additional areas of opportunity where engineering solutions can benefit treatment of patients with aortic aneurysms.

**TABLE 1. Critical path opportunities list**

1. Better evaluation tools
2. Streamlining clinical trials
3. Harnessing bioinformatics
4. Moving manufacturing into the 21st century

## COMPUTER-AIDED DESIGN AND COMPUTER-AIDED MANUFACTURE (CADCAM)

Fenestrated and branched endografts are under clinical trial at a few U.S. institutions. Successful development will obviously increase the population of aneurysm patients who are candidates for endografts. Yet, because of natural variation in branch vessel anatomy as well as because of distortions in branch artery anatomy imposed by the elongation and kinking of the aneurysmal aorta, considerable variation in aortic and arterial anatomy is encountered in clinical practice. The manufacturers of the test device have elected to accommodate this anatomic variation by means of an endograft built to individual patient specification. The anatomical details of a given aneurysm and design of the matching endograft can be specified with great precision by means of several commercial rendering-software packages. A company spokesman estimated (in a personal communication) that building such a device required 20 h of labor by hand (FIG. 5). The device is, therefore, built with the help of computer-aided design and, literally, manufactured; it is a child of the 21st and 19th centuries. The real cost of building such a device is proprietary information. The 20 h of hand labor severely limits turnaround between device specification and shipping. Clearly, however, to extend the benefit of this device to a larger group of patients, to allow emergency use of the device on patients presenting with symptomatic aneurysms, and to extend use of the device to patients with marginal anatomy, it will be necessary to replace manual fabrication with computer-aided manufacture.

**TABLE 2. Better tools for evaluating medical innovations***

6. Surrogate outcomes for cardiovascular drug eluting stents
7. Circulating biomarkers in cardiovascular diseases
22. Using medical imaging as a product development tool
23. Imaging biomarkers in cardiovascular disease
29. Imaging implanted devices
30. Improving extrapolation from animal data to human experience

*Numbers correspond to itemized list in the Critical Path document.

**TABLE 3. Streamlining clinical trials***

34. Design of active controlled trials
36. Use of prior experience of accumulated information in trial design
44. Development of data standards
45. Consensus on standards for case report forms

*Numbers correspond to itemized list in the Critical Path document.

## MICRO-ELECTRO-MECHANICAL SYSTEMS (MEMS)

According to a web site dedicated to this technology, micro-electro-mechanical systems (MEMS) comprise "the integration of mechanical elements, sensors, actuators, and electronics on a common silicon substrate through microfabrication technology."[6] One realization of this technology is the pressure sensor, marketed by CardioMEMS, Inc., designed to be implanted in the aneurysm sac after deployment of an aortic endograft. The device itself is several centimeters long. The "micro" in the name refers to the manufacturing technique used in fabricating the induction coil of the sensor. The resonant frequency of the device is determined by the ambient pressure. By interrogating the device externally and measuring the frequency of induced signal, the pressure in the sac surrounding the sensor can be determined.

In designing systems such as this, several constraints have to be considered. The actuator, which in this case is pressure within the aneurysm sac, must be a surrogate that reliably predicts the desired (or undesirable) endpoint. Implicit in choosing sac-pressure as a surrogate for a stable treated aorta are the following assumptions: rising sac pressure predicts an unstable aneurysm in time to treat the patient, and a single sac pressure is representative of pressure throughout the aneurysm sac. The second assumption is equivalent to treating the sac as a single compartment filled with a liquid. The clinical experience with the device will settle the question whether these assumptions are adequate for reliable patient follow-up, and what pressure change within the sac is clinically significant.

Actuators responding to shear stress or temperature could be developed if needed. All these devices have to be enclosed in a biocompatible package.

**TABLE 4. Harnessing bioinformatics***

47. Virtual control groups in clinical trials
49. Multiple complex therapies
50. Modeling device performance
51. Clinical trial simulation
52. Failure analysis

*Numbers correspond to itemized list in the Critical Path document.

**TABLE 5. Moving manufacturing into the 21st century***

61. Device interaction with blood flow
62. Development of a biocompatibility database
66. Characterizing and qualifying nanotechnologies

*Numbers correspond to itemized list in the Critical Path document.

This packaging requirement does not interfere with measuring ambient pressure using the technique of the CardioMEMS device, which transduces minute physical deformations of the gap between the membranes. However, a sensor that responded to levels of a protein or other molecular species needs to interact with its medium without eliciting an allergic, antigenic, foreign-body, or nonspecific inflammatory reaction that might interfere with sampling of its biochemical environment.

Extensions of the MEMS technology include Micro-Optical-Electro-Mechanical Systems (MOEMS) and Nano-Electro-Mechanical Systems (NEMS). As noted above, the CardioMEMS EndoSure™ Wireless AAA Pressure Measurement System is a macrodevice that is constructed using microtechniques. It is a macrosensor, and, when implanted, sits side-by-side with the endograft, a macrodevice. But it is clear, from examples in the space and automobile industries, that sensors can be incorporated in the construction of a device such as an airbag accelerometer, fuel tank sensor, or tire pressure monitor. An endograft so constructed would have, embedded in its construction, micro or nanodevices that monitored surrogates for device integrity and aneurysm stability.

## ARTIFICIAL ARTERIES

Vascular graft material is needed for coronary artery and lower extremity bypasses, dialysis conduits, and repair of abdominal aortic aneurysms. The diameter of these conduits ranges from 3 mm to 10 mm for arterial bypasses and dialysis grafts, to 15–40 mm for aortic grafts. The ideal conduit resists thrombosis and infection, does not incite an inflammatory or antigenic response, and responds to vasoactive stimuli. It should have compliance, resistance to

**TABLE 6. Challenges to conducting device trials in high risk medical conditions**

1. Design of a device trial when the test device removes clinical equipoise relative to standard treatment
2. Execution of a device trial when the test device is available commercially for a different indication, and off-label treatment of the test condition competes with the trial for patient accrual
3. Execution of a device trial when a new device competes with approved devices for patient accrual

**TABLE 7. FDA 2006 Centennial science forum: Breakout sessions[a]**

1. FDA science at the centennial: History and perspective
2. Seafood safety: From algae to aquaculture
3. Preparing for and preventing a modern plague: Focus on avian flu
4. **Nanotechnology**
5. **Clinical trials & statistics: A glance at the past and present & a look to the future**
6. Omics along the critical path to new medical products
7. Body marking: Tattoos, permanent make-up and laser removal
8. **Partnering on the critical path to new products**
9. Rapid detection of multiple pathogens
10. Bioinformatics
11. **Risk-based inspections and surveillance**
12. Personalized medicine
13. Obesity
14. Bringing home biomarkers: Science, regulation and common sense
15. Current challenges in the treatment of parasitic diseases in humans and animals
16. **Combination products**
17. **Advances and frontiers in using records databases for surveillance of medical products**
18. Pediatric experience with the FDA: Where we have been and where we are going
19. Public health preparedness
20. Blood and tissue safety
21. Public health during natural disasters: The FDA Katrina-Rita experience
22. **Minimally invasive devices**
23. **Managing uncertainty in risk assessment: Probabilistic approaches**
24. Novel approaches to cancer therapy and monitoring

[a]Sessions in bold font discuss Critical Path research relevant to medical device development.

kinking, and tensile strength similar to native vessels. For use as a surgical implant, it should be easy to process and handle, capable of holding sutures without tearing, and available in a suitable range of diameters and lengths.

Synthetic conduits like Dacron and PTFE have limited patency, especially for smaller diameters and longer lengths. They may kink if extended across joints of the upper or lower extremity. The patient's own vessels present a limited source of autologous vascular "grafts," including the great saphenous vein, radial and internal mammary artery, and superficial veins in the forearm used *in situ* in an arteriovenous shunt for dialysis access. Medicare figures from 1996 suggest significant potential application of a biological graft that combines the advantages of the autologous material to the availability of the synthetic graft. Per 1,000 Medicare enrollees in 1996, there were 6.5 coronary artery bypass procedures (70% using the internal mammary artery), 2.0 infrainguinal bypass procedures (39% using synthetic conduits), 1.6 major amputations, and 1.6 initial vascular access procedures for hemodialysis (83% using synthetic conduits).[7] Several centers have been exploring ways to construct biological implants.[8,9] These efforts have resulted in successful implants in nonprimate mammals but not, to my knowledge, in humans. This work has obvious importance in this era of growing prevalence of patients with type II

**TABLE 8. FDA 2006 Centennial science forum: Focus on devices**

1. Quantum dots: Emerging applications in biology, imaging and medicine
2. The toxicology of nanomaterials: Size, number and surface as determinants of toxicity
3. Preclinical characterization of nanomaterials intended for cancer diagnostics and therapeutics
4. From microscopy toward nanoscopy and nanobiosensing: How to break the diffraction barrier in subwavelength nanoscale
5. A history of clinical trials from post Harris Kefauver, 1962 , to present
6. The future of clinical trials – informatics
7. The future of clinical trials – clinical medicine
8. The future of clinical trials – industry
9. CPath Institute – Cross-validation of genomic biomarkers and the community pharmacy program for drug safety
10. Imaging as a Biomarker – FDG-PET in non-Hodgkin's lymphoma
11. Numerical models and tools – "The virtual family"
12. Utilization of FDA's ECG warehouse for monitoring cardiac safety in medical product development
13. Case study: Cordis cypher sirolimus-eluting stent
14. Case study: Boston scientific taxus paclitaxel-eluting stent
15. Regulatory challenges
16. Drug-eluting stents: Pharmaceutical challenges
17. Beyond drug-eluting stents: The next frontier in drug delivery
18. Drug safety in the Department of Veterans Affairs
19. Frontiers in surveillance of medical devices
20. Prompt, active identification of ADR signals using population-based data
21. Medications – adverse events, unanticipated benefits and what to do about them – the Indiana experience
22. Optical coherence tomography for detection of atherosclerotic plaque
23. High intensity focused ultrasound surgery and extracorporeal shock wave therapy
24. Recent advances in medical imaging
25. Image-guided surgery and drug therapy

diabetes, in whom coronary, lower extremity, and dialysis conduits are needed. A smaller group of patients in whom biological grafts might be used are those with abdominal aortic aneurysms (1.09 repairs per 1,000 Medicare enrollees[7]), where autologous biological graft might offer advantages over fabric for composite endografts in reducing endoleaks and inducing perigraft thrombosis and aneurysm shrinkage.

## CONCLUSION

There is no shortage of engineering challenges in endovascular treatment of aneurysm and other vascular disease. Focusing specifically on treatment of aortic aneurysms, these include MEMS and related technologies for smart devices to monitor device integrity and complications, artificial vascular tissue as biofabrics for endografts or branch artery prostheses, and biocompatible coatings for stents, valves, and vascular access devices. However, in the excitement of exploring these technical paths of research, the vascular community must keep in mind the sobering reminder from the FDA: IND applications are diminishing, and costs are expanding. Critical path research, as outlined above, while less glamorous than basic or translational research, may actually benefit more patients sooner.

## REFERENCES

1. Innovation or Stagnation? 2004. *Challenge and Opportunity on the Critical Path to New Medical Products.* U.S. Department of Health and Human Services, Food and Drug Administration, Washington, D.C. Accessed October 20, 2006: http://www.fda.gov/oc/initiatives/criticalpath/whitepaper.html
2. *Office of Device Evaluation Annual Report Fiscal Year 2004.* March 2005. U.S. Department of Health and Human Services, Washington, D.C. Accessed October 20, 2006: http://www.fda.gov/cdrh/annual/fy2004/ode/part3.html
3. Korn D., Stanski D.R., Eds. *Drug Development Science: Obstacles and Opportunities for Collaboration Among Academia, Industry and Government.* Association of American Medical Colleges, AAMC-FDA Conference on Drug Development Science Report, January, 2005. Accessed October 20, 2006: https://services.aamc.org/Publications/index.cfm?fuseaction=Product.displayForm&prd_id=135&prv_id=159
4. Innovation or Stagnation? *Critical Path Opportunities List.* U.S. Department of Health and Human Services, Food and Drug Administration, Washington, D.C. March 2006. Accessed October 20, 2006: http://www.fda.gov/oc/initiatives/criticalpath/reports/opp_list.pdf
5. FDA's Science Forum Centennial Home Page. U.S. Department of Health and Human Services, Food and Drug Administration, Washington, D.C. Accessed October 20, 2006: http://www.fda.gov/scienceforum/
6. What is MEMS Technology. MEMS and Nanotechnology Clearinghouse. Accessed October 20, 2006: http://www.memsnet.org/mems/what-is.html
7. Figures for vascular access, lower extremity bypass, and abdominal aortic aneurysm repair procedures are available *In* The Dartmouth Atlas of Vascular Health Care. J.L. Cronenwett & J.D. Birkmeyer, Eds.: 8, 122, 142. AHA Press. Chicago. http://www.dartmouthatlas.org/atlases/atlas˙series.shtm. (accessed May 3, 2006).
8. POH, M., M. BOYER, A. SOLAN, *et al.* 2005. Blood vessels engineered from human cells. Lancet. **365:** 2122–2124.
9. HOENIG, M.R., G.R. CAMPBELL, B.E. ROLFE & J.H. CAMPBELL. 2005. Tissue-engineered blood vessels: alternative to autologous grafts? Arterioscler. Thromb. Vasc. Biol. **25:** 1128–1134.

# Abdominal Aortic Aneurysm Is a Specific Antigen-Driven T Cell Disease

CHRIS D. PLATSOUCAS,[a] SONG LU,[a] IFEYINWA NWANESHIUDU,[a]
CHARALAMBOS SOLOMIDES,[b] ALEXIS AGELAN,[a]
NEKTARIA NTAOULA,[a] ENKHTUYA PUREV,[a] LI PING LI,[a]
PASCHALIS KRATSIOS,[a] EFSTRATIOS MYLONAS,[a] WEON-JU JUNG,[a]
KYLE EVANS,[a] SEAN ROBERTS,[a] YANDI LU,[a] RICARDO LAYVI,[a]
WAN LU LIN,[a] XIAOYING ZHANG,[a] JOHN GAUGHAN,[c]
DIMITRIOS S. MONOS,[d] EMILIA L. OLESZAK,[e] AND JOHN V. WHITE[f]

[a]*Departments of Microbiology and Immunology, Temple University School
of Medicine, Philadelphia, Pennsylvania, USA*

[b]*Departments of Pathology and Laboratory Medicine, Temple University School
of Medicine, Philadelphia, Pennsylvania, USA*

[c]*Department of Physiology (Biostatistics), Temple University School
of Medicine, Philadelphia, Pennsylvania, USA*

[d]*Department of Pediatrics, University of Pennsylvania School of Medicine, and
Department of Pathology and Laboratory Medicine, Children's Hospital of
Philadelphia, Philadelphia, Pennsylvania, USA*

[e]*Department of Anatomy and Cell Biology, Temple University School
of Medicine, Philadelphia, Pennsylvania, USA*

[f]*Department of Surgery, Advocate-Lutheran General Hospital, University of
Illinois School of Medicine, Park Ridge, Illinois, USA*

ABSTRACT: To determine whether monoclonal/oligoclonal T cells are
present in abdominal aortic aneurysm (AAA) lesions, we amplified
β-chain T cell receptor (TCR) transcripts from these lesions by the
nonpalindromic adaptor (NPA)-polymerase chain reaction (PCR)/V-β-
specific PCR followed by cloning and sequencing. Sequence analysis revealed the presence of substantial proportions of identical β-chain TCR
transcripts in AAA lesions in 9 of 10 patients examined, strongly suggesting the presence of oligoclonal populations of αβ TCR+ T cells. We have
also shown the presence of oligoclonal populations of γδ TCR+ T cells
in AAA lesions. Sequence analysis after appropriate PCR amplification
and cloning revealed the presence of substantial proportions of identical
VγI and VγII TCR transcripts in 15 of 15 patients examined, and of Vδ1

Address for correspondence: Chris D. Platsoucas, Ph.D., Department of Microbiology and Immunology, Temple University School of Medicine, 3400 North Broad Street, Philadelphia, PA 19140. Voice:
215-707-7929; fax: 215-829-1320.
e-mail: Chris.Platsoucas@temple.edu

Ann. N.Y. Acad. Sci. 1085: 224–235 (2006). © 2006 New York Academy of Sciences.
doi: 10.1196/annals.1383.019

and Vδ2 TCR transcripts in 12 of 12 patients. These clonal expansions were very strong. All these clonal expansions were statistically significant by the binomial distribution. In other studies, we determined that mononuclear cells infiltrating AAA lesions express early- (CD69), intermediate- (CD25, CD38), and late- (CD45RO, HLA class II) activation antigens. These findings suggest that active ongoing inflammation is present in the aortic wall of patients with AAA. These results demonstrate that oligoclonal αβ TCR+ and γδ TCR+T cells are present in AAA lesions. These oligoclonal T cells have been clonally expanded *in vivo* in response to yet unidentified antigens. Although the antigenic specificity of these T cells remains to be determined, these T cells may play a significant role in the initiation and/or the propagation of the AAA. It appears that AAA is a specific antigen-driven T cell disease.

KEYWORDS: abdominal aortic aneurysm; T cell mononuclear infiltrates; alpha/beta T cell receptor; gamma/delta T cell receptor; clonal expansions of T cells; oligoclonal T cells; expression of early-, intermediate-, and late-activation antigens

## INTRODUCTION

The etiology and pathogenesis of abdominal aortic aneurysm (AAA) are poorly understood. AAA is one of the first 10 causes of death in men 55–74 years of age and is responsible for 1–2% of all deaths of men in that age range.[1–3] The mortality of ruptured AAA is very high, in the range of 80–90%.[4] Genetic and environmental factors are involved in the pathogenesis of AAA.

Autoimmunity may be responsible for the pathogenesis of AAA. This is supported by: (a) the presence of inflammatory infiltrates in AAA lesions, particularly in the adventitia, comprising T, B, and plasma cells, and monocytes;[5–7] (b) an association between particular HLA alleles and AAA;[8–10] (c) the presence of autoantibodies in AAA lesions.[11–13] Purified IgG antibody from the wall of AAA aorta recognized proteins isolated from normal aortic tissue demonstrating the presence of an autoimmune antibody response in AAA lesions;[11–13] (d) oligoclonal expansions of infiltrating T cells found in the aortas of patients with giant cell arteritis (GCA)[14] and Takayasu arteritis.[15,16] Both diseases are related to AAA; and (e) the fact that cytokines play an important role in the pathogenesis of AAA. Both Th1 and Th2 cytokines have been reported in human AAAs and in animal models.[17–23] CD4+ Th1 cells may be predominant in human AAA lesions.[21]

However, many questions remain to be answered to determine whether AAA is an autoimmune disease. It is not known whether the inflammatory response is antigen-driven, although a number of putative self- and nonself antigens have been suggested including elastin and elastin fragments,[24–27] oxidized low-density lipoprotein (LDL),[28,29] aortic aneurysm antigenic protein-40 (AAA-P), also known as human microbial-associated glycoprotein 36 (MAGP-36),[11–13] collagen types 1 and 3,[30–33] *Chlamydia pneumoniae*,[34–37] cytomegalovirus,[38] and *Treponema palladium*.[39] Molecular mimicry (Oleszak *et al*.[40]) may be responsible for the induction of T cell inflammatory responses in AAA lesions. Molecular mimicry is defined as sharing of common antigenic epitopes between microorganisms such as bacteria or viruses, and host antigens. An immune response of the host induced by a virus and directed against a viral epitope may recognize as nonself a host (self) epitope that shares structural or conformational similarities with the viral epitope that induced the response long after the virus is gone. Molecular mimicry may lead to autoimmune disease. It appears to be responsible for a number of autoimmune diseases (Oleszak *et al*.). Although it is well documented that infiltrating T cells are essentially always present in AAA lesions, very little is known about the role of T cells in the initiation and propagation of the disease.

*Active ongoing inflammation is present in the aortic wall of patients with AAA:* Expression of early-, intermediate-, and late-activation antigens are expressed on mononuclear cells infiltrating AAA lesions. We have carried out immunohistochemical studies (TABLE 1) to characterize the mononuclear cells infiltrating AAA lesions using a panel of monoclonal antibodies (mAbs) recognizing differentiation antigens expressed on leukocytes (LCA), T cells (CD3, CD4, and CD8), monocytes (CD68), B cells (CD20), naive lymphocytes, and other cells (CD45RA) as well as early- (CD69),[41,42] intermediate- (CD25, CD38),[43] and late- (CD45RO, HLA class II)[44] activation antigens. Nine of 11 AAA specimens demonstrated mild to heavy CD3+ T cell infiltration. Substantial numbers of monocyte/macrophages and B cells/plasma cells were co-localized with the CD3+ T cell infiltrates. Mononuclear cells, including T lymphocytes, expressing early- (CD69), intermediate- (CD25, CD38), and late- (CD45RO HLA class II) activation antigens are present in AAA lesions. The majority of specimens demonstrate more widespread immunoreactivity with mAbs to late-activation antigens than to early and intermediate antigens. The presence of early-, intermediate-, and late-activation antigens in AAA lesions suggests active ongoing inflammation in these lesions. While it could be argued[45] that a portion of CD45RO+ memory T cells may infiltrate AAA lesions from the peripheral blood, the presence of CD69+ T cells in these lesions strongly suggests that activation is occurring *in situ* in these lesions. CD69 is expressed on the surface of T cells very early upon activation and has been reported to be responsible for T cell interactions requiring cell–cell contact with cells of the monocyte/macrophage lineage leading to the production of IL-1.[41,42] The results described below strongly suggest that these T cell responses are specific antigen-driven.

*Mononuclear cells infiltrating AAA lesions contain monoclonal/oligoclonal populations of* αβ *T cell receptor (TCR)+ T cells:* T cells recognize through their αβ TCR small peptides in association, in general, with major histocompatibility complex (MHC) class I or II. In addition, certain αβ TCR+ T cell clones recognize in an MHC-independent manner, peptides presented by CD1 molecules, carbohydrates, lipids, glycolipids, and other molecules.

**TABLE 1. Cell-surface antigen expression**

| Antigen | Number of positive cells (range) per high power field ($\times 400$) |
| --- | --- |
| LCA | 34.7–1108.3 |
| CD3 | 19.9–317.5 |
| CD4 | 6.2–269.9 |
| CD8 | 12.7–209.2 |
| CD68 | 27.5–158.2 |
| CD20 | 10.8–535.2 |
| CD45RA | 12.7–661.30 |
| CD69 | 11.30–103.40 |
| CD25 | 3.20–190.50 |
| CD38 | 7.30–362.90 |
| CD45RO | 18.90–395.90 |

T cells comprise many different T cell clones. Each T cell clone recognizes a different antigenic epitope and expresses a different TCR. Each TCR serves as a unique fingerprint of that T cell clone.[46–48] The T cell repertoire is very large and it is acquired in the thymus. TCRs are highly polymorphic molecules generated by several diversity mechanisms. The maximum theoretical number of different $\alpha\beta$ TCR+ T cell clones have been estimated[46] to be on the order of $10^{18}$ and that of the $\beta$-chain TCR transcripts on the order of 10.[12] However, because of thymic selection, most of the thymocytes are eliminated in the thymus, and only a small proportion ($<10\%$) of them survive to became postthymic mature T lymphocytes.[46–48] The actual size of the T cell repertoire in the peripheral blood of normal donors has been estimated to use $10^6$ different $\beta$-chain TCR transcripts and each one is pairing, on the average, with 25 or more different $\alpha$-chains.[49] These numbers of different T cell clones are still very large and clearly sufficient to recognize any conceivable antigenic epitope. In consideration of the above, the probability of finding by chance multiple identical copies of a particular $\alpha$- or $\beta$-chain TCR transcript in an independent sample of T cells is negligible. Therefore, the appearance of multiple identical copies of one or few $\alpha$- or $\beta$-chain TCR transcripts must be the result of specific antigen-driven activation, proliferation, and clonal expansion of particular T cell clones in response to the antigen that they recognize. Thus, a specific antigen-driven T cell response elicits monoclonal/oligoclonal T cell expansion(s), identified by the presence of multiple identical TCR transcripts.

To determine whether T cells infiltrating AAA lesions contain clonally expanded T cells, we employed nonpalindromic adaptor (NPA)-polymerase chain reaction (PCR)/V $\beta$-specific PCR amplification, followed by cloning and sequencing. The NPA-PCR method has been previously developed in our laboratory for the amplification of transcripts with unknown or variable 5' end such as the TCR and Igs[45,50–54] and has certain distinct advantages over classical PCR techniques. The major advantage of this technique is that only one

**TABLE 2. Clonal expansions of α- and β-chain TCR transcripts in AAA lesions**

| Patients with AAA | Clonal expansion(s) | |
|---|---|---|
| | β-chain | α-chain |
| AAA09 | Yes | Yes |
| AAA03 | Yes | Yes |
| AAA06 | Yes | Not done |
| AAA00 | Yes | Yes |
| AAA10 | Yes | Yes |
| AAA12 | Polyclonal | Polyclonal |
| AAA04 | Yes | Not done |
| AAA07 | Yes | Not done |
| AAA02 | Yes | Not done |
| AAA14 | CD4: Yes | Not done |
| | CD8: polyclonal | |

amplification is needed for the α-chain TCR transcripts and a second amplification for the β-chain TCR transcripts.

Sequence analysis of β-chain TCR transcripts from AAA lesions after NPA-PCR/Vβ-specific PCR amplification and cloning revealed the presence of substantial proportions of identical β-chain TCR transcripts in AAA lesions in 9 out of 10 patients examined, strongly suggesting the presence of oligoclonal populations of αβ TCR+ T cells (TABLE 2). These clonal expansions were statistically significant by the binomial distribution. In certain patients, these clonal expansions were very strong and identical β-chain TCR transcripts accounted for as high as 60% of the transcripts sequenced. Clonal expansions identified by NPA-PCR amplification followed by cloning and sequencing were confirmed in certain patients by Vβ-specific PCR amplification from the same RNA preparation, followed by cloning and sequencing and yielded clonally expanded TCR transcripts identical to those that were found to be clonally expanded after NPA-PCR amplification. The use of two different PCR amplification methods, which yielded identical results, is an advantage and demonstrates beyond doubt that monoclonal/oligoclonal T cells are present in AAA lesions. Two typical examples are listed below:

(a) *Patient AAA09.* Amplification by NPA-PCR/Vβ-specific PCR of β-chain PCR transcripts from AAA lesion of this patient followed by cloning and sequencing revealed a clonal expansion (clone AAA09-02; Vβ14.1Dβ2.1Jβ2.3) that accounted for 8 out of 38 (21%) β-chain PCR transcripts sequenced ($P < 0.0001$). To obtain independent confirmation of this clonal expansion, we amplified by Vβ14-specific PCR β-chain TCR transcripts from cDNA from AAA lesion of patient AAA09. The amplified transcripts were cloned and sequenced. Sequence analysis revealed that 12 out of 21 (57%) ($P < 0.0001$) β-chain PCR transcripts sequenced were identical to clone AAA09-02 (Vβ14.1Dβ2.1Jβ2.3) that was found to be clonally expanded in AAA lesions of patient AAA09 after NPA-PCR/Vβ-specific PCR amplification followed by cloning and sequencing.

(b) *Patient AAA03.* Sequence analysis of β-chain PCR transcripts from AAA lesion of patient AAA03 after NPA-PCR/Vβ-specific PCR amplification, cloning, and sequencing revealed a possible clonal expansion. Clone AAA03-11 (Vβ24.1Dβ1.1Jβ1.3) accounted for 3 out of 24 (13%) β-chain PCR transcripts sequenced. Vβ24 transcripts were amplified by Vβ24-specific PCR followed by cloning and sequencing. Sequence analysis revealed that 17 out of 20 (85%, $P < 0.0001$) transcripts sequenced were identical to clone AAA03-11 (Vβ24.1Dβ1.1 Jβ1.3) that was found to be expressed in triplicate in AAA lesions of patient AAA03.

Peripheral blood mononuclear cells (PBMC) from normal donors were used as methodological controls. Amplification of β-chain TCR transcripts from PBMC from normal donors by the approaches mentioned above followed by cloning and sequencing revealed unique transcripts when compared to each other, typical of polyclonal populations of T cells.[45,50–54]

Six of the 10 AAA patients were typed by DNA-based methodologies for HLA-DRB1, -DQA1, and -DQB1 loci, as previously described.[55] Interestingly, all 6 patients were characterized by the presence of the DRβGln(70) amino acid residue that has been previously reported to be associated with AAA.[9] Even though this is a small sample for evaluating the significance of the Gln 70 amino acid residue as a risk factor for AAA, it forms a basis for identifying the specific molecular entities that may participate in this process, namely the clonally expanded α- and β-chain TCR transcripts and the DRβGln(70)-carrying HLA.

Amplification by NPA-PCR of α-chain TCR transcripts from AAA lesions followed by cloning and sequencing revealed clonally expanded T cells in 4 of 5 patients with AAA (TABLE 2). β-chain TCR transcripts were also clonally expanded in these AAA lesions.

*Mononuclear cells infiltrating AAA lesions contain monoclonal/oligoclonal populations of γδ TCR+ T–cells. Multiple copies of identical γ- and δ-chain TCR transcripts are present in AAA lesions:* The second TCR comprises a γ- and δ-chain heterodimer and it is expressed on a small proportion (3–10%) of peripheral blood mononuclear cells. γδ TCR+ T cells are also expressed on a number of lymphoid peripheral tissues. In contrast to αβ TCR+ T cells, most of which recognize peptides in association with MHC, most of the γδ TCR+ T cells recognize whole proteins in a manner independent of MHC (Platsoucas *et al.*[56]). Other γδ TCR+ T cells have been reported to recognize lipids, carbohydrates, glycolipids, and other ligands in an MHC-independent manner.[56]

We have shown the presence of oligoclonal populations of γδ TCR+ T cells in AAA lesions. VγI and VγII subgroup TCR transcripts as well as Vδ1 and

TABLE 3. γ- and δ-chain T cell receptor transcripts from AAA lesions are clonally expanded

| Patients with AAA | Clonal expansion(s) | | | |
|---|---|---|---|---|
| | γ-chain | | δ- chain | |
| | V γ I | V γ II | V δ 1 | V δ 2 |
| JW5 | yes | yes | yes | yes |
| AAA58 | yes | yes | yes | yes |
| JW10 | yes | yes | yes | yes |
| JW7 | yes | yes | yes | yes |
| JW6 | yes | yes | yes | yes |
| JW2 | yes | yes | ND* | ND |
| JW12 | yes | yes | ND | ND |
| JW9 | yes | yes | yes | yes |
| JW4 | yes | yes | yes | yes |
| JW3 | yes | yes | ND | ND |
| JW00 | yes | yes | ND | ND |
| JWE | yes | yes | yes | yes |
| JWD | yes | yes | yes | yes |
| JWC | yes | yes | ND | ND |
| AAA88 | yes | yes | yes | yes |

Vδ2 TCR transcripts were amplified by two-sided subgroup- or V-specific PCR using the appropriate primers for each amplification.[57,58] The amplified transcripts were cloned and sequenced. Sequence analysis revealed the presence of multiple identical copies of VγI transcripts in 15 of 15 patients examined (30% to 80% of the VγI TCR transcripts sequenced were identical) and of VγII TCR transcripts in 15 of 15 patients examined (39% to 80% of the VγII TCR transcripts sequenced were identical). These results were statistically significant by the binomial distribution (TABLE 3). Similarly, sequence analysis revealed the presence of multiple identical copies of Vδ1 TCR transcripts in 12 of 12 patients examined (29% to 94% of the Vδ1 TCR transcripts sequenced were identical), and of Vδ2 TCR transcripts in 10 of 10 patients examined (40% to 91% of the Vδ2 TCR transcripts sequenced were identical). These results were also statistically significant by the binomial distribution (TABLE 3). These clonal expansions were very strong.

PBMCs from normal donors were also used as methodological controls. Amplification of VγI, VγII, and Vδ2 TCR transcripts from PBMCs from normal donors by two-sided PCR followed by cloning and sequencing revealed almost entirely unique transcripts when compared to each other, typical of polyclonal populations of T cells. Sequence analysis of Vδ1 TCR transcripts from PBMCs from normal donors revealed the presence of statistically significant clonal expansions in two of three normal donors in agreement with previous reports in the literature.[59,60] These clonal expansions of Vδ1 TCR transcripts in PBMCs from normal donors, although well documented, are poorly understood.

**TABLE 4. Evidence supporting the view that AAA is a specific antigen-driven T cell disease**

1. Mononuclear inflammatory infiltrates comprised primarily of T, B, and plasma cells, and monocytes are present in AAA lesions.
2. Mononuclear cells infiltrating AAA lesions express early- (CD69), intermediate- (CD25, CD38), and late- (CD45RO, HLA class II) activation antigens.
3. There is an association between particular HLA alleles with AAA.
4. Autoantibodies are present in AAA lesions.
5. Th1 and Th2 cytokines have been reported in AAA lesions.
6. Putative self- and nonself antigens have been suggested in AAA including elastin and elastin fragments, oxidized LDL, AAA-P (also known as MAGP-36), collagen types 1 and 3, chlamydia, cytomegalovirus, and others.
7. Monoclonal/oligoclonal $\alpha\beta$ TCR+ and $\gamma\delta$ TCR+T cells are present in AAA lesions.
8. Molecular mimicry may be responsible for the induction of T cell inflammatory responses in AAA lesions.

## CONCLUSIONS

These results demonstrate that monoclonal/oligoclonal T cells are present in AAA lesions. These monoclonal/oligoclonal T cells have been clonally expanded *in vivo* in response to yet unidentified antigens. These clonally expanded T cells may recognize certain putative AAA antigens. Although the antigenic specificity of these T cells remains to be determined, they may play an important role in the initiation and/or the propagation of the disease. These T cells may recognize host antigens by molecular mimicry. It is likely that the disease is initiated by a T cell response to a specific antigen. Damage to the aortic wall is very likely the far-reaching consequence of this immune response. Both T cells and activated macrophages recruited to the site of inflammation produce, directly or indirectly, products (such as NO, MMPs) noxious to the aortic wall resulting in aneurysmal disease. These findings provide compelling evidence that AAA is a specific antigen-driven T cell disease (TABLE 4). These results permit for the first time the development of a clear and unified hypothesis for the pathogenesis of the disease and the identification of the antigens responsible for inducing the chronic inflammation in AAA.

## ACKNOWLEDGMENTS

This work was supported in part by Grant RO1 HL64340 from NIH.

## REFERENCES

1. BICKERSTAFF, L.K., L.H. HOLLIER, H.J. VAN PEENEN, *et al.* 1984. Abdominal aortic aneurysms: the changing natural history. J. Vasc. Surg. **1:** 6–12.

2. MELTON, L.J., L.K. BICKERSTAFF, L.H. HOLLIER, *et al.*1984. Changing incidence of abdominal aortic aneurysms: a population-based study. Am. J. Epidemiol. **120:** 379–386.
3. VAN DER VLIET, J.A. & A.P. BOLL. 1997. Abdominal aortic aneurysm. Lancet **349:** 863–866.
4. LINDHOLT, J.S. 2001. Screening for abdominal aortic aneurysm. Br. J. Surg. **88:** 625–626.
5. PEARCE, W.H. & A.E. KOCH. 1996. Cellular components and features of immune response in abdominal aortic aneurysms. Ann. N.Y. Acad. Sci. **800:** 175–185.
6. KOCH, A.E., G.K. HAINES, R.J. RIZZO, *et al.*1990. Human abdominal aortic aneurysms. Immunophenotypic analysis suggesting an immune-mediated response. Am. J. Pathol. **137:** 1199–1213.
7. HANSSON, G.K., L. JONASSON, J. HOLM & L. CLAESSON-WELSH. 1986. Class II MHC antigen expression in the atherosclerotic plaque: smooth muscle cells express HLA-DR, HLA-DQ and the invariant gamma chain. Clin. Exp. Immunol. **64:** 261–268.
8. TILSON, M.D., K.J. OZSVATH, H. HIROSE & S. XIA. 1996. A genetic basis for autoimmune manifestations in the abdominal aortic aneurysm resides in the MHC class II locus DR-beta-1. Ann. N. Y. Acad. Sci. **800:** 208–215.
9. RASMUSSEN, T.E., J.W. HALLETT, JR., R.L. METZGER, *et al.* 1997. Genetic risk factors in inflammatory abdominal aortic aneurysms: polymorphic residue 70 in the HLA-DR B1 gene as a key genetic element. J. Vasc. Surg. **25:** 356–364.
10. HIROSE, H., M. TAKAGI, N. MIYAGAWA, *et al.* 1998. Genetic risk factor for abdominal aortic aneurysm: HLA-DR2(15), a Japanese study. J. Vasc. Surg. **27:** 500–503.
11. TILSON, M.D. 1995. Similarities of an autoantigen in aneurysmal disease of the human abdominal aorta to a 36-kDa microfibril-associated bovine aortic glycoprotein. Biochem. Biophys. Res. Commun. **213:** 40–43.
12. GREGORY, A.K., N.X. YIN, J. CAPELLA, *et al.* 1996. Features of autoimmunity in the abdominal aortic aneurysm. Arch. Surg. **131:** 85–88.
13. XIA, S., K. OZSVATH, H. HIROSE & M.D. TILSON. 1996. Partial amino acid sequence of a novel 40-kDa human aortic protein, with vitronectin-like, fibrinogen-like, and calcium binding domains: aortic aneurysm-associated protein-40 (AAAP-40) [human MAGP-3, proposed]. Biochem. Biophys. Res. Commun. **219:** 36–39.
14. WEYAND, C.M., J. SCHONBERGER, U. OPPITZ, *et al.* 1994. Distinct vascular lesions in giant cell arteritis share identical T-cell clonotypes. J. Exp. Med. **179:** 951–960.
15. SEKO, Y., O. SATO, A. TAKAGI, *et al.* 1996. Restricted usage of T-cell receptor Valpha-Vbeta genes in infiltrating cells in aortic tissue of patients with Takayasu's arteritis. Circulation **93:** 1788–1790.
16. NITYANAND, S., R. GISCOMBE, S. SRIVASTAVA, *et al.* 1997. A bias in the alphabeta T-cell receptor variable region gene usage in Takayasu's arteritis. Clin. Exp. Immunol. **107:** 261–268.
17. SCHONBECK, U., G.K. SUKHOVA, N. GERDES & P. LIBBY. 2002. T(H)2 predominant immune responses prevail in human abdominal aortic aneurysm. Am. J. Pathol. **16:** 499–506.
18. XIONG, W.Y. Zhao, A. PRALL, T.C. GREINER & B.T. BAXTER. 2004. Key roles of CD4+ T-cells and IFN-gamma in the development of abdominal aortic aneurysms in a murine model. J. Immunol. **273:** 2607–2612.
19. SHIMIZU, K., M. SHICHIRI, P. LIBBY, *et al.* 2004. Th2-predominant inflammation and blockade of IFN-gamma signaling induce aneurysms in allografted aortas. J. Clin. Invest. **114:** 300–308.

20. DUFTNER, C., R. SELLER, P. KLEIN-WEIGEL, *et al.* 2005. High prevalence of circulating CD4+CD28- T-cells in patients with small abdominal aortic aneurysms. Arterioscler. Thromb. Vasc. Biol. **25:** 1347–1352.

21. GALLE, C., L. SCHANDENE, P. STORDEUR, *et al.* 2005. Predominance of type 1 CD4+ T-cells in human abdominal aortic aneurysm. Clin. Exp. Immunol. **142:** 519–527.

22. LINDHOLT, J.S. & G.P. SHI. 2006. Chronic inflammation, immune response, and infection in abdominal aortic aneuysms. Eur. J. Vasc. Endovasc. Surg. **31(5):** 453–463.

23. SHIRMIZU, K., R.N. MITCHELL & P. LIBBY. 2006. Inflammation and cellular immune responses in abdominal aortic aneurysms. Arterioscler. Thromb. Vasc. Biol. **26(5):** 987–994.

24. WHITE, J.V., K. HAAS, S. PHILLIPS & A.J. COMEROTA. 1993. Adventitial elastolysis is a primary event in aneurysm formation. J. Vasc. Surg. **17:** 371–380.

25. BAXTER, B.T., G.S. MCGEE, V.P. SHIVELY, *et al.* 1992. Elastin content, cross-links, and mRNA in normal and aneurysmal human aorta. J. Vasc. Surg. **16:** 192–200.

26. GANDHI, R.H., E. IRIZARRY, J.O. CANTOR, *et al.* 2004. Analysis of elastin cross-linking and the connective tissue matrix of abdominal aortic aneurysms. Surgery **115:** 617–620.

27. REILLY, J.M., C.M. BROPHY & M.D. TILSON. 1992. Characterization of an elastase from aneurysmal aorta which degrades intact aortic elastin. Ann. Vasc. Surg. **6:** 499–502.

28. STEMME, S., B. FABER, J. HOLM, *et al.* 1995. T lymphocytes from human atherosclerotic plaques recognize oxidized low density lipoprotein. Proc. Natl. Acad. Sci. USA **92:** 3893–3897.

29. MATTHYS, K., C.E. VANHOVE, M.M. KOCKX, *et al.* 1997. Local application of LDL promotes intimal thickening in the collared carotid artery of the rabbit. Arterio. Throm. Vasc. Biol. **17:** 2423–2429.

30. MENASHI, S., J.S. CAMPA, R.M. GREENHALGH & J.T. POWELL. 1987. Collagen in abdominal aortic aneurysm: typing, content, and degradation. J. Vasc. Surg. **6:** 578–582.

31. TROMP, G., Y. WU, D.J. PROCKOP, *et al.* 1993. Sequencing of cDNA from 50 unrelated patients reveals that mutations in the triple-helical domain of type III procollagen are an infrequent cause of aortic aneurysms. J. Clin. Invest. **91:** 2539–2542.

32. KONTUSAARI, S., G. TROMP, H. KUIVANIEMI, *et al.* 1990. A mutation in the gene for type III procollagen (COL3A1) in a family with aortic aneurysms. J. Clin. Invest. **86:** 1465–1473.

33. ANDERSON, D.W., T.K. EDWARDS, M.H. RICKETTS, *et al.* 1996. Multiple defects in type III collagen synthesis are associated with the pathogenesis of abdominal aortic aneurysms. Ann. N. Y. Acad. Sci. **800:** 216–228.

34. JUVONEN, J., T. JUVONEN, A. LAURILA, *et al.* 1997. Demonstration of Chlamydia pneumoniae in the walls of abdominal aortic aneurysms. J. Vasc. Surg. **25:** 499–505.

35. HALME, S., T. JUVONEN, A. LAURILA, *et al.* 1999. Chlamydia pneumoniae reactive T lymphocytes in the walls of abdominal aortic aneurysms. Eur. J. Clin. Invest. **29:** 546–552.

36. KARLSSON, L., J. GNARPE, J. NAAS, *et al.* 2000. Detection of viable Chlamydia pneumoniae in abdominal aortic aneurysms. Eur. J. Vasc. Endovasc. Surg. **19:** 630–635.

37. LINDHOLT, J.S., H.A. ASHTON & R.A. SCOTT. 2001. Indicators of infection with Chlamydia pneumoniae are associated with expansion of abdominal aortic aneurysms. J. Vasc. Surg. **34:** 212–215.

38. TANAKA, S., K. KOMORI, K. OKADOME, et al. 1994. Detection of active cytomegalovirus infection in inflammatory aortic aneurysms with RNA polymerase chain reaction. J. Vasc. Surg. **20:** 235–243.

39. OZSVATH, K.J., H. HIROSE, S. XIA & M.D. TILSON. 1996. Molecular mimicry in human aortic aneurysmal diseases. Ann. N. Y. Acad. Sci. **800:** 288–893.

40. OLESZAK, E.L., J.R. CHANG, H. FRIEDMAN, et al. 2004. Theiler's virus infection: a model for multiple sclerosis. Clin. Microbiol. Rev. **17:** 174–207.

41. TESTI, R., J.H. PHILLIPS & L.L. LANIER. 1989. Leu 23 induction as an early marker of functional CD3/T-cell antigen receptor triggering. J. Immunol. **142:** 1854–1860.

42. ISLER, P., E. VEU, J.H. ZHANG & J.M. DAYER. 1993. Cell surface glycoproteins expressed on activated human T-cells induce production of interleukin-1 beta by monocytic cells: a possible role of CD69. Eur. Cytokine Net. **4:** 15–23.

43. JACKSON, D.G. & J.I. BELL. 1990. Isolation of a cDNA encoding the human CD38(T10) molecule, a cell surface glycoprotein with an unusual discontinuous pattern of expression during lymphocyte differentiation. J. Immunol. **144:** 2811–2815.

44. AKBAR, A.N., L. TERRY, A. TIMMS, et al. 1986. Loss of CD45R and gain of UCHLI reactivity is a feature of primed T-cells. J. Immunol. **140:** 2171–2178.

45. LIN, W.L., J.E. FINCKE, L.R. SHARER, et al. 2005. Oligoclonal T-cells are infiltrating the brains of children with AIDS: sequence analysis reveals high proportions of identical beta-chain T-cell receptor transcripts. Clin. Exp. Immunol. **141:** 338–356.

46. BOEHM, T. & T.H. RABBITTS. 1989. The human T-cell receptor genes are targets for chromosomal abnormalities in T-cell tumors. FASEB J. **3:** 2344–2359.

47. ARDEN, B., S.P. CLARK, D. KABELITZ & T.W. MAK. 1995. Human T-cell receptor variable gene segment families. Immunogenetics **42:** 455–500.

48. SLANSKY, J.E. 2003. Antigen-specific T-cells: analyses of the needles in the haystack. PLoS Biol. **1:** 329.

49. ARSTILA, T.P., A. CASROUGE, V. BARON, et al. 1999. A direct estimate of the human alphabeta T cell receptor diversity. Science. **286:** 958–961.

50. SLACHTA, C.A., V. JEEVANANDAM, B. GOLDMAN, et al. 2000. Coronary arteries from human cardiac allografts with chronic rejection contain oligoclonal T-cells: persistence of identical clonally expanded TCR transcripts from the early post-transplantation period (endomyocardial biopsies) to chronic rejection (coronary arteries). J. Immunol. **165:** 3469–3483.

51. OLESZAK, E.L., W.L. LIN, A. LEGIDO, et al. 2001. Presence of oligoclonal T-cells in cerebrospinal fluid of a child with multiphasic disseminated encephalomyelitis following hepatitis A virus infection. Clin. Diagn. Lab. Immunol. **8:** 984–992.

52. SAKKAS, L.I., B. XU, C.M. ARTLETT, et al. 2002. Oligoclonal T-cell expansion in the skin of patients with systemic sclerosis. J. Immunol. **168:** 3649–3659.

53. XU, B., L.I. SAKKAS, B.I. GOLDMAN, et al. 2003. Identical alpha-chain T-cell receptor transcripts are present on T-cells infiltrating coronary arteries of human cardiac allografts with chronic rejection. Transplantation **225:** 75–90.

54. PAPPAS, J. W.J. JUNG, A.K. BARDA, et al. 2005. Substantial proportions of identical beta-chain T-cell receptor transcripts are present in epithelial ovarian carcinoma tumors. Cell. Immunol. **234:** 81–101.

55. MONOS, D.S., J. PAPPAS, E.E. MAGIRA, *et al*. 2005. Identification of HLA-DQalpha and –DRbeta residues associated with susceptibility and protection to epithelial ovarian cancer. Hum. Immunol. **66:** 554–562.
56. PLATSOUCAS, C.D., J.E. FINCKE, J. PAPPAS, *et al*. 2003. Immune responses to human tumors: development of tumor vaccines. Anticancer Res. **23:** 1969–1996.
57. MATHIOUDAKIS, G., P.-F. CHEN, Y. LI, *et al*. 1993. Preferential rearrangements of the V gamma I subgroup of the gamma-chain of the T-cell antigen receptor to J gamma 2 C gamma 2 gene segments in peripheral blood lymphocyte transcripts from normal donors. Scand. J. Immunol. **38:** 31–36.
58. MATHIOUDAKIS, G., R.A. GOOD, Y. CHERNAJOVSKY, *et al*. 1996. Selective γ-chain T-cell receptor gene rearrangements in a patient with Omenn's Syndrome: absence of V-II subgroup (Vγ9) transcripts. Clin. Diagn. Lab. Immunol. **3:** 616–619.
59. BELDJORD, K., C. BELDJORD, E. MACINTYRE, *et al*. 1993. Peripheral selection of V delta 1+ cells with restricted T-cell receptor delta gene junctional repertoire in the peripheral blood of healthy donors. J. Exp. Med. **178:** 121–127.
60. BOULLIER, S., M. COCHET, F. POCCIA & M.L. GOUGEON. 1995. CDR3-independent gamma delta Vdelta1+ T-cell expansion in the peripheral blood of HIV-infected persons. J. Immunol. **154:** 1418–1431.

# Genes Predisposing to Rapid Aneurysm Growth

J.T. POWELL

*Imperial College, London, UK*

ABSTRACT: The aim of the study was to investigate the effect of functional polymorphisms in promoters of the MMP-2 ($-1306$ C > T), MMP-3 ($-1171$ 5A > 6A), MMP-9 ($-1562$ C > T), MMP-12 ($-82$ A > G), TIMP-1 ($-372$ C > T), and PAI-1 ($-675$ 4G > 5G and $-847$ A > G) genes on the growth rate of small abdominal aortic aneurysms. The patients with small aneurysms were recruited from the surveillance arm of the U.K. Small Aneurysm Trial and monitored for aneurysm growth, mean follow-up 2.6 years. Mean linear aneurysm growth rates were calculated by flexible modeling. For MMP-2, MMP-3, MMP-9, MMP-12, and TIMP-1 polymorphisms there were no clear associations with aneurysm growth. The increased growth rates for patients of 5G5G PAI-1 genotype were of borderline significance ($P = 0.06$). However, PAI-1 haplotype analysis showed that 5G5G/GG patients had significantly faster aneurysm growth (mean 0.46 mm/year faster). There was no evidence that any specific MMP polymorphism had a clinically significant effect on aneurysm growth. However the plasminogen system (via PAI-1) appears to have a small, but clinically significant, role in aneurysm growth.

KEYWORDS: aneurysm; proteases; anti-proteases

## INTRODUCTION

Abdominal aortic aneurysm (AAA) is a common degenerative vascular disease present in 5% of men over the age of 60 years. The epidemiology of AAA reveals subtly different risk factors in comparison to coronary heart disease; for instance, smoking is much more important for AAA. The high sensitivity and specificity of ultrasonography for the detection of AAA has been essential to revealing the familial aggregation of this disorder. Apart from these interests AAA and its treatment is a major health concern for patients, clinicians, and health service providers. Contemporary issues include the outcome and cost-effectiveness of endovascular and open repair. The study of genetic polymorphisms has an important role in furthering our understanding of the

Address for correspondence: J.T. Powell, Imperial College, Charing Cross Campus, St. Dunstan's Rd., London W6 8RP, UK. Voice: 44-208-846-7312; fax: 44-208-846-7330.

e-mail: j.powell@imperial.ac.uk

Ann. N.Y. Acad. Sci. 1085: 236–241 (2006). © 2006 New York Academy of Sciences.

doi: 10.1196/annals.1383.042

etiology and prognosis of AAA. Whether these polymorphisms are used to study genes causing AAA, genes associated with the progression of AAA, or genes associated with patient prognosis before and after intervention, the crucial issues are common; the need for unbiased accumulation of study cohorts, sufficiently powered studies, and accurate description (or phenotyping) of the outcome measure.[1]

There are two types of study that should be used to assess the role of specific genes in contributing to the causation of a disease. The first of these is the study of affected families to identify the mode of transmission with the use of genetic markers (principally microsatellites) to identify specific chromosomal areas associated with the disease. Kuivaniemi and colleagues have used this approach to show that the transmission of AAA is heterogeneous and to identify a region on chromosome 19 (19q13) that could be important to disease development.[2] Others have used the same approach to implicate regions on at least three different chromosomes (3, 5, and 11) in the causation of familial thoracic aortic aneurysm.[3] The second type of study requires the prior identification of candidate genes and should be conducted on a population basis. The literature suggests a large number of candidate genes for AAA including the matrix metalloproteinases (MMPs),[4] but there have been no properly powered population studies. The numerous case–control studies are flawed by the selection procedure for cases and controls, small size, and publication bias.[1] This means that the results are unlikely to be reproducible in a second study.[5,6] A recent review of the influence of polymorphisms in the MMP genes on cardiovascular disease exemplifies this problem clearly.[7]

There are two types of polymorphisms that can be used in association studies: neutral polymorphisms that do not influence gene expression and functional polymorphisms that influence gene expression. This latter type of polymorphism is often to be found in the gene promoter, where it influences the binding of activators or repressors of gene expression. For instance the $-1612$ 5A > 6A polymorphism of the MMP-3 gene is located within an interleukin-1 (IL-1) responsive element of the gene promoter and the 5A allele is associated with higher gene expression *in vitro* and *in vivo*.[7]

The effect of functional polymorphisms of protease and protease inhibitor genes on aneurysm growth has been studied recently.[8] Here, the difficulty has been using an unbiased method to evaluate aneurysm growth and even large studies (500 patients) are only capable of discerning associations with polymorphisms that have a large functional effect, about 20% or more, on gene expression.

## METHODS

All studies had approval from local ethical committees. Patients with abdominal aortic aneurysm (AAA) referred to vascular surgeons at 93 U.K. hospitals were entered into the U.K. Small Aneurysm Trial, although some with initial AAA diameter <4.0 cm were first followed up in the associated study.[9] There were 527 patients randomized to ultrasonographic surveillance for AAA growth with a baseline blood sample for plasma and extraction of DNA: plasma was stored in aliquots at −70°C. Polymerase chain reaction quality DNA was extracted for 455 (86%) patients, DNA was of poor quality for 23 patients (residual salts, protein or PCR inhibitors), and there were insufficient blood cells available for the remainder. Plasma PAI-1 measurements (TintElize®, Biopool, Umea, Sweden) were available for 256 unselected patients out of the total 455 (56%). Plasma PAI-1 was the last in a sequence of assays and no further plasma aliquots were available for the remaining patients: there was no difference in age, sex, initial AAA diameter, or smoking status between patients with plasma samples for PAI-1 assay and those with no remaining plasma sample. Details of patient surveillance and follow-up and flexible hierarchical modeling to estimate AAA growth rates have been described previously.[10] The repeatability of the measurement of the aneurysm diameter was ± 0.2 cm. Adjustment for smoking and other variables was performed by entering them into the model as fixed effects allowed to influence the linear component of growth. All parameter estimates reported are medians of the relevant posterior distributions and 95% credible intervals (CI) were constructed from the 2.5 and 97.5 percentiles of the posterior distributions.

### Genotyping

DNA was prepared from peripheral blood cells and stored in 96-well arrays at −20°C. Determination of MMP-2 −1306 C > T and MMP-3 −1171 5A > 6A genotypes was performed with real-time sequencing using the Pyrosequencing equipment and protocol (Pyrosequencing AB, Uppsala, Sweden).

Genotyping for MMP-9 −1562C > T, MMP-12 −82A > G, TIMP-1 −372 C > T (men only), and PAI-1 −675 4G > 5G and −847 A > G was performed using standard methods.

### Statistical Considerations

With 400 patients, the study had 90% power to detect a true difference in AAA growth rate of 0.7 mm/year (with 5% significance). A $\chi^2$ test was used to compare the observed numbers of each genotype with those expected for a population in the Hardy–Weinberg equilibrium. All growth rates were adjusted for initial AAA diameter and the frequently observed acceleration of growth with increasing diameter. The most abundant genotype provided the reference group against which to compare growth rate in other genotypes.

**TABLE 1. Estimated AAA growth by functional polymorphisms of selected genes**

| Gene | N* | Mean baseline diameter, mm | Linear growth rate (mm/year) | | |
|---|---|---|---|---|---|
| | | | Average | Difference† (95% CI) | Difference‡ (95% CI) |
| MMP-2 | | | | | |
| CC | 257 | 44.1 | 3.05 | Reference | Reference |
| CT (163 + 27TT) | 190 | 45.6 | 3.12 | 0.13 (−0.32 to 0.63) | 0.16 (−0.24 to 0.57) |
| MMP-3 | | | | | |
| 5A5A 5A6A | 129 | 45.4 | 3.05 | −0.05 (−0.54 to 0.45) | 0.01 (−0.50 to 0.40) |
| 6A6A | 201 | 44.8 | 3.19 | Reference | Reference |
| | 95 | 44.9 | 2.90 | −0.32 (−0.88 to 0.18) | −0.29 (−0.85 to 0.26) |
| MMP-9 | | | | | |
| CC | 333 | 45.1 | 3.15 | Reference | Reference |
| CT (107 + 8TT) | 115 | 44.6 | 2.90 | −0.12 (−0.61 to 0.39) | −0.09 (−0.65 to 0.37) |
| MMP-12 | | | | | |
| AA | 358 | 44.9 | 3.10 | Reference | Reference |
| AG (37 + 1GG) | 88 | 45.6 | 3.09 | 0.08 (−0.54 to 0.63) | −0.003 (−0.56 to 0.54) |
| TIMP-1 372 men | | | | | |
| C | 284 | 45.3 | 3.10 | 0.00 (−0.11 to 0.09) | 0.00 (−0.12 to 0.09) |
| T | 175 | 45.4 | 3.08 | | |
| PAI-1 −675 | | | | | |
| 1 (4G4G) | 141 | 45.1 | 3.05 | 0.07 (−0.43 to 0.52) | 0.09 (−0.37 to 0.55) |
| 2 (4G5G) | 231 | 44.6 | 2.92 | Reference | Reference |
| 3 (5G5G) | 76 | 46.2 | 3.47 | 0.40 (−0.02 to 0.98) | 0.43 (−0.02 to 1.07) |
| PAI-1 −675/847 | | | | | |
| 1 (4G4Gaa) | 132 | 45.1 | 3.18 | 0.07 (−0.40 to 0.51) | 0.10 (−0.32 to 0.52) |
| 2 (4G5Gag) | 219 | 44.8 | 2.92 | Reference | Reference |
| 3 (5G5Ggg) | 66 | 46.4 | 3.47 | 0.40 (0.05 to 0.93) | 0.46 (0.06 to 0.97) |

*Add to less than 455 since genes not typed on all patients.
† Adjusted for baseline diameter and curvature in growth pattern.
‡ Adjusted for age, sex, smoking status, baseline diameter, and curvature in growth pattern.

## RESULTS

The mean follow up was 2.6 years with a mean of 7.4 AAA diameter measurements per patient. The mean linear growth rate was 3.08 mm/year. The success of genotyping ranged from 99% for *MMP-9* and *PAI-1* to 93% for the final polymorphism analyzed, *MMP-3*. The genotype distributions and growth rates are shown in Table 1.

There were no significant associations between genotype and aneurysm growth rate for any of the polymorphisms analyzed. Baseline plasma PAI-1 concentrations varied with the *PAI-1* polymorphism: 4G4G ($n = 85$) 31 ± 3 ng/mL, 4G5G ($n = 129$) 29 ± 2 ng/mL and 5G5G ($n = 44$) 25 ± 4 ng/mL, ANOVA $P = 0.018$. The *PAI-1* polymorphism appeared to have an effect on aneurysm growth, those of 5G5G had faster AAA growth by 0.4 mm/year, a 15–20% increase, but this difference did not quite achieve statistical significance ($P = 0.06$). After adjustment for smoking, the magnitude of the effect of *PAI-1* 5G5G genotype was very similar, but the association remained nonsignificant (Table 1); further adjustment for diabetes did not alter the growth rates. However, when the two separate PAI-1 polymorphisms were assessed together, there was a significant association between haplotype and aneurysm growth, $P = 0.02$. We also observed a significant relationship of *PAI-1* with the initial AAA diameter, patients of PAI-1 5G5G genotype presented with larger AAA, ANOVA $P = 0.03$.

## DISCUSSION

In this study, variability in the PAI-1 gene was associated with AAA growth rate. It is likely that the MMP polymorphisms we studied did not influence tissue gene expression by a sufficient margin to permit an effect on AAA growth in a study of this size, although it is possible that another of the known polymorphisms in the MMP genes would have had greater effect. It is rare that nonpathological polymorphisms have a very strong effect on gene expression *in vivo*, but PAI-1 is one example. However, it is more likely that several factors or genes contribute to AAA growth rates and this underscores the difficulty of a possible future medical therapy based on selective protease inhibition. There remains an urgent need to identify new medical therapies and to add justification to the role of population screening programs, and it would be helpful to confirm the role of PAI-1 in a larger study.

## ACKNOWLEDGMENTS

I would like to thank the many collaborators who have contributed to these findings and funding for this research from the British Heart Foundation.

# REFERENCES

1. DAVEY SMITH, G., S. EBRAHIM, S. LEWIS, *et al.* 2005. Genetic epidemiology and public health: hope, hype and future prospects. Lancet **366:** 1484–1498.
2. SHIBAMURA, H., J.M. OLSON, C. VAN VLIJMEN-VAN KEULEN, *et al.* 2004. Genome scan from familial abdominal aortic aneurysm using sex and family history as covariates suggests genetic heterogeneity and identifies linkage to chromosome 19q13. Circulation **2103:** 2103–2108.
3. HASHAM, S.N., M.C. WILLING, D.C. GUO, *et al.* 2003. Mapping a locus for familial thoracic aortic aneurysms and dissections (TAAD2) to chromosome 3p24-25. Circulation **107:** 3184–3190.
4. STRAUSS, E., K. WALISZEWSKI, M. GABRIEL, *et al.* 2003. Increased risk of abdominal aortic aneurysm in carriers of the MTHFR 677T allele. J. Appl. Genet **44:** 85–93.
5. JONES, G.T., E.L. HARRIS, L.V. PHILLIPS & A.M. VAN RIJ. 2005. The methylenetetrahydrofolate reductase C677T polymorphism does not associate with susceptibility to abdominal aortic aneurysm. Eur. J. Vasc. Endovasc. Surg. **30:** 137–142.
6. CHOKE, E., G. COCKERILL, W.R. WILSON, *et al.* 2005. A review of biological factors implicated in abdominal aortic aneurysm rupture. Eur. J. Vasc. Endovasc. Surg. **30:** 227–244.
7. YE, S. 2006. Influence of matrix metalloproteinase genotype on cardiovascular disease susceptibility and outcome. Cardiovasc. Res. **69:** 636–645.
8. ERIKSSON, P., S. JORMSJO-PETTERSSON, A.R. BRADY, *et al.* 2005. Genotype-phenotype relationships to investigate the role of proteases in abdominal aortic aneurysm expansion. Br. J. Surg. **92:** 1372–1376.
9. U.K. Small Aneurysm Trial Participants. 2002. Long-term outcomes of immediate repair compared with surveillance for small abdominal aortic aneurysm. N. Engl. J. Med. **346:** 1445–1452.
10. BRADY, A.R., S.G. THOMPSON, F.G.R. FOWKES, *et al.* 2004. Abdominal aortic aneurysm expansion: risk factors and time intervals for surveillance. Circulation **110:** 16–21.

# Genetic Basis of Thoracic Aortic Aneurysms and Dissections

## Potential Relevance to Abdominal Aortic Aneurysms

HARIYADARSHI PANNU, NILI AVIDAN, VAN TRAN-FADULU, AND DIANNA M. MILEWICZ

*Department of Internal Medicine and Institute of Molecular Medicine, The University of Texas Health Science Center, Houston, Texas, USA*

ABSTRACT: Ascending thoracic aortic aneurysms leading to type A dissections (TAAD) have long been known to occur in association with a genetic syndrome such as Marfan syndrome (MFS). More recently, TAAD has also been demonstrated to occur as an autosomal dominant disorder in the absence of syndromic features, termed *familial TAAD*. Familial TAAD demonstrates genetic heterogeneity, and linkage studies have identified TAAD loci at 5q13-14 (*TAAD1*), 11q23 (*FAA1*), 3p24-25 (*TAAD2*), and 16p12.2-13.13. The genetic heterogeneity of TAAD is reflected by variation in disease in terms of the age of onset, progression, penetrance, and association with additional cardiac and vascular features. The underlying genetic heterogeneity of TAAD is reflected in the phenotypic variation associated with familial TAAD with respect to age of onset, progression, penetrance, and association with additional cardiac and vascular features. Mutations in the *TGFBR2* gene have been identified as the cause of disease linked to the 3p24-25 locus, implicating dysregulation of TGF-β signaling in TAAD. Mutations in myosin heavy chain (*MYH11*), a smooth muscle cell-specific contractile protein, have been identified in familial TAAD associated with patent ductus arteriosus (PDA) linked to 16p12.2-12.13. The identification of these novel disease pathways has led to new directions for future research addressing the pathology and treatment of TAAD.

KEYWORDS: aneurysms; dissections; aorta; aortic disease; transforming growth factor-β; *TGFBR1*; *TGFBR2*; *FBN1*; *MYH11*

## INTRODUCTION

Aortic aneurysms and dissections are the major diseases affecting the aorta, and a leading cause of morbidity and mortality in the United States.[1,2] The

Address for correspondence: Dr. D.M. Milewicz, 6431 Fannin, Department of Internal Medicine and Institute of Molecular Medicine, The University of Texas Health Science Center, MSB 6.100, Houston, TX, 77030. Voice: 713-500-6725 ; fax: 713-500-0693.
e-mail: Dianna.M.Milewicz@uth.tmc.edu

Ann. N.Y. Acad. Sci. 1085: 242–255 (2006). © 2006 New York Academy of Sciences.
doi: 10.1196/annals.1383.024

most common location for aneurysms is the infrarenal abdominal aorta (abdominal aortic aneurysms, AAAs), followed by aneurysms of the ascending thoracic aorta (thoracic aortic aneurysms, TAAs) (FIG. 1A). Aortic dissections typically begin with a tear in the aortic inner layer, the intima, and then blood penetrates the diseased medial layer and dissects along the plane of the aortic wall. The dissection usually proceeds antegrade from the site of the intimal tear, but can also proceed retrograde. Like aortic aneurysms, aortic dissections are classified based on location and the extent of the dissection (FIG. 1B). More than 95% of aortic dissections originate either in the ascending aorta within several centimeters of the aortic valve (type A dissections) or in the descending aorta just distal to the origin of the left subclavian artery (type B dissections). Ascending thoracic aortic aneurysms and type A dissections (TAAD) are related conditions as indicated by the fact that progressive enlargement of the ascending aorta leads to type A dissections in the absence of prophylactic surgical repair of the aneurysm.

The average age of patients with AAAs is 75 years and the affected men to women ratio as high as 6:1.[3] Pathologic examination of the aorta indicates that atherosclerosis is associated with AAAs. These lesions are associated with intimal atherosclerosis, medial destruction of the elastic lamellae, medial neovascularization, a decrease in vascular smooth muscle cells, and a chronic immune/inflammatory response.[4,5] In contrast, the average age of patients with TAAs is 65 years, and men are at a slightly increased risk compared to women (1.7:1).[6] The pathology associated with TAAs is typically medial degeneration, a poorly understood pathologic process previously termed *cystic medial necrosis* by Erdheim.[7] Medial degeneration is characterized by degeneration and fragmentation of elastic fibers, loss of smooth muscle cells with evidence of apoptosis of these cells, and interstitial collection of proteoglycans. Therefore, the epidemiology and pathology associated with AAAs and TAAs differ, suggesting that different genes and environmental factors play a role in these diseases.

Studies have indicated that genetic factors play a role in the pathogenesis of AAAs with segregation analysis suggesting the most likely genetic model to be a major autosomal allele for a recessively inherited gene.[8–13] Currently, studies are in progress to determine the genetic basis for AAAs using an affected relative pair analysis.[14]

In contrast to studies addressing the genetic basis of AAAs, the genetic basis of TAAs and aortic dissections has relatively recently begun to be investigated. It has been recognized for several years that TAAD occurs in conjunction with several genetic syndromes, in particular Marfan syndrome (MFS), and research initially focused on the genetic basis of syndromic TAAD. More recently, research has focused on defining the genetic component for nonsyndromic TAAD, and mapping and identifying genes for this condition. The mapping and identification of disease genes causing both syndromic and nonsyndromic TAAD have progressed rapidly and outpaced the progress in the understanding

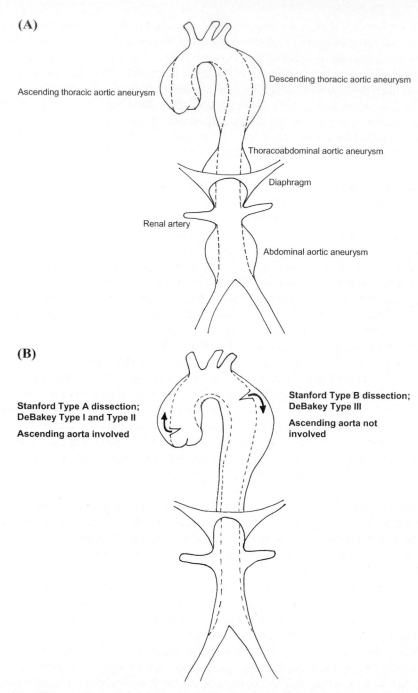

**FIGURE 1.** Classification of aortic aneurysms (**A**) and dissections (**B**) according to anatomical location.

of the genetic basis of AAAs. This article will discuss genetic predisposition to thoracic aortic aneurysms leading to type A dissections (TAAD), highlight how these gene discoveries have increased our understanding of the molecular defects leading to this disease, and identify factors that have allowed for the rapid mapping and identification of disease genes.

## GENETIC SYNDROMES WITH TAAD AS A MAJOR MANIFESTATION

TAAD is the major cardiovascular complication associated with the well-known genetic syndrome MFS (OMIM No. 154700), a disorder with cardio-vascular, skeletal, and ocular manifestations that is inherited in an autosomal dominant manner. The progressive dilation of the aortic root culminating in dissection is a major cause of morbidity and mortality in MFS patients.[15–17] Aortic disease in MFS is the result of defects in the fibrillin-1 (*FBN1*) gene that localizes to chromosome 15q15-31.[18] *FBN1* is a large 350-kDa cysteine-rich glycoprotein that is a major component of the 10 nm microfibrils that make up the elastic fiber and has a repetitive domain structure containing calcium-binding epidermal growth factor precursor-like and transforming growth factor-β-binding 8-cysteine motifs.[19,20] Over 600 mutations in the *FBN1* gene have been identified to date (http://www.umd.be:2030/). In addition to MFS, *FBN1* mutations may also result in a range of clinical manifestations including isolated ocular, skeletal defects, or cardiovascular features of MFS.[21–26]

Immunohistochemical studies and metabolic labeling studies have shown that the majority of fibroblast cells explanted from MFS patients have a decrease in fibrillin-1-containing microfibrils in the extracellular matrix far below the 50% level predicted by a heterozygous *FBN1* mutation.[26–28] Analysis of the *FBN1*-deficient mouse models of MFS has provided a connecting pathway between decreased formation of microfibrils and the manifestations of MFS. Fibrillin-1-deficient mice demonstrated increased active TGF-β in tissues when compared with wild-type mice, suggesting that diminished microfibrils increased the bioavailability of active TGF-β in tissues.[29] Furthermore, antagonism of TGF-β signaling prevented the pulmonary parenchymal abnormalities, mitral valve abnormalities, and aortic dilatation observed in mouse models of MFS, suggesting a critical role for TGF-β signaling in MFS.[29–31]

More than a decade ago, genetic heterogeneity for MFS was proposed and a second locus for MFS, termed the *MFS2* locus, was mapped to chromosome 3p25-24.2.[32] This locus was identified using a single large family and whether the affected family members met the diagnostic criteria for MFS was controversial.[33,34] Recently, a heterozygous mutation in *TGFBR2* leading to a splicing error in the kinase domain was identified as the cause of disease in this family.[35] DNA from nine MFS families with no identified mutations in

*FBN1* was also sequenced, and *TGFBR2* missense mutations were identified in three of these families. These *TGFBR2* mutations in MFS patients all involved the intracellular serine-threonine kinase domain of the receptor, and have been determined to diminish receptor signaling induced by TGF-β when coexpressed with a TGF-β responsive promoter in an *in vitro* assay system.

*TGFBR1* and *TGFBR2* mutations have also been reported in a syndrome with craniosynostosis, cleft palate, congenital heart disease, arterial aneurysms, and mental retardation as part of the phenotype, termed *Loeys-Dietz Aortic Aneurysm Syndrome* (LDS, OMIM #609192)[36] (FIG. 2). With the exception of one mutation affecting splicing of the extracellular region of *TGFBR2* and one mutation affecting an amino acid distal to the intracellular kinase domain of *TGFBR1*, all mutations observed were germline heterozygous missense mutations affecting amino acids in the functionally critical intracellular kinase domain of the proteins. Surprisingly, tissues from affected individuals showed increased expression of collagen and connective tissue growth factor as well as nuclear enrichment of phosphorylated Smad2, both observations suggesting increased TGF-β signaling in these tissues.

This suggests a common theme of dysregulated TGF-β signaling in aortic disease pathogenesis, either due to the presence of increased active TGF-β as observed in MFS or by disruptions in signaling due to mutations in the receptors for TGF-β (FIG. 3). The bioavailability of active TGF-β ligand is known to be tightly regulated and dependent on its release from a large latent complex to which TGF-β is noncovalently associated with its propeptide fragment,

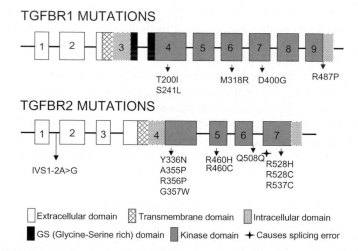

**FIGURE 2.** Heterozygous germline *TGFBR1* and *TGFBR2* mutations in syndromic and nonsyndromic aortic disease. Genomic and protein structure of the *TGFBR1* and *TGFBR2* genes showing known mutations previously identified in MFS, LDS, Furlong syndrome, and TAAD.[35,36,47,65–67]

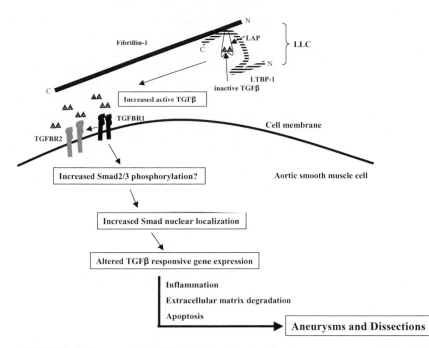

**FIGURE 3. Dysregulated TGF-β signaling leading to aneurysms and dissections.** Transforming growth factor-β (TGF-β) is secreted in a biologically inactive form and stored in the extracellular matrix in a complex termed the large latent TGF-β complex (LLC), consisting of a TGF-β homodimer associated with the latency-associated peptide (LAP) and the latent TGF-β-binding protein-1 (LTBP-1). Dysregulated TGF-β signaling results from mutations in fibrillin-1, *TGFBR1*, or *TGFBR2*, leading to altered transcription of TGF-β-responsive genes, resulting in medial degeneration leading to aneurysms and dissections.

the latency-associated peptide, and covalently linked to latent TGFβ-binding protein (LTBP) (FIG. 3). This complex associates with fibrillin-1-containing extracellular microfibrils and mutations in fibrillin-1 lead to diminished amounts of microfibrils in the extracellular matrix, and thereby to increased amounts of bioavailable TGF-β in the tissues of patients with *FBN1* mutations. This mechanism of enhanced TGF-β signaling caused by *FBN1* mutations, while difficult to reconcile with the putatively kinase-inactivating *TGFBR1* and *TGFBR2* mutations identified in LDS, appears to be the basis of aortic disease in both these syndromes as increased TGF-β signaling is also observed in aortic tissue from LDS patients.[36] These observations are strikingly similar to previous research demonstrating fibroblast-specific expression of a kinase-deficient *TGFBR2* in a transgenic mouse model leads to the paradoxical upregulation of the TGF-β signaling pathway.[37,38] The biological mechanism behind the TGF-β signaling upregulation observed in aortic disease remains to be elucidated.

## Familial TAAD

Although it has been recognized for some time that TAAD occurs in association with known genetic syndromes, a genetic basis of TAAD in individuals who do not have a known genetic syndrome has only relatively recently been investigated. Although families with multiple members with TAAD were described in the literature, only a few of these reports excluded MFS as the cause of disease.[39] In the past decade, familial aggregation studies of patients referred for repair of ascending aneurysms or dissections who did not have an associated genetic syndrome have indicated that between 11–19% of these patients have a first-degree relative with TAAD, providing evidence that genetic predisposition plays a significant role in the etiology of this disease.[40,41] Furthermore, patients with a family history of TAAD present with aortic disease at a mean age of 56.8 years, which is significantly younger than that for patients with sporadic TAAD (64.3 years) and older than patients with MFS (24.8 years). In contrast to AAAs in which segregation studies have suggested an autosomal recessive mode of inheritance of predisposing genes, studies of families with multiple members with TAAD have established that the disease segregates predominantly as an autosomal dominant disorder.[13,42] Aortic imaging of individuals at risk for inheriting the defective gene often identifies individuals with asymptomatic ascending aortic aneurysms and aids in the confirmation of autosomal dominant inheritance of the disease. Families with inherited forms of TAAD demonstrate a wide range of onset of the familial disease (variable expression); the age of acute dissections has ranged from 19 to 81 years of age with a single family.[43] In addition, this disorder demonstrates decreased penetrance of the phenotype (someone inherits the defective gene but does not develop aortic disease) and the decreased penetrance has been documented primarily in women. In families with inherited forms of TAAD, the pathology in the aortic wall of aneurysms and dissection is medial degeneration.

Families identified for genetic mapping studies have been used to identify the chromosomal location of genes that predispose individuals to TAAD. The fact that one of many genes can be mutated leading to this disease (termed genetic heterogeneity) was recognized early for familial TAAD. Despite this complicating factor, four loci have been identified through genetic mapping studies. The success of these genetic studies has been dependent on the use of a mapping strategy that focuses on a single large family to initially map the chromosomal location of novel genes causing this disease, thus reducing the effect of genetic heterogeneity on mapping TAAD genes. This strategy has allowed for the successful mapping of genes despite the significant genetic heterogeneity extant in TAAD.

The first locus to be mapped for familial TAAD was the *TAAD1* locus at 5q13-14.[44] The initial genetic screen to identify the location of the defective gene used two families with a similar phenotype for the mapping. Subsequent to mapping the locus, 15 families in which TAAD segregated as an autosomal dominant disease with reduced penetrance were studied and the linkage analysis was used to establish linkage of 9 of these families to 5q13-14. *TAAD1* has been confirmed as a major predisposition locus for TAAD by a subsequent study showing evidence for linkage of disease in 7 of 11 Finnish families to markers at the *TAAD1* locus.[45]

A locus for familial aortic aneurysms, designated *FAA1*, was mapped to 11q23-24.[46] Linkage to this region was established using a single large family. In contrast to *TAAD1*, the disease associated with *FAA1* is characterized by a more diffuse vascular disease with aneurysms affecting both the thoracic and abdominal aorta as well as other arteries in affected individuals. This locus appears to be a rare cause of TAAD since no additional families with disease linked to the *FAA1* locus have been described.

A second locus predisposing to TAAD, *TAAD2*, was mapped to 3p24-25, and it has recently been determined that *TGFBR2* is the mutant gene at this locus.[43,47] The *TGFBR2* gene was screened for missense, nonsense, and exon splicing errors and mutations were found in 4 out of 80 unrelated families (5%) with familial TAAD indicating that *TGFBR2* mutations are a relatively rare cause of familial TAAD. Although the majority of vascular disease in these families involved ascending aortic aneurysms leading to type A dissections, affected family members also had descending aortic disease and aneurysms of other arteries including cerebral, carotid, and popliteal aneurysms. Strikingly, all 4 families carried mutations that affected arginine at amino acid 460 in the intracellular domain, suggesting a mutation "hot-spot" for familial TAAD and establishing a strong genotype–phenotype correlation between familial TAAD and mutations at this location. Polymorphic markers flanking the *TGFBR2* mutation indicated that the families do not share a common haplotype, providing further evidence of a "hot-spot" for mutations causing this disease. Structural analysis of the *TGFBR2* serine/threonine kinase domain revealed that R460 is strategically located within a highly conserved region of this domain and that the amino acid substitutions resulting from these mutations will interfere with the receptor's ability to transduce signals. A surprising observation in these families was that there is no evidence of an increased susceptibility to cancer in families with germline *TGFBR2* mutations (Milewicz, unpublished data), despite evidence in the literature that somatic *TGFBR2* mutations occur in a variety of cancers.[48]

A fourth locus was mapped at 16p12.2-13.13 in a large French family with TAAD associated with patent ductus arteriosus (PDA).[49] In addition to the large French family, an American family has been described with TAAD associated with PDA.[50] The defective gene at the 16p locus was identified as the smooth muscle cell myosin heavy chain 11 (*MYH11*).[51] *MYH11* is a major contractile protein specific to the smooth muscle cells. Affected individuals heterozygous for *MYH11* mutations marked aortic stiffness with a substantial decrease in aortic compliance and increase in pulse wave velocity. On pathological examination of these aortas, large areas of medial degeneration were found with very low SMC content. Comparable to the PDA as a consequence of the *MYH11* mutation in human disease, mice deficient in *MYH11* demonstrate delayed closure of the ductus arteriosus. Appropriate development and closing of the ductus arteriosus requires apposite smooth muscle cell migration, proliferation, contraction, and differentiation. Thus the pathogenic mechanism of aneurysms caused by heterozygous *MYH11* mutations will require insight into both the structural and functional roles of this contractile protein in smooth muscle cells. A parallel for the disease process may be sought in cardiomyopathies caused by mutations in *MYH6* or *MYH7*, where pathological sequelae develop secondarily to functional defects in specific MYH proteins.[52]

More recently, we have used a large TAAD family comprising 134 individuals to map a fourth locus. This family presented with a unique aortic phenotype of dissections involving both the ascending and descending aorta along with AAAs.[53] After determining that the phenotype was not linked to any of the known TAAD loci, a genome-wide linkage analysis was completed and significant linkage to markers on chromosome 15q was found.[54] A shared 15q haplotype was found in 14 affected individuals and a maximum multipoint LOD score of 4.0 was obtained. Subsequently, 16 families with 3 or more affected individuals were studied and we found 2 additional families linked to this locus with an increase in the overall LOD score to 5.0. A detailed analysis of the clinical features of individuals in these families demonstrated some unique features associated with this novel locus.[53] Unlike the majority of TAAD families, penetrance of aortic disease was equal between genders. Of 14 males and 19 females who inherited the affected haplotype at this locus imaged for aortic disease, 11 males (78%) and 15 females (80%) had aortic disease. The equal penetrance in both genders was also supported by the Kaplan-Meier survival curve that indicates no difference in survival between the genders ($p = 0.123$). In addition, women ($n = 11$) and men ($n = 11$) dissected on average at similar ages ($36.6 \pm 13.7$ vs. $39.6 \pm 21.8$ years, respectively, $p$-value = 0.703). Additionally, aortic dissections (type A or B) occurred in a subset of family members at a young age with type A dissections that were often fatal and documented to cause death as young as 14 years of age. Four individuals had type B dissections with one of these individuals initially presenting with type B dissection, subsequently followed by a type A dissection. Three affected women presented with AAAs; all of these individuals also had ascending aortic aneurysms or subsequently had type A dissections, suggesting that the defective gene leads to a considerably diffuse aortic pathology.

Despite the identification of these aortic aneurysm loci, the occurrence of TAAD families that are not linked to genetic markers at any of the known loci suggests that there is at least one additional major TAAD predisposition locus to be identified (Milewicz, unpublished data). Reflecting this underlying genetic heterogeneity, TAAD families are observed to exhibit considerable clinical heterogeneity in the age of onset, penetrance, and associated features.

In addition to the TAAD families described above, there are TAAD families described with associated features such as bicuspid aortic valve (BAV), cervicocephalic arterial dissections, cerebral aneurysms, and coarctation of the aorta, suggesting that these malformations result from a single developmental diathesis and potentially due to different genes for each familial form of TAAD associated with a specific defect.[55–59] The successful identification of *MYH11* as the gene responsible for PDA in conjunction with TAAD lends support to this hypothesis. In addition, familial aggregation studies have established the cosegregation of TAAD and BAV, and an increased prevalence of aortic root enlargement has been noted in patients with BAV further suggesting a common genetic basis for TAAD and BAV.[60–63]

The aortic valvular cusps and the arterial media of the ascending aorta and its branches are derived from neural crest cells, raising the possibility that a defect in the neural crest-derived cells may be the cause of the cardiovascular disease in these families.[64] Thus, investigation into the dysregulation of TGF-β signaling in these cells could potentially provide insight into pathways leading to TAAs and dissections.

## SUMMARY AND CONCLUSIONS

In summary, research addressing the genetic basis of TAAD has progressed substantially over the past decade. One reason for the greater success in disease gene mapping and identification for TAAD as compared to studies for AAA has been the aggressive pursuit of large families to map genes that cause the TAAD and using single families to definitively map novel disease loci. The identification of these disease genes has highlighted significant pathways that lead to TAAD. Studies of fibrillin-deficient mouse models as well as initial molecular evidence from studies of *TGFBR1* and *TGFBR2* mutations identified in TAAD underscore the critical role of the TGF-β pathway in aortic disease. The identification of *MYH11* mutations suggests that viable contractile machinery in smooth muscle cells is also essential to prevent aortic disease. Although current evidence suggests that distinct genetic and environmental mechanisms lead to TAAD and AAA, it is anticipated that there will be some overlap of genes that lead to TAAD and AAA. This may be minimal and primarily observed in individuals with early onset of AAA, who might also exhibit involvement of the ascending aorta.

Continuing advances in research addressing the molecular pathogenesis of aortic disease will be useful in informing improved clinical management of patients. The observed heterogeneity in aortic disease onset, presentation, and progression may be attributed in part to the underlying genetic mutation and the functional consequence of this mutation on protein function. Therefore, recommendations for the extent of imaging of the vasculature, medical management, and appropriate timing for surgery may be evolved from a greater understanding of the pathways leading to aortic disease.

## ACKNOWLEDGMENTS

The authors thank all the patients and families who have participated in these studies.

## REFERENCES

1. LILIENFELD, D.E., P.D. GUNDERSON, J.M. SPRAFKA & C. VARGAS. 1987. Epidemiology of aortic aneurysms: I. Mortality trends in the United States, 1951 to 1981. Arteriosclerosis **7:** 637–643.
2. LINDSAY, J., JR. 1997. Diagnosis and treatment of diseases of the aorta. Curr. Probl. Cardiol. **22:** 485–542.
3. PLEUMEEKERS, H.J., A.W. HOES, D.E. VAN DER, et al.1995. Aneurysms of the abdominal aorta in older adults. The Rotterdam Study. Am. J. Epidemiol. **142:** 1291–1299.
4. THOMPSON, R.W., D.R. HOLMES, R.A. MERTENS, et al.1995. Production and localization of 92-kilodalton gelatinase in abdominal aortic aneurysms. An elastolytic metalloproteinase expressed by aneurysm-infiltrating macrophages. J. Clin. Invest. **96:** 318–326.
5. PYO, R., J.K. LEE, J.M. SHIPLEY, et al. 2000. Targeted gene disruption of matrix metalloproteinase-9 (gelatinase B) suppresses development of experimental abdominal aortic aneurysms. J. Clin. Invest. **105:** 1641–1649.
6. BICKERSTAFF, L.K., P.C. PAIROLERO, L.H. HOLLIER, et al.1982. Thoracic aortic aneurysms: a population-based study. Surgery **92:** 1103–1108.
7. ERDHEIM, J. 1930. Medionecrosis aortae idiopathica cystica. Virchows Arch. Path. Anat. **276:** 187–229.
8. TILSON, M.D. & M.R. SEASHORE. 1984. Fifty families with abdominal aortic aneurysms in two or more first-order relatives. Am. J. Surg. **147:** 551–553.
9. WEBSTER, M.W., P.L. ST. JEAN, D.L. STEED, et al. 1991. Abdominal aortic aneurysm: results of a family study. J. Vasc. Surg. **13:** 366–372.
10. COLLIN, J. 1996. The oxford screening program for aortic aneurysm and screening first-order male siblings of probands with abdominal aortic aneurysm. Ann. N. Y. Acad. Sci. **800:** 36–43.
11. VERLOES, A., N. SAKALIHASAN, R. LIMET & L. KOULISCHER. 1996. Genetic aspects of abdominal aortic aneurysm. Ann. N. Y. Acad. Sci. **800:** 44–55.
12. NORRGARD, O., O. RAIS & K.A. ANGQUIST. 1984. Familial occurrence of abdominal aortic aneurysms. Surgery **95:** 650–656.
13. MAJUMDER, P.P., P.L. ST. JEAN, R.E. FERRELL, et al. 1991. On the inheritance of abdominal aortic aneurysm. Am. J. Hum. Genet. **48:** 164–170.
14. SHIBAMURA, H., J.M. OLSON, C. VAN VLIJMEN-VAN KEULEN, et al. 2004. Genome scan for familial abdominal aortic aneurysm using sex and family history as covariates suggests genetic heterogeneity and identifies linkage to chromosome 19q13. Circulation **109:** 2103–2108.
15. FINKBOHNER, R., D. JOHNSTON, E.S. CRAWFORD, et al.1995. Marfan syndrome. Long-term survival and complications after aortic aneurysm repair. Circulation **91:** 728–733.
16. SILVERMAN, D.I., K.J. BURTON, J. GRAY, et al. 1995. Life expectancy in the Marfan syndrome. Am. J. Cardiol. **75:** 157–160.

17. VAN KARNEBEEK, C.D., M.S. NAEFF, B.J. MULDER, *et al.* 2001. Natural history of cardiovascular manifestations in Marfan syndrome. Arch. Dis. Child **84:** 129–137.

18. LEE, B., M. GODFREY, E. VITALE, *et al.* 1991. Linkage of Marfan syndrome and a phenotypically related disorder to two different fibrillin genes. Nature **352:** 330–334.

19. CORSON, G.M., S.C. CHALBERG, H.C. DIETZ, *et al.* 1993. Fibrillin binds calcium and is coded by cDNAs that reveal a multidomain structure and alternatively spliced exons at the 5′ end. Genomics **17:** 476–484.

20. PEREIRA, L., M. D'ALESSIO, F. RAMIREZ, *et al.* 1993. Genomic organization of the sequence coding for fibrillin, the defective gene product in Marfan syndrome. Hum. Mol. Genet. **2:** 961–968.

21. MILEWICZ, D.M., J. GROSSFIELD, S.N. CAO, *et al.* 1995. A mutation in FBN1 disrupts profibrillin processing and results in isolated skeletal features of the Marfan syndrome. J. Clin. Invest. **95:** 2373–2378.

22. MILEWICZ, D.M., K. MICHAEL, N. FISHER, *et al.* 1996. Fibrillin-1 (FBN1) mutations in patients with thoracic aortic aneurysms. Circulation **94:** 2708–2711.

23. FRANCKE, U., M.A. BERG, K. TYNAN, *et al.* 1995. A Gly1127Ser mutation in An Egf-like domain of the fibrillin-1 gene is a risk factor for ascending aortic aneurysm and dissection. Am. J. Hum. Genet. **56:** 1287–1296.

24. ADES, L.C., D. SREETHARAN, E. ONIKUL, *et al.* 2002. Segregation of a novel FBN1 gene mutation, G1796E, with kyphoscoliosis and radiographic evidence of vertebral dysplasia in three generations. Am. J. Med. Genet **109:** 261–270.

25. FAIVRE, L., R.J. GORLIN, M.K. WIRTZ, *et al.* 2003. In frame fibrillin-1 gene deletion in autosomal dominant Weill-Marchesani syndrome. J Med. Genet. **40:** 34–36.

26. KATZKE, S., P. BOOMS, F. TIECKE, *et al.* 2002. TGGE screening of the entire FBN1 coding sequence in 126 individuals with Marfan syndrome and related fibrillinopathies. Hum. Mutat. **20:** 197–208.

27. HOLLISTER, D.W., M. GODFREY, L.Y. SAKAI & R.E. PYERITZ. 1990. Immunohistologic abnormalities of the microfibrillar-fiber system in the Marfan syndrome. N. Engl. J. Med. **323:** 152–159.

28. MILEWICZ, D.M., R.E. PYERITZ, E.S. CRAWFORD & P.H. BYERS. 1992. Marfan syndrome: defective synthesis, secretion, and extracellular matrix formation of fibrillin by cultured dermal fibroblasts. J. Clin. Invest. **89:** 79–86.

29. AOYAMA, T., U. FRANCKE, H.C. DIETZ & H. FURTHMAYR. 1994. Quantitative differences in biosynthesis and extracellular deposition of fibrillin in cultured fibroblasts distinguish five groups of Marfan syndrome patients and suggest distinct pathogenetic mechanisms. J. Clin. Invest. **94:** 130–137.

30. NEPTUNE, E.R., P.A. FRISCHMEYER, D.E. ARKING, *et al.* 2003. Dysregulation of TGFbeta activation contributes to pathogenesis in Marfan syndrome. Nat. Genet. **33:** 407–411.

31. NG, C.M., A. CHENG, L.A. MYERS, *et al.* 2004. TGF beta-dependent pathogenesis of mitral valve prolapse in a mouse model of Marfan syndrome. J. Clin. Invest. **114:** 1586–1592.

32. HABASHI, J.P., D.P. JUDGE, T.M. HOLM, *et al.* 2006. Losartan, an AT1 antagonist, prevents aortic aneurysm in a mouse model of Marfan syndrome. Science **312:** 117–121.

33. COLLOD, G., M.C. BABRON, G. JONDEAU, *et al.* 1994. A second locus for Marfan syndrome maps to chromosome 3p24.2-p25. Nat. Genet. **8:** 264–268.

34. BOILEAU, C., G. JONDEAU, M.C. BABRON, *et al.*1993. Autosomal dominant Marfan-like connective-tissue disorder with aortic dilation and skeletal anomalies not linked to the fibrillin genes. Am. J. Hum. Genet. **53:** 46–54.
35. DIETZ, H., U. FRANCKE, H. FURTHMAYR, *et al.*1995. The question of heterogeneity in Marfan syndrome. Nat. Genet. **9:** 228–231.
36. MIZUGUCHI, T., G. COLLOD-BEROUD, T. AKIYAMA, *et al.* 2004. Heterozygous TGFBR2 mutations in Marfan syndrome. Nat. Genet. **36:** 855–860.
37. LOEYS, B.L., J. CHEN, E.R. NEPTUNE, *et al.* 2005. A syndrome of altered cardiovascular, craniofacial, neurocognitive and skeletal development caused by mutations in TGFBR1 or TGFBR2. Nat. Genet. **37:** 275–281.
38. DENTON, C.P., B. ZHENG, L.A. EVANS, *et al.* 2003. Fibroblast-specific expression of a kinase-deficient type II transforming growth factor beta (TGFbeta) receptor leads to paradoxical activation of TGFbeta signaling pathways with fibrosis in transgenic mice. J. Biol. Chem. **278:** 25109–25119.
39. DENTON, C.P., G.E. LINDAHL, K. KHAN, *et al.* 2005. Activation of 78II transforming growth factor-{beta} receptor (T{beta}RII{Delta}k). J. Biol. Chem. **280:** 16053–16065.
40. NICOD, P., C. BLOOR, M. GODFREY, *et al.*1989. Familial aortic dissecting aneurysm. J. Am. Coll. Cardiol. **13:** 811–819.
41. BIDDINGER, A., M. ROCKLIN, J. COSELLI & D.M. MILEWICZ. 1997. Familial thoracic aortic dilatations and dissections: a case control study. J. Vasc. Surg. **25:** 506–511.
42. COADY, M.A., R.R. DAVIES, M. ROBERTS, *et al.* 1999. Familial patterns of thoracic aortic aneurysms. Arch. Surg. **134:** 361–367.
43. MILEWICZ, D.M., H. CHEN, E.S. PARK, *et al.*1998. Reduced penetrance and variable expressivity of familial thoracic aortic aneurysms/dissections. Am. J. Cardiol. **82:** 474–479.
44. HASHAM, S.N., M.C. WILLING, D.C. GUO, *et al.* 2003. Mapping a locus for familial thoracic aortic aneurysms and dissections (TAAD2) to 3p24-25. Circulation **107:** 3184–3190.
45. GUO, D., S. HASHAM, S.Q. KUANG, *et al.*2001. Familial thoracic aortic aneurysms and dissections: genetic heterogeneity with a major locus mapping to 5q13-14. Circulation **103:** 2461–2468.
46. KAKKO, S., T. RAISANEN, M. TAMMINEN, *et al.* 2003. Candidate locus analysis of familial ascending aortic aneurysms and dissections confirms the linkage to the chromosome 5q13-14 in Finnish families. J. Thorac. Cardiovasc. Surg. **126:** 106–113.
47. VAUGHAN, C.J., M. CASEY, J. HE, *et al.* 2001. Identification of a chromosome 11q23.2-q24 locus for familial aortic aneurysm disease, a genetically heterogeneous disorder. Circulation **103:** 2469–2475.
48. PANNU, H., V. FADULU, J. CHANG, *et al.* 2005. Mutations in transforming growth factor-beta receptor type II cause familial thoracic aortic aneurysms and dissections. Circulation **112:** 513–520.
49. KIM, S.J., Y.H. IM, S.D. MARKOWITZ & Y.J. BANG. 2000. Molecular mechanisms of inactivation of TGFbeta receptors during carcinogenesis. Cytokine Growth Factor Rev. **11:** 159–168.
50. VAN KIEN, P.K., J.E. WOLF, F. MATHIEU, *et al.* 2004. Familial thoracic aortic aneurysm/dissection with patent ductus arteriosus: genetic arguments for a particular pathophysiological entity. Eur. J. Hum. Genet. **12:** 173–180.
51. GLANCY, D.L., M. WEGMANN & R.W. DHURANDHAR. 2001. Aortic dissection and patent ductus arteriosus in three generations. Am. J. Cardiol. **87:** 813–815, A9.

52. ZHU, L., R. VRANCKX, P.K. VAN KIEN, *et al.* 2006. Mutations in myosin heavy chain 11 cause a syndrome associating thoracic aortic aneurysm/aortic dissection and patent ductus arteriosus. Nat. Genet. **38:** 343–349.

53. AHMAD, F., J.G. SEIDMAN & C.E. SEIDMAN. 2005. The genetic basis for cardiac remodeling. Annu. Rev. Genomics Hum. Genet. **6:** 185–216.

54. TRAN-FADULU, V.T., J. CHEN, D. LEMUTH, *et al.* 2006. Syndrome of ascending and descending aortic dissections due to novel locus: variable expression in momozygotic twins and evidence for *de novo* mutations. Am. J. Med. Genet. **140:** 1196–1202.

55. AVIDAN, N., V. TRAN-FADULU, J. CHEN, *et al.* 2006. A novel locus for familial thoracic aortic aneurysms and dissection mapped to 15q24-26 (*TAAD3*): locus specific phenotypes for familial aortic disease.Submitted.

56. MCKUSICK, V.A. 1972. Association of congenital bicuspid aortic valve and Erdheim's cystic medial necrosis. Lancet **1:** 1026–1027.

57. MCKUSICK, V.A., R.B. LOGUE & H.T. BAHSON. 1957. Association of aortic valvular disease and cystic medial necrosis of the ascending aorta. Circulation **16:** 188–194.

58. LINDSAY, J., JR. 1988. Coarctation of the aorta, bicuspid aortic valve and abnormal ascending aortic wall. Am. J. Cardiol. **61:** 182–184.

59. SCHIEVINK, W.I. & B. MOKRI. 1995. Familial aorto-cervicocephalic arterial dissections and congenitally bicuspid aortic valve. Stroke **26:** 1935–1940.

60. KIM, D.H., G. VAN GINHOVEN & D.M. MILEWICZ. 2005. Familial aggregation of both aortic and cerebral aneurysms: evidence for a common genetic basis in a subset of families. Neurosurgery **56:** 655–661.

61. HAHN, R.T., M.J. ROMAN, A.H. MOGTADER & R.B. DEVEREUX. 1992. Association of aortic dilation with regurgitant, stenotic and functionally normal bicuspid aortic valves. J. Am. Coll. Cardiol. **19:** 283–288.

62. GLICK, B.N. & W.C. ROBERTS. 1994. Congenitally bicuspid aortic valve in multiple family members. Am. J. Cardiol. **73:** 400–404.

63. CLEMENTI, M., L. NOTARI, A. BORGHI & R. TENCONI. 1996. Familial congenital bicuspid aortic valve: a disorder of uncertain inheritance. Am. J. Med. Genet. **62:** 336–338.

64. HUNTINGTON, K., A.G. HUNTER & K.L. CHAN. 1997. A prospective study to assess the frequency of familial clustering of congenital bicuspid aortic valve. J. Am. Coll. Cardiol. **30:** 1809–1812.

65. ROSENQUIST, T.H. & A.C. BEALL. 1990. Elastogenic cells in the developing cardiovascular system. Smooth muscle, nonmuscle, and cardiac neural crest. Ann. N. Y. Acad. Sci. **588:** 106–119.

66. ADES, L.C., K. SULLIVAN, A. BIGGIN, *et al.* 2006. FBN1, TGFBR1, and the Marfancraniosynostosis/mental retardation disorders revisited. Am. J. Med. Genet. **140A:** 1047–1058.

67. KI, C.S., D.K. JIN, S.H. CHANG, *et al.* 2005. Identification of a novel TGFBR2 gene mutation in a Korean patient with Loeys-Dietz aortic aneurysm syndrome; no mutation in TGFBR2 gene in 30 patients with classic Marfan's syndrome. Clin. Genet. **68:** 561–563.

68. DISABELLA, E., M. GRASSO, N. MARZILIANO, *et al.* 2006. Two novel and one known mutation of the TGFBR2 gene in Marfan syndrome not associated with FBN1 gene defects Eur. J. Hum. Genet. **14:** 34–38.

# Structural and Functional Genetic Disorders of the Great Vessels and Outflow Tracts

KATHARINE J. BEE,[a] DAVID WILKES,[a] RICHARD B. DEVEREUX,[a] BRUCE B. LERMAN,[a] HARRY C. DIETZ,[b] AND CRAIG T. BASSON[a]

[a]Center for Molecular Cardiology, Greenberg Division of Cardiology, Department of Medicine, Weill Medical College of Cornell University, New York, New York 10021, USA

[b]Institute of Genetic Medicine, Howard Hughes Medical Institute, Johns Hopkins School of Medicine, Baltimore, Maryland 21205, USA

ABSTRACT: Development of the aorta and pulmonary artery is a complex process involving multiple molecular genetic pathways that modulate morphogenesis of the outflow tracts and the anastomosis of branch vessels. Recent genetic studies of the cardiovascular system demonstrate that congenital and adult onset progressive disorders of the great vessels such as aneurysms are components of generalized vascular, cardiac, and extracardiovascular syndromes. Current paradigms suggest that aortic disease is founded in patterning anomalies of the conotruncus that occur *in utero*. These aberrations can be consequences of genetic aberrations in transcriptional regulation of signal transduction both within and outside the developing great vessels.

KEYWORDS: aneurysm; *in utero*; conotruncus; genetic; signal transduction; great vessels

## INTRODUCTION

Aortic aneurysm is a common progressive disorder in which, beginning at birth, the aorta progressively dilates over the course of life.[1–4] At some stage, the dilated aorta is unable to withstand the shear forces produced by the hemodynamic stresses on the blood vessel, and it either ruptures or dissects. Despite advances in surgical and percutaneous approaches to aortic disease, aortic rupture is usually a fatal event, and all too often the disorder is clinically silent and unsuspected until aortic dissection or rupture occurs.[3] Although aortic

Address for correspondence: Craig T. Basson, M.D., Ph.D., Director, Cardiovascular Research, Greenberg Cardiology Division, Department of Medicine, Weill Medical College of Cornell University, 525 E. 68th Street, New York, NY 10021. Voice: 212-746-2201; fax: 212-746-2222.
e-mail: ctbasson@med.cornell.edu

Ann. N.Y. Acad. Sci. 1085: 256–269 (2006). © 2006 New York Academy of Sciences.
doi: 10.1196/annals.1383.002

aneurysm is a feature of complex connective tissue syndromes such as Marfan and Ehlers–Danlos type IV,[5–8] most aortic aneurysms occur as isolated entities or features of diffuse arteriopathy (affecting multiple aortic segments and even blood vessels other than the aorta) without manifestations outside the vasculature. Although most individuals with familial aortic disease present with dilatation restricted to the thoracic ascending, thoracic descending, or abdominal aortic segments, such individuals may often have disease that extends throughout multiple aortic segments. Even in Marfan syndrome where aortic root aneurysms are the rule, 4% of patients will have primary presentations with abdominal disease and nearly one-fourth of the patients will have abdominal disease in the setting of concurrent or prior thoracic aortic disease (Devereux, unpublished data).

## Clinical Strategies for Phenotyping

Methods of accurately assessing thoracic aortic dilatation prior to true aneurysm formation (i.e., "preaneurysmal dilatation") and certainly prior to clinically evident rupture or dissection have been the key to the recognition that nearly one-fifth of thoracic aortic aneurysms are inherited familial traits.[5,6,9] Roman and Devereux used echocardiography in cohorts of "normal" individuals to define the relationship between aortic root size and an individual's body size and age.[10] They developed a series of nomograms that allow physicians to define the upper limit of normal for aortic root size based on the individual's age and body surface area. Thus, echocardiography and these nomograms can be used to analyze aortic measurements at specific anatomic locations (aortic valve annulus, widest point in the sinuses of Valsalva, the sinotubular junction, and the proximal ascending aorta) in first-degree relatives of individuals with known aortic disease to determine familial risk (FIG. 1A). Such accurate phenotyping is key for appreciation of assignment of diagnoses in familial aortic aneurysm (FAA) disease and for appreciation of modes of inheritance. The absence of such standardized assessment of preaneurysmal dilatation in the abdominal aorta is one factor that hampers genetic analyses of kindreds with abdominal aortic disease.

To assign affected status in the absence of frank aneurysm and/or dissection in our genetic studies of aortic aneurysms, we define preaneurysmal aortic dilatation consistent with an affected status as aortic measurements that exceed the 95% confidence limits for maximal aortic dimensions relative to those predicted by the age and body surface area-specific nomograms (FIG. 1B). In addition, for individuals with preaneurysmal dilatation, we have now had the opportunity to follow individuals in our familial cohorts in many cases for several years with annual echocardiography. We have come to recognize that, in rare cases, initial determination of affected status may be erroneous when based on analysis of aortic measurements made at a single time point. This is

(A)                                                    (B)

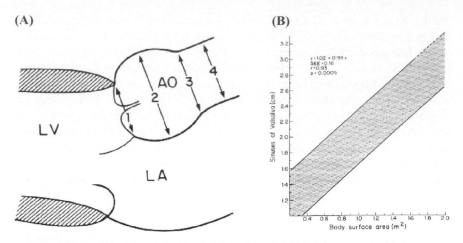

**FIGURE 1.** (**A**) Schematic illustration of the aortic root in the two-dimensional parasternal long-axis view. Measurements are obtained at four levels including the annulus, sinuses of Valsalva, supraaortic ridge, and proximal ascending aorta. (**B**) Nomogram showing 95% normal confidence limits for aortic root diameter at the sinuses of Valsalva in relation to body surface area in infants and children. (Adapted from Roman *et al.* 1989).[10]

usually the result of dramatic, rapid changes in body surface area (e.g., due to dietary changes, intercurrent severe illness, or pubertal growth spurts) that obfuscate not the accuracy of the measurement but rather the interpretation of the measurement with respect to the age and body surface area-dependent nomograms. Accordingly, whenever feasible, we define affected status as aortic dimensions that exceed age and body surface area-specific normative values persistently on two consecutive annual echocardiograms.

## Genetic Bases of FAA

Linkage analysis of families affected by thoracic aneurysms/dissections has led to the identification of several monogenic aortic aneurysm loci. Linkage to the *FBN1* gene is seen in 25–30% of families with FAA but who do not meet diagnostic criteria for Marfan syndrome (Wilkes, Bee, and Basson, unpublished data). These data reinforce the major role of fibrillin-1 dependent biology in the integrity of the aortic wall even outside the context of Marfan syndrome. An additional 5–10% of FAA families (without obvious Ehlers–Danlos syndrome) exhibit linkage to the *COL3A1* gene on chromosome 2, a finding that lends further credence to the contribution of matrix integrity to aortic aneurysm pathogenesis. More recently, thoracic aortic aneurysms associated with patent ductus arteriosus have been linked to mutations in the chromosome 16p12.2 myosin heavy chain 11 *(MYH11)* gene.[11] Thus, the intracellular cytoskeleton appears to play a critical role in aneurysm pathogenesis just like the extracellular matrix.

A fourth locus, FAA1, is located on chromosome 11q23-q24.[12] Analyses of families with multiple members having thoracic aortic aneurysms and dissections (TAAD) revealed evidence of linkage to a locus, TAAD1, on chromosome 5q13-q14. [13,14] An additional TAA locus, TAAD2, now known to be the *TGFBR2* gene, is located on chromosome 3p25-24.2.[15] Linkage to chromosome 15q has been suggested in TAA associated with bicuspid aortic valve.[16] Similarly, bicuspid aortic valve as well as aortic root dilatation and coarctation is often seen in Turner syndrome, a genetic disorder resulting from a lack of all or part of an X chromosome.[17,18] Finally, abdominal aortic aneurysms (AAA) have been linked to chromosome 16 and loci on chromosomes 4 (AAA2) and 19 (AAA1).[19,20]

Nonetheless, the gene defects underlying most aortic aneurysms (thoracic or abdominal) remain to be identified. We demonstrated that an as yet unidentified gene defect at a locus (FAA1) on chromosome 11q23 causes autosomal dominant FAA in a large FAA family (ANA).[12] Although the FAA trait in this family exhibits a high degree of penetrance, affected members of family ANA have a variable age of onset as well as a variable rate of aortic dilatation and incidence of dissection. Importantly, some members of family ANA exhibit abdominal aortic dilatation as well as thoracic aortic dilatation (FIG. 2). Thus,

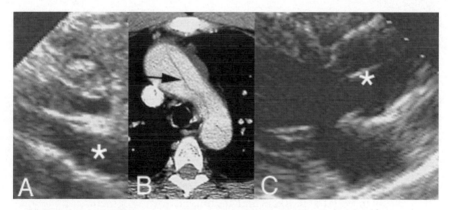

**FIGURE 2.** Clinical features of FAA aortic disease in family ANA. FAA can affect all aortic segments in family ANA individuals. (**A**) Abdominal ultrasound of an affected individual II-10 demonstrates fusiform preaneurysmal dilatation of abdominal aorta (*) at level of celiac axis. Aortic diameter at this level was 20 mm, 125% of upper limits of normal. (**B**) Affected individual II-2 exhibited aneurysmal dilatation of all aorta segments that ultimately resulted in dissections of thoracic and abdominal aorta. CT scan shows aortic arch dissection flap (arrow). (**C**) Echocardiography of an affected individual II-10 demonstrates that proximal aortic root is dilated as well as abdominal aorta. Sinuses of Valsalva (*) are 38 mm in diameter, 112% of upper limits of normal. (Adapted from Vaughan *et al.* 2001).[12]

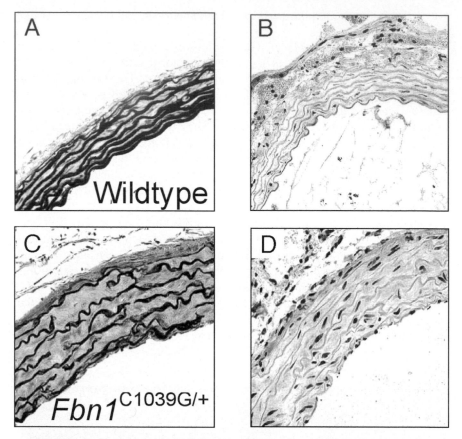

**FIGURE 3.** Characterization of the ascending aortic wall in wild-type (**A, B**) and $Fbn1^{C1039G/+}$ (**C, D**) mice. (**A, C**) Verhoeff-Van Gieson (VVG) stain for elastin demonstrating diffuse disruption of elastic lamellae in $Fbn1^{C1039G/+}$ mice. (**B, D**) Nuclear pSmad2, a marker of TGFB signaling demonstrating markedly increased pSmad2 in the $Fbn1^{C1039G/+}$ mice. (Adapted with permission from Habashi et al. 2006).[26]

evaluation of family ANA supports potential relationships between aneurysm pathogenesis in both the thoracic and abdominal aortic segments.

Our linkage analyses of family ANA revealed a maximum LOD score of 4.4 on the long arm of chromosome 11, located near to, but excluding, a cluster of matrix metalloproteinase (MMP) genes. Given the prominent role that has been hypothesized for MMPs in aortic aneurysms,[22] we also sequenced all the coding regions of genes in this MMP cluster in affected ANA family members and found no evidence of mutation. That the FAA trait is concordant with *FAA1* genotypes in two additional families also supports a role for a gene at FAA1 in aneurysm pathogenesis (Wilkes, Bee, & Basson, unpublished data and ref. 13).

Initial studies defined the interval as a 2.3 cM locus at chromosome 11q23-q24 based on flanking recombination events in the proband and another affected family member.[12] However, our subsequent serial echocardiographic analyses of this other family member and his two potentially affected children revealed that the initial measurements of marginally enlarged aortic roots did not persist over five subsequent years as these individuals' body surface area changed with weight loss and puberty. Therefore, ongoing studies have regarded these individuals as having an indeterminate diagnosis and have focused on an expanded 5-megabase interval for the FAA1 locus defined by recombination events at D11S1792 and rs675873.

Certainly, FAA is a highly genetically heterogeneous disorder. For instance, Guo *et al.* proposed a locus for thoracic aortic aneurysm and dissection (TAAD) on chromosome 5q.[13] In their study, in 9 of 15 families the aneurysm trait was concordant with polymorphisms on chromosome 5q, and aggregation of individual family LOD scores produced a combined maximum LOD score of 4.74 at this locus. Like families linked to FAA1, these families transmitted TAAD in an autosomal dominant fashion with variable expressivity, but they also exhibited marked incomplete penetrance. Kakko *et al.* suggested that two additional families were also linked to this TAAD locus; the most significant linkage was seen in one family with a LOD score of 2.65.[14] Affected members in these families varied in the severity of their condition (from asymptomatic aortic root dilatation to fatal aortic dissection), but several individuals predicted to be affected based on chromosome 5q genotypes showed no sign of aortic root dilatation.

### Genetic Analyses and TGF-β Signaling in Aortic Disease

Further evidence of the ability of aortic aneurysm syndromes to affect multiple aortic segments is supported by recent data demonstrating that mutations in the transforming growth factor β-type II receptor (*TGFBR2*) gene at chromosome 3p24-25 are associated with both thoracic and abdominal aortic dilatation in a syndrome that somewhat resembles Marfan syndrome.[23] Pannu *et al.* demonstrated that four families with autosomal dominant thoracic aortic disease had mutations in *TGFBR2,* which resulted in alterations of the Arg460 residue.[23] Individuals in these families did not meet criteria for Marfan syndrome but did have evidence of a disseminated connective tissue disorder including high arched palate, arachnodactyly, pectus deformity, and mitral valve prolapse. We have recently screened a cohort of 50 FAA families for mutations in *TGFBR1* and *TGFBR2* and have only found a *TGFBR2* mutation in a single proband who also had connective tissue anomalies (Bee & Basson, in preparation). Our findings suggest that *TGFBR2* mutations are not a common cause of isolated FAA without disseminated connective tissue anomalies.

In fact, mutations in the *TGFBR1* and *TGFBR2* genes are now thought to cause a newly defined aortic aneurysm—connective tissue syndrome associated with developmental defects. This syndrome, known as Loeys–Dietz syndrome (LDS), is characterized by hypertelorism, bifid uvula and/or cleft palate, and generalized arterial tortuosity with ascending aortic aneurysm and dissection.[26] Minor features of LDS include exotropia, craniosyostosis, Chiari I malformation, dural ectasia, mental retardation, and congenital heart disease (patent ductus arteriosus, atrial septal defects, and bicuspid aortic valve). Although LDS patients most often exhibit proximal ascending aortic dilatation, AAA and pathology of other aortic segments and vascular structures are commonly observed as well. Sequencing of both the *TGFBR1* and *TGFBR2* genes in a cohort of 52 families showing features suggestive of LDS revealed 42 mutations in all, including the R460 mutation previously associated with familial TAAD.[25] In both genes, the majority of the mutations cluster in the kinase domain, and biochemical analyses of the mutations suggest that they cause loss-of-function. However, cell culture and histologic analyses of patient samples demonstrate a paradoxical enhancement of TGF-β signaling. These findings as well as recent genetic analyses of genetically engineered models of Marfan syndrome have established a new TGF-β signaling-based paradigm for aortic aneurysm and dissection.

Though distinct disorders, MFS and LDS both affect the normal propagation of TGF-β signaling. MFS is a connective tissue disorder caused by mutations in *FBN1*, the gene encoding fibrillin-1, a major component of the extracellular matrix microfibril.[7] Fibrillin-1 is thought to play a role in the TGF-β signaling cascade via its interaction with a latent TGF-β-binding protein (LTBP). LTBP binds TGF-β via an LTBP-associated protein (LAP), forming what is known as the large latent complex. Defects in *FBN1* likely disrupt the targeting and sequestration of the large latent complex due to an inability of LTBP to bind to the microfibrils. This leads to an increase in TGF-β activity due to a higher than normal level of available TGF-β. Heterozygous LDS mutations appear to amplify TGF-β signaling by as yet unidentified compensatory mechanisms.

Histologic studies of the aortic wall in both MFS and LDS reveal loss of elastin content and disarray of elastic fibers compared to control samples along with increased collagen deposition. Increased interstitial collagen deposition is likely a consequence of TGF-β activity, and increased TGF-β activity can be directly measured. Binding of TGF-β to its receptor results in the phosphorylation of Smad2, one of several Smad proteins necessary for TGF-β signal propagation. Therefore, Loeys *et al.* evaluated phosphorylation of Smad2 as a measure of TGF-β signaling in primary dermal fibroblasts heterozygous for mutations in TGFBR1 or TGFBR2.[26] Cells lines from affected individuals exhibited mild elevations of pSmad2 at baseline, but maintain persistently elevated levels of pSmad2 even several hours after TGF-β stimulation compared to the control cells. Such persistent evidence of TGF-β activity was also evident *in vivo*, where aortic walls of MFS and LDS patients exhibited increased nuclear staining of pSmad2 compared with unaffected individuals.

Murine models of MFS have similarly highlighted a critical role of TGF-β signaling in aortic aneurysms as well as other features of MFS (and presumably LDS). Mouse models of MFS with genetically engineered mutation of FBN1 exhibit both disorganization of elastin in the aortic wall as well as increased levels of pSmad2 consistent with elevated TGF-β signaling (FIG. 3).[27] Importantly, such signaling is abrogated by treatment of the mice with neutralizing antibodies to TGF-β, and in this setting, aortic root dilatation is prevented. Thus, these findings suggested that pharmacologic antagonism of TGF-β signaling may prove to be an effective strategy for treatment of MFS patients as well as other aortic aneurysm patients.

Manipulation of the renin-angiotensin system for control of hypertension may be useful in the management of both thoracic and AAA. However, independent of hemodynamic effects, pharmacologic manipulation of this system may also provide benefits for aortic aneurysm patients by altering TGF-β signaling. Activation of the angiotensin II type I receptor (AT1) increases the expression of TGF-β ligands and receptors as well as inducing the expression of thrombospondin-1, an activator of TGF-β. Therefore, losartan, an antihypertensive AT1 antagonist, might be useful to correct aberrant TGF-β signaling in disorders such as MFS or LDS. Dietz and colleagues compared the effects of losartan to the β-adrenergic blocker propranolol and to placebo in mice heterozygous for *Fbn1* mutations.[27] Strikingly, unlike propanolol or placebo, losartan impaired TGF-β signaling and not only retarded aortic dilatation but actually reversed aortic pathology. Thus, these studies hold great promise for new pharmacologic strategies that can effectively treat patients with MFS and other aortic aneurysm disorders.

## *Development of the Heart and Outflow Tract*

The recognition that aortic aneurysms can be associated with both defective regulation of TGF-β signaling and a wide array of congenital cardiac malformations mandates a careful consideration of the intersection of aortic aneurysms with outflow tract development during embryogenesis. During early development, cardiac precursor cells are located in two fields on either side of the primitive streak. As cells migrate to the anterior region of the mesoderm, their anteroposterior polarity has already been established and corresponds to their lineage fates; the anterior cells contribute to the future truncus, the posterior cells of the future atria, and lying in between are the ventricular precursors. Critical to the specification of the cardiac progenitor cells is signaling from both bone morphogenetic protein (BMP2) and fibroblast growth factor-4 (FGF4). After cell lineages are specified, the cells within the heart fields divide into two separate populations of cells, those fated to become endocardium and those which will become myocardial cells. This is followed by the fusion of the heart fields along the anteroposterior axis to form the heart tube. During this process, the relative positions of precardiac cells in the primitive streak are maintained.

Critical to midline fusion of the heart tube is the transcription factor GATA-4. GATA-4 regulates expression of several cardiac-specific genes such as the α- and β-type myosin heavy chains and cardiac troponin C, and this factor interacts with NKX2.5 and TBX5, two other cardiogenic transcription factors. Mutations in both *GATA-4* and *NKX2.5* have been shown to cause congenital heart defects that reflect these transcription factors' contributions both at this early stage of cardiogenesis as well as at later stages, such as chamber septation.[28–30] Once the heart tube has formed, it is repositioned via cardiac looping such that the atrial pole is anterior to the ventricular pole. Essential to the proper positioning of the heart tube is the transcription factor PITX2, which is involved in establishing the left-right axis around which the heart tube rotates. Mutations in the PITX2 gene are associated with Axenfeld-Rieger syndrome, which is characterized by ocular, craniofacial, and umbilical abnormalities.[31]

The venous pole of the primary heart tube lengthens as myocardium is added from the paired heart-forming fields, and this segment eventually differentiates into the atrioventricular, atrial, and inflow regions of the heart. By contrast, recent studies reveal that the arterial pole, which contributes to the right ventricle and outflow tract, expands by addition of cells originating from the secondary (or anterior) heart field, a distinct population of myocardial precursor cells located anterior to the primitive heart tube.[32] Recruitment of cells from the anterior heart field to the growing outflow tract is thought to be a result of short-range inductive signaling, possibly via BMPs, from differentiated arterial pole myocardium.[33] The existence of two sources of myocardial precursor cells implies that there are transcription factors and other regulatory proteins that have activities unique to each heart field, and this is currently an area of intense investigation.

Throughout looping, the heart tube undergoes morphological changes that begin to define the specific structural segments that will make up the atria, atrioventricular canal, ventricles, and the outflow tract. Abnormal looping of the heart is associated with a failure of "wedging"—a process in which the outflow tract moves to a position wedged between the two developing ventricular chambers. Nonwedging of the aorta is a major feature of tetralogy of Fallot and other aortic arch disorders such as DiGeorge syndrome. DiGeorge syndrome is associated with deletions at chromosome 22q11 as well as mutations in the TBX1 gene located at 22q11.2.[7] TBX1 encodes a transcription factor involved in growth and septation of the outflow tract. Tetralogy of Fallot, which is also seen in Alagille syndrome, is an autosomal dominant disorder involving various cardiac outflow tract defects (e.g., peripheral pulmonic arterial stenosis) and which is caused by mutations in the *JAG1* gene encoding Jagged-1.[34] Jagged-1 is a member of the Notch signaling pathway and is expressed in a specific population of endocardial cells of the outflow tract that undergo epithelial to mesenchymal transformation. Interestingly, NOTCH1 mutations have also been associated with bicuspid aortic valve.[35]

During the later stages of cardiac looping, cells from the proepicardial organ migrate as an epithelial sheet to the heart, where they envelop the myocardium to form the epicardium. The epicardial cells migrate into the myocardium where they undergo an epithelial-to-mesenchymal transformation to form the primitive coronary vasculature including endothelium, smooth muscle, and fibroblasts. Involved in this transition are several signaling factors such as endothelin, FGF isoforms, BMPs, and TGF-β. Defects of the coronary vasculature such as aneurysms of the coronary arteries have been linked to abnormalities in various MMPs, proteins responsible for the degradation of the extracellular matrix. In addition, mutations in Tbx5 that have been associated with Holt-Oram syndrome can also produce epicardial and coronary vessel defects in both humans and experimental animal models.[36,37] The contribution of these participants in coronary vasculogenesis to the anastomosis of the coronary vessels to the conotruncus remains to be determined.

As the heart continues to develop, the conotruncus, which initially connects the ventricles with the aortic arch arteries, is remodeled into the ascending aorta and the pulmonary trunk. Morphogenesis of the endocardial cushions that contribute to septation of the conotruncus into the ventricular outflow tracts as well as formation of the atrioventricular valves is critically dependent upon the activity of TGF-β and its signaling cousins, the BMPs. In addition to the myocardium and vascular smooth muscle originating from the anterior heart field found at the base of the aortic root, cardiac neural crest cells add to the developing aortic arches and migrate into the areas of the outflow tract undergoing septation. Therefore, two outflow tract interfaces exist at which different cell types originating from various sources meet. One junction involves the transition between myocardium from the secondary heart field and vascular smooth muscle cells of the same origin. The second junction is between the secondary heart field-derived smooth muscle cells and smooth muscle cells from the cardiac neural crest.[32] These interfaces are the locations of aneurysms often seen in Marfan syndrome and stenosis in Noonan syndrome. Similar interfaces exist in the pulmonary veins, and the anastomosis of the pulmonary veins with the atria are often foci for aberrant cardiac conduction that results in atrial fibrillation. Thus, it is critical to recognize that defects in developmental cascades that lead to structural anomalies of the great vessels and outflow tracts may also lead to functional abnormalities of the cardiovascular system.

### *Electrophysiologic Disorders of the Outflow Tracts*

Electrophysiologic abnormalities including predisposition to ventricular tachycardia (VT) may be one functional manifestation of defective outflow tract integrity. VT can arise from foci in various intracardiac locations. Those that arise from the ventricular outflow tracts have distinctive electrophysiologic features including their sensitivity to drugs such as verapamil and adenosine, two agents that do not terminate most tachycardias that arise from ventricular myocardium. Recent clinical studies reveal that there are no clinical or electrophysiologic features that distinguish between VT arising from the left versus the right outflow tract suggesting that the underlying abnormality is one of outflow tract morphogenesis.

Why are outflow tract tachycardias terminated by verapamil? VTs in this region are related to intracellular calcium overload and triggered activity. In outflow tract myocardium, activation of the β-adrenergic receptor, a G-protein-coupled receptor, leads to activation of the stimulatory G-protein G-αs with consequent generation of cAMP via adenyl cyclase. cAMP in turn triggers the release of calcium from the sarcoplasmic reticulum via PKA-dependent phosphorylation of the ryanodine receptor. Verapamil, an L-type calcium channel blocker, impairs calcium entry into the cell and calcium-induced calcium release from the sarcoplasmic reticulum. Adenosine acts to terminate these tachycardias via a different mechanism. It acts through its A1 receptor to activate the inhibitory G-protein G-αI that inhibits cAMP generation by adenyl cyclase. The result is that adenosine blocks the triggered release of calcium from the sarcoplasmic reticulum even in the face of normal calcium stores. In the case of either verapamil or adenosine, the tachycardia terminates due to attenuation of sarcoplasmic calcium release.

An unusual subset of outflow tract tachycardias is sensitive to verapamil but insensitive to adenosine. Such electrophysiologic characteristics suggest a defect may exist in this setting in the G-αI-dependent inhibitory limb of the cAMP signaling pathway. Lerman and colleagues tested this hypothesis.[35] They mapped the focus of such a tachycardia from an individual with an adenosine-insensitive outflow tract VT and then performed an endomyocardial biopsy at this location. Biopsies were also performed at the right ventricular apex in normal myocardium that did not participate in the genesis of the arrhythmia. Genomic DNA was prepared from these biopsy samples as well as from peripheral lymphocytes, and the *GNAI2* gene for the inhibitory G-protein G-αi2 was PCR amplified from all DNA samples and sequenced. These analyses demonstrated a *GNAI2* missense mutation (F200L) in the DNA from the arrhythmia focus, and this mutation was determined to be somatic since it was not present in DNA from either the right ventricular apex or peripheral lymphocytes. *In vitro* analyses of the F200L *GNAI2* mutation demonstrated that the encoded mutant G-αi2 produced increased intracellular cAMP and impaired adenosine-mediated cAMP suppression. Thus, intact genetic regulation of outflow tract integrity is critical for the maintenance of cardiovascular physiology. Combined with recent evidence that *MYH11* mutations in aortic aneurysm syndromes can manifest as abnormal vasomotor tone even when aortic dilatation is not present,[11] these findings demonstrate that investigation of outflow tract anomalies needs to encompass both structural and functional assessments in patients and experimental models.

As we look to the future, key paradigms in outflow tract and great vessel disorders are emerging. Along with an increasing awareness of common mechanisms underlying both adult onset and developmental disorders, we see the integration of extracellular matrix, cytokine signaling, and transcriptional regulation into a unified paradigm of pathogenesis. Such a paradigm will set the stage to target novel therapies such as TGF-β antagonists at genetically defined patient populations. As patients are counseled about their own risk and the risk of disease transmission, physicians needs to recognize the extensive familial nature of these disorders but at the same time acknowledge the potentially large contribution of somatic mutations that are patient specific. In aggregate, the future holds rich opportunities for significant improvements in the management of great vessel and outflow tract disorders.

## ACKNOWLEDGMENTS

CTB is supported by NIH R01-HL66214, NIH R01-HL80663, the Snart Cardiovascular Fund, and an Established Investigator Award of the American Heart Association. HCD is supported by the Howard Hughes Medical Institute.

## REFERENCES

1. BICKERSTAFF, L.K., P.C. PAIROLERO, L.H. HOLLIER, *et al.* 1982. Thoracic aortic aneurysms: a population-based study. Surgery **92:** 1103–1108.
2. BICKERSTAFF, L.K., L.H. HOLLIER, H.J. VAN PEENEN, *et al.* 1984. Abdominal aortic aneurysms: the changing natural history. J. Vasc. Surg. **1:** 6–12.
3. MELTON, L.J., L.K. BICKERSTAFF, L.H. HOLLIER, *et al.* 1984. Changing incidence of abdominal aortic aneurysms: a population based study. Am. J. Epidemiol. **120:** 379–386.
4. POWELL, J.T., S.T.R. MACSWEENEY & R.M. GREENHALGH. 1994. The spontaneous course of small aortic aneurysm. *In* Aneurysms: New Findings and Treatments. J.S.T. Yao & W.H. Pearce, Eds.: 71–78. Appleton and Lange. Norwalk, CT.
5. JOHANSEN, K. & T. KOEPSELL. 1986. Familial tendency for abdominal aortic aneurysms. JAMA **256:** 1934–1936.
6. KUIVANIEMI, H., G. TROMP & D.J. PROCKOP. 1991. Genetic causes of aortic aneurysms. J. Clin. Invest. **88:** 1441–1444.
7. ONLINE MENDELIAN INHERITANCE IN MAN, OMIM™. 1996. Center for Medical Genetics, Johns Hopkins University (Baltimore, MD) and National Center for Biotechnology Information, National Library of Medicine (Bethesda, MD), World Wide Web URL: http://www.ncbi.nlm.nih.gov/omim/.
8. SERRY, C., O.S. AGOMUOH & M.D. GOLDIN. 1988. Review of Ehlers-Danlos syndrome. J. Cardiovasc. Surg. **29:** 530–534.

9. VERLOES, A., N. SAKALIHASAN, L. KOULISCHER, *et al*. 1995. Aneurysms of the abdominal aorta: familial and genetic aspects in three hundred thirteen pedigrees. J. Vasc. Surg. **21:** 646–655.
10. ROMAN, M.J., R.B. DEVEREUX, R. KRAMER-FOX, *et al*. 1989. Two-dimensional echocardiographic aortic root dimension in normal children and adults. Am. J. Cardiol. **64:** 507–512.
11. ZHU, L., R. VRANCKX, P.D. VAN KIEN, *et al*. 2006. Mutations in myosin heavy chain 11 cause a syndrome associating thoracic aortic aneurysm/aortic dissection and patent ductus arteriosis. Nat. Genet. **38:** 343–349.
12. VAUGHAN, C.J., M. CASEY, J. HE, *et al*. 2001. Identification of a chromosome 11q23.2-q24 locus for familial aortic aneurysm disease, a genetically heterogeneous disorder. Circulation **103:** 2469–2475.
13. GUO, D., S. HASHAM, S. KUANG, *et al*. 2001. Familial thoracic aortic aneurysms and dissections: genetic heterogeneity with a major locus mapping to 5q13-14. Circulation **103:** 2461–2468.
14. KAKKO, S., T. RAISANEN, M. TAMMINEN, *et al*. 2003. Candidate locus analysis of familial ascending aortic aneurysms and dissections confirms the linkage to the chromosome 5q13-14 in Finnish families. J. Thorac. Cardiovasc. Surg. **126:** 106–113.
15. HASHAM, S.N., M.C. WILLING, D. GUO, *et al*. 2003. Mapping a locus for familial thoracic aortic aneurysms and dissections (TAAD2) to 3p24-25. Circulation **107:** 3184–3190.
16. GOH, D.L., L.F. HAN, D.P. JUDGE, *et al*. 2002. Linkage of familial bicuspid aortic valve with aortic aneurysm to chromosome 15q. Presented at the 52nd Annual Meeting of The American Society of Human Genetics. Baltimore, MD. October 19.
17. MILLLER, M.J., M.E. GEFFNER, B.M. LIPPE, *et al*. 1983. Echocardiography reveals a high incidence of bicuspid aortic valve in Turner syndrome. J. Pediat. **102:** 47–50.
18. OSTBERG, J.E., J.A. BROOKES, C. MCCARTHY, *et al*. 2004. A comparison of echocardiography and magnetic resonance imaging in cardiovascular screening of adults with Turner syndrome. J. Clin. Endocrinol. Metab. **89:** 5966–5971.
19. Powell, J.T., A. BASHIR, S. DAWSON, *et al*. 1990. Genetic variation on chromosome 16 is associated with adbominal aortic aneurysm. Clin. Sci. (Lond.) **78:** 13–16.
20. Shibamura, H., J.M. OLSON, C. VAN VLIJMEN-VAN KEULEN, *et al*. 2004. Genome scan for familial abdominal aortic aneurysm using sex and family history as covariates suggests genetic heterogeneity and identifies linkage to chromosome 19q13. Circulation **109:** 2103–2108.
21. KADOGLOU, N.P. & C.D. LIAPIS. 2004. Matrix metalloproteinases: contribution to pathogenesis, diagnosis, surveillance and treatment of abdominal aortic aneurysms. Curr. Med. Res. Opin. **20:** 419–432.
22. MIZUGUCHI, T., G. COLLOD-BEROUD, T. AKIYAMA, *et al*. 2004. Heterozygous TGFBR2 mutations in Marfan syndrome. Nat. Genet. **36:** 855–860.
23. PANNU, H., V.T. FADULU, J. CHANG, *et al*. 2005. Mutations in transforming growth factor-β receptor type II cause familial thoracic aortic aneurysms and dissections. Circulation **112:** 513–520.
24. LOEYS, B.L., J. CHEN, E.R. NEPTUNE, *et al*. 2005. A syndrome of altered cardiovascular, craniofacial, neurocognitive and skeletal development caused by mutations in TGFBR1 or TGFBR2. Nat. Gen. **37:** 275–281.

25. LOEYS, B.L., U. SCHWARZE, T. HOLM, *et al.* 2006. Aneurysm syndromes caused by mutations in the TGF-β receptor. NEJM **355:** 788–798.

26. HABASHI, J.P., D.P. JUDGE, T.M. HOLM, *et al.* 2006. Losartan, an AT1 antagonist, prevents aortic aneurysm in a mouse model of Marfan syndrome. Science **312:** 117–121.

27. GARG, V., I.S. KATHIRIYA, R. BARNES, *et al.* 2003. GATA4 mutations cause human congenital heart defects and reveal an interaction with TBX5. Nature **424:** 443–447.

28. SCHOTT, J.J., D.W. BENSON, C.T. BASSON, *et al.* 1998. Congenital heart disease caused by mutations in the transcription factor NKX2-5. Science **281:** 108–111.

29. HATCHER, C.J., N.Y. DIMAN, M.S. KIM, *et al.* 2004. A role for Tbx5 in proepicardial cell migration during cardiogenesis. Physiol. Genomics **18:** 129–140.

30. FRANCO, D. & M. CAMPIONE. 2003. The role of Pitx2 during cardiac development. Linking left-right signaling and congenital heart diseases. Trends Cardiovasc. Med. **13:** 157–163.

31. WALDO, K.L., M.R. HUTSON, C.C. WARD, *et al.* 2005. Secondary heart field contributes myocardium and smooth muscle to the arterial pole of the developing heart. Dev. Biol. **281:** 78–90.

32. MJAATVEDT, C.H., T. NAKAOKA, R. MORENO-RODRIGUEZ, *et al.* 2001. The outflow tract of the heart is recruited from a novel heart-forming field. Dev. Biol. **238:** 97–109.

33. LOOMES, K.M., L.A. UNDERKOFFLER, J. MORABITO, *et al.* 1999. The expression of Jagged1 in the developing mammalian heart correlates with cardiovascular disease in Alagille syndrome. Hum. Mol. Genet. **8:** 2443–2449.

34. GARG, V., A.N. MUTH, J.F. RANSOM, *et al.* 2005. Mutations in *NOTCH1* cause aortic valve disease. Nature **437:** 270–274.

35. BASSON, C.T., D.R. BACHINSKY, R.C. LIN, *et al.* 1997. Mutations in human *TBX5* cause limb and cardiac malformation in Holt-Oram syndrome. Nat. Genet. **15:** 30–35.

36. DIAS, R.R., J.M. ALBUQUERQUE, A.C. PEREIRA, *et al.* 2005. Holt-Oram syndrome presenting as agenesis of the left pericardium. Int. J. Cardiol. In press.

37. LERMAN, B.B., B. DONG, K.M. STEIN, *et al.* 1998. Right ventricular outflow tract tachycardia due to a somatic cell mutation in G protein subunit alphai2. J. Clin. Invest. **101:** 2862–2868.

# Genome-Wide Approach to Finding Abdominal Aortic Aneurysm Susceptibility Genes in Humans

HELENA KUIVANIEMI,[a,b] YOSHIKI KYO,[a] GUY LENK,[a] AND GERARD TROMP[a]

[a] Center for Molecular Medicine and Genetics, Wayne State University School of Medicine, Detroit, MI, USA

[b] Department of Surgery, Wayne State University School of Medicine, Detroit, MI, USA

ABSTRACT: Familial aggregation of abdominal aortic aneurysms (AAAs) is now widely recognized, however, susceptibility genes have not yet been identified. Our approach to find susceptibility genes has been to collect families with AAAs and to perform DNA linkage analyses to identify regions on the human chromosomes that are linked to AAAs and could harbor susceptibility genes for AAAs. We identified 233 families with at least two individuals diagnosed with AAAs. These families had 653 AAA patients and an average of 2.8 cases per family. When evaluating mode of inheritance, 167 (72%) families were consistent with autosomal recessive inheritance, whereas 58 (25%) families were consistent with autosomal dominant inheritance and in 8 families the familial aggregation could be explained by autosomal dominant inheritance with incomplete penetrance. Blood samples from 235 affected relative pairs (ARPs) and their unaffected relatives were collected for DNA isolation and the DNA used for genotyping with highly variable microsatellite markers. We included covariates in the statistical analyses to allow for genetic heterogeneity. The results for chromosomes 19g13 and 4q31 were significant with sex, number of affected first-degree relatives, and their interaction as covariates. These chromosomal regions contain many plausible candidate genes, and the future research will include more detailed analyses of these positional candidate genes.

KEYWORDS: genetics of abdominal aortic aneurysm; chromosome 19g13; DNA linkage analysis

Address for correspondence: Helena Kuivaniemi, M.D., Ph.D., Center for Molecular Medicine and Genetics and Department of Surgery, Wayne State University School of Medicine, 3317 Gordon H. Scott Hall of Basic Medical Sciences, 540 E. Canfield Ave., Detroit, MI 48201, USA. Voice: 313-577-8733; fax: 313-577-5218.

e-mail: kuivan@sanger.med.wayne.edu

Ann. N.Y. Acad. Sci. 1085: 270–281 (2006). © 2006 New York Academy of Sciences.
doi: 10.1196/annals.1383.022

# INTRODUCTION

Abdominal aortic aneurysms (AAAs) are frequently familial, even when they are not associated with heritable disorders such as the Marfan syndrome or the type IV variant of the Ehlers–Danlos syndrome. Based on interviews of the patients and ultrasonography examinations of first-degree family members, approximately 15% of AAA patients have at least one first-degree relative with AAA[1,2] (TABLES 1 and 2). Examination of altogether 666 brothers and 523 sisters of AAA patients by ultrasonography showed that 17.2% of brothers and 4.2% of sisters had AAA (TABLE 2). In addition, many characteristics of AAA patients are consistent with AAA being a genetic disease: (1) statistical evaluation of the available family data using an approach called segregation analysis suggests that AAAs are caused by genetic defects;[3,4] (2) operative mortality for intact and ruptured AAA is higher among female patients as compared to male patients;[5,6] (3) the prevalence of AAA is about six times higher in men than in women; (4) incidence of rupture is higher in familial cases;[7] and (5) prevalence of AAA varies between ethnic groups.[8] It would be expected that when the disease does occur in females, it is due to the presence of a larger number of liabilities, a phenomenon characteristic to multifactorial diseases with a threshold effect.[9] Female AAA patients would then represent the more severe spectrum of the aneurysmal disease and their offspring would be expected to be at higher risk for AAAs. In a study in which the family histories of 542 AAA patients were collected, 82 (15.1%) patients had a positive family

TABLE 1. Familial prevalence of AAA based on interviews

| Authors | Patients surveyed (N) | Patients with positive history (N) | Familial prevalence (%) |
|---|---|---|---|
| Norrgård et al., 1984[12] | 87 | 16 | 18.4 |
| Johansen and Koepsell, 1986[13] | 250 | 48 | 19.2 |
| Powell and Greenhalgh, 1987[14] | 56 | 20 | 35.7 |
| Johnston and Scobie, 1988[15] | 666 | 41 | 6.1 |
| Cole et al., 1989[16] | 305 | 34 | 11.1 |
| Darling et al., 1989[10] | 542 | 82 | 15.1 |
| Majumder et al., 1991[3] | 91 | 13 | 14.3 |
| Verloes et al., 1995[4] | 313 | 39 | 12.5 |
| Lederle et al., 1997[17] | 985 | 91 | 9.2 |
| Lawrence et al., 1998[18] | 86 | 19 | 22.1 |
| Salkowski et al., 1999[19] | 72 | 19 | 26.4 |
| Rossaak et al., 2001[20] | 248 | 48 | 19.4 |
| Total | 3,701 | 470 | |
| Combined prevalence | | | 12.7 |

Modified with permission from Kuivaniemi and Tromp, 2000.[2]

**TABLE 2. Prevalence of AAA among first-degree family members based on ultrasonography screening**

| Authors | Country | Brothers[a](%) | Sisters[a](%) | Other[a](%) |
|---|---|---|---|---|
| Bengtsson et al., 1989[21] | Sweden | 10/35 (28.6) | 3/52 (5.8) | |
| Collin and Walton, 1989[22] | UK | 4/16 (25.0) | 0/15 (0) | |
| Webster et al., 1991[23] | USA | 5/24 (20.8) | 2/30 (6.7) | 7/103 (6.8) |
| Adamson et al., 1992[24] | UK | 5/25 (20.0) | 3/28 (10.7) | |
| Bengtsson et al., 1992[25] | Sweden | | | 9/62 (14.5) |
| van der Lugt et al., 1992[26] | Netherlands | 16/56 (28.6) | 3/52 (5.8) | |
| Adams et al., 1993[27] | UK | 4/23 (17.4) | 1/28 (3.6) | 6/23 (26.1) |
| Moher et al., 1994[28] | Canada | 9/48 (18.8) | | |
| Fitzgerald et al., 1995[29] | Ireland | 13/60 (21.7) | 2/65 (3.1) | |
| Larcos et al., 1995[30] | Australia | | | 0/52 (0) |
| Baird et al., 1995[31] | Canada | 7/26 (26.9) | 3/28 (10.7) | |
| Jaakkola et al., 1996[32] | Finland | 4/45 (8.9) | 1/78 (1.3) | |
| van der Graaf et al., 1998[33] | Netherlands | 26/210 (12.4) | | |
| Salo et al., 1999[34] | Finland | | | 11/238 (4.6) |
| Rossaak et al., 2001[20] | New Zealand | | | 4/49 (8.2) |
| Ogata et al., 2005[35] | Canada | 11/98 (11.2) | 4/147(2.7) | 0/31 (0) |
| Total | | 114/666 (17.2) | 22/523 (4.2) | 37/558 (6.6) |

[a]Number of individuals identified with AAA/number of individuals examined by ultrasonography. Other refers to relatives other than sisters and brothers of the AAA patient, or the categories of relatives were not specified. Modified with permission from Kuivaniemi and Tromp, 2000.[2]

history for AAA and 460 were sporadic cases.[10] Out of the sporadic cases, 86% were males and 14% females, whereas in the familial AAA group 65% were males and 35% were females. Also, male patients in the familial AAA group were significantly younger than in the sporadic AAA group. There was no difference in smoking, hypertension, or presence of coronary artery disease between the familial and sporadic AAA groups.[10] The patients who had a positive family history and their first-degree relatives had altogether 209 AAAs, 45 of which had ruptured and 164 were unruptured AAAs. Female patients had 73 of the AAAs and male patients 136 AAAs. Altogether 22 (30.1%) AAAs among the female patients had ruptured, whereas only 23 (16.9%) of the AAAs among the male patients had ruptured. The authors called this phenomenon "black widow syndrome" after the New World black widow spider to describe the fatal trait of female AAA patients and the increased risk to her relatives.[10] Given the strong evidence that AAA is a genetic disorder, it is important to identify the genetic risk factors for AAA. The approaches to identify the susceptibility gene(s) for AAA are summarized in TABLE 3. In this article, we will concentrate on the DNA linkage analyses.

**TABLE 3. Different approaches to identify susceptibility gene(s) for AAA**

| Approach | Advantages | Disadvantages |
|---|---|---|
| **1.** DNA linkage analysis<br>a) ASPs<br>b) Other affected pedigree members (ARP)<br>c) Family based | (1) No prior knowledge needed<br>(2) Unbiased<br><br>(3) DNA can be isolated from blood<br><br>(4) No diagnostic uncertainty with ASP and ARP<br>(5) Best statistical power with family based | (1) Large number of cases and family members<br>(2) Lower statistical power with ASP and ARP<br>(3) Diagnostic uncertainty gives misleading results with family-based study<br>(4) Family based is difficult, since AAA has a late-age-at-onset |
| **2.** Candidate gene analysis<br>(a) Screen for mutations<br>(b) Association studies with known or new polymorphisms | (1) Samples from cases are sufficient for screening<br>(2) Relatively small number of cases for screening<br><br>(3) Association is cheap and technically simple | (1) Prior knowledge about pathogenesis needed<br>(2) Screening is labor intensive and expensive<br><br>(3) Structure and sequence of the gene required<br>(4) Large number of cases and matched controls |
| **3.** Search for differences in expression profiles<br>(a) Differential display PCR<br>(b) Subtraction hybridization<br>(c) Microarrays | (1) No prior knowledge needed<br>(2) Unbiased | (1) Labor intensive<br><br>(2) Expensive<br><br>(3) Technically difficult<br><br>(4) Analysis of a large number of samples is time consuming<br>(5) Aortic tissue samples from cases and matched controls needed |

Modified with permission from Kuivaniemi and Shibamura, 2003.[36]

# DNA LINKAGE ANALYSES

## *Family-Based Analyses*

Linkage is a term in genetics that indicates that a marker, a polymorphic DNA marker, a variation in the DNA sequence, is in families coinherited with a phenotype, the disease.[11] Linkage of a disease phenotype and a marker means that the two are located closely on the same physical piece of DNA. The closer the disease and the marker occur on a piece of DNA, the less frequent crossovers are between them, and the more tightly the two are linked. Establishing linkage with the conventional family-based approaches requires large families with affected individuals in at least three generations and available for the study (alive and willing to give a blood sample for DNA isolation). The larger the number of offspring in each generation, the more meioses and, therefore, the more useful the family is for linkage studies. Large families are needed also because of the possibility that different families do not share the same genetic component, a phenomenon known as heterogeneity of the disease. Another requirement is that the disease is diagnosed accurately because an undiagnosed individual will result, at best, in data that suggest a larger distance between the marker and the disease locus, and at worst, in data that suggest lack of linkage or exclusion of the gene in that family. It is desirable to obtain samples from as many as possible affected and unaffected individuals. For the above-mentioned reasons, family-based linkage studies of late-onset diseases such as AAAs are difficult, if not impossible. It is rare to find large families that have more than two generations of living individuals diagnosed with AAA so that blood samples can be obtained for isolating genetic material. By the time an individual has been diagnosed with an aneurysm, his or her parents have died and the children of the AAA patient are still too young to have aneurysms. Diagnosis is also a problem since few individuals develop AAAs before the age of 50 years. Therefore, an individual who is currently between the ages of 50 and 55 years and unaffected may develop an AAA by the age of 65 years and linkage data obtained from such an individual's family would be skewed toward nonlinkage.

### Sib Pair Approach

Another approach, namely the sib-pair approach, of genetic linkage is suitable for diseases in which identifying large families is a difficult task. Sib pairs are extremely useful in genetic studies of complex traits because of a feature that is unique to sib relationships (brother–brother; brother–sister; sister–sister): sibs can share 0, 1, or 2 alleles identical by descent at any given locus. For example, if sibs do not share any alleles, sib 1 has alleles A and C, whereas sib 2 has alleles B and D for a particular marker. If sibs share 1 allele, sib 1 has alleles A and C, whereas sib 2 has alleles A and D for the same marker. If sibs share 2 alleles, sib 1 has alleles A and C and sib 2 has alleles A and C for the same marker. The distribution of the alleles expected by chance is simple and leads to predictions that can be tested without specifying the mode of inheritance that makes this approach a so-called model-free method. The sib-pair linkage approach is, however, less powerful than the extended pedigree approach and a large number of sib pairs are needed to identify susceptibility loci. There are two major types of sib-pair analyses: affected sib-pair analysis (ASP, both sibs have AAA), and discordant sib-pair analysis (one sib has AAA and the other does not). ASP approach is the most appropriate for AAA since it is not possible to say with certainty that a person is unaffected (has no AAA and will not get AAA later). The genetic term for this phenomenon is called age-dependent penetrance. It is also possible that the disease shows incomplete penetrance meaning that an individual has the gene, but does not show the disease and has an affected offspring and an affected parent, which is demonstrated by the fact that the disease skips a generation. With the ASP approach, the penetrance issue becomes irrelevant since there is 100% penetrance in the pool of individuals used for the analyses. The only complications left to deal with are phenocopies (which means that AAA can also be caused by other than genetic, for example, by environmental factors) and heterogeneity (AAA caused by defects in multiple genes at the population level and each of the genes contributing to varying degrees in individual AAA patients).

Use of linkage analysis to identify the genetic causes of late-onset, lethal diseases such as AAA was until recently difficult at best. Several technological advantages have drastically changed the outlook. First, the interest in carrying out noninvasive diagnostic imaging such as ultrasonography screening studies on relatives of AAA patients has made it possible to detect far more family members with AAA prior to rupture (TABLE 2). As a result, there are far more live, affected members available for genetic studies. Second, the development of highly informative markers that can be easily analyzed using polymerase chain reaction (PCR) has greatly enhanced the power of any linkage study. Third, the large number of linkage studies being performed on complex human diseases has refined and advanced the methods and models for linkage analyses. Fourth, there have been theoretical and applied advances in the linkage methodology itself.[11]

## *Collection of 233 Families with AAA*

We collected families with AAA (FIG. 1) and performed DNA linkage analyses to identify regions on the human chromosomes, which are linked to AAAs and could, therefore, harbor susceptibility genes for AAAs. Families for the study were recruited through various vascular surgery centers in the USA, Finland, Belgium, Canada, the Netherlands, Sweden, and the UK as well as through our patient recruitment web site[37] (http://www.genetics.wayne.edu/ags). We identified 233 families that had at least two individuals diagnosed with AAAs.[38] These families had 653 patients with a confirmed diagnosis of AAA, an average of 2.8 cases per family. The majority of the probands (82%) and affected relatives (77%) were males and the most common relationship to the proband was that of brother. When evaluating the mode of inheritance, 167 (72%) families were consistent with autosomal recessive inheritance, whereas 58 (25%) families were consistent with autosomal dominant inheritance and in 8 families the familial aggregation could be

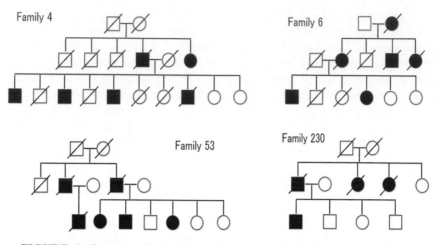

**FIGURE 1.** Representative AAA families from our collection of 233 families. *Slash* across symbol means death. *Black squares* and *circles* indicate male and female members, respectively, diagnosed with AAA.

explained by autosomal dominant inheritance with incomplete penetrance. In the 66 families where AAAs appeared to be inherited in a dominant manner, 141 transmissions of the disease from one generation to another were identified. We asked two questions about these apparently dominant transmissions: (1) Was there any difference in the frequency with which AAAs were inherited from a mother or a father? and (2) Did both daughters and sons inherit AAAs from their parents? Altogether 46% of the 141 transmissions were from father to son, 11% were from father to daughter, 32% from mother to son, and 11% from mother to daughter. This preliminary analysis suggested that it was more likely that a son than a daughter inherited an AAA from the parents.

## Results of a Genome-Wide Screen for AAA

For our genetic studies (FIG. 2), blood samples from altogether 235 affected relative pairs (ARPs) and their unaffected relatives, if available, were collected for DNA isolation and the DNA used for genotyping with highly variable microsatellite markers.[39] We included covariates in the statistical analyses to allow for genetic heterogeneity. Such statistical approaches have been successful in dissecting the genetic components in other complex diseases such as prostate cancer, Alzheimer's disease, and systemic lupus erythematosus.[39] We carried out the study in two phases to reduce the amount of genotyping. In the first phase, 75 ARPs from 36 families were used for a whole genome scan with approximately 400 microsatellite markers and five chromosomal regions exceeded our set threshold logarithm of odds (lod) score of 0.8. A region on

AAA-PATIENTS AND THEIR RELATIVES

↓

COLLECT FAMILY TREE, CLINICAL DATA AND BLOOD

↓

ISOLATE TOTAL GENOMIC DNA FROM BLOOD

↓

WHOLE GENOME SCAN WITH 10 cM DENSITY (400 MARKERS)

↓

AFFECTED RELATIVE-PAIR LINKAGE ANALYSIS

↓

IDENTIFY CHROMOSOMAL REGIONS LINKED TO AAA

↓

GENOTYPE ADDITIONAL MARKERS (2 cM density) IN CANDIDATE
INTERVALS at Chr. 4p12, Chr. 4q31 and Chr. 19q13

↓

IDENTIFY CANDIDATE GENES
Chr. 4: PDGFRA, SPINK2, GAB1 and ENDRA
Chr. 19: HPN, PDCD5, TGFB1, PEPD and LRP3

↓

SCREEN FOR MUTATIONS

↓

DIAGNOSTIC GENETIC TEST

**FIGURE 2.** Outline of steps needed to identify susceptibility genes(s) for AAA using ARP-DNA linkage analysis. As discussed in the text, including only the relatives who have been diagnosed with AAA will improve the accuracy of the analysis since AAA is a late-age-at-onset disease. For details, see Shibamura *et al*., 2004.[39]

chromosome 19 had a lod score of 4.64 with covariate analyses and was studied further with 160 additional ARPs from 83 families. The results remained significant with a lod score of 4 in this larger sample. In combined analyses with a total of 119 families, the results were significant with sex, number of affected first-degree relatives, and their interaction as covariates. We also identified a region on chromosome 4 with a lod score of 3.73 using the same covariate model as for chromosome 19. The chromosome 19 and 4 loci have been designated as the AAA1 and AAA2 loci in the Online Mendelian Inheritance in Man database (OMIM,  http://www.ncbi.nlm.nih.gov/entrez/dispomim.cgi?id=609781  and http://www.ncbi.nlm.nih.gov/entrez/dispomim.cgi?id=609782).

The chromosome 4 and 19 regions contain many plausible candidate genes whose protein products are important in the physiology of arteries such as PDGFRA (platelet-derived growth factor receptor, alpha polypeptide),

SPINK2 (serine peptidase inhibitor, Kazal type 2), GAB1 (GRB2-associated binding protein 1; an important mediator of branching tubulogenesis and a central protein in cellular growth response, transformation, and apoptosis), and EDNRA (endothelin receptor type A; an endothelin-1 receptor expressed in many human tissues with the highest level in the aorta) on chromosome 4 as well as LRP3 (LDL receptor-related protein 3), HPN (transmembrane protease, serine 1; a serine-type peptidase involved in cell growth and maintenance), TGF-β1 (transforming growth factor, beta 1), PDCD5 (programmed cell death 5; a protein expressed in tumor cells during apoptosis independent of the apoptosis-inducing stimuli), and PEPD (peptidase D; an Xaa-Pro dipeptidase important in collagen catabolism) on chromosome 19 (http://www.ncbi.nlm.nih.gov/, http://www.gene.ucl.ac.uk/nomenclature/). LRP3 is particularly interesting because conditional knockout mice for LRP1, another member of the gene family, developed arterial aneurysms and atherosclerosis.[40] Our future research will include more detailed studies of these positional candidate genes in the pathogenesis of AAAs.

## CONCLUSIONS

AAA is a complex genetic disorder with so far unknown causes. Approaches like the DNA linkage analyses discussed above and genetic association studies require a collection of DNA samples from a large number of AAA patients and their family members. For example, for the ARP approach, samples from at least 200 relative pairs are needed. To succeed in collecting samples from 200 ARPs, the initial AAA patient pool from which to gather these samples has to be in the order of 2,000–3,000 AAA patients when assuming that about 15% (300–450) of the patients have a positive family history for AAA, about 50% of the affected relatives are alive, and that only some of the affected relatives are sisters or brothers. Therefore, it would be important to examine with ultrasonography all the sisters and brothers that are over 55 years of age to detect unruptured, asymptomatic AAAs. Identification of silent AAAs would increase the number of sibs known to have an AAA and available for genetic studies. After the genome scan-using ASPs have revealed possible suggestive genetic loci, biologically and physiologically relevant candidate genes located in the candidate intervals can be screened for mutations (FIG. 2). This is called the positional candidate gene approach. Additional knowledge gained from expression studies using aortic tissue samples and differential display PCR,[41] subtraction hybridization or microarray expression profiling[42] to identify those genes that are specific to aortic wall and whose expression is altered in aneurysmal aorta will help identify pathways involved in the development of AAAs. The final goal is to identify risk factors that would help us predict who is at risk for developing an AAA. Based on the identified risk factors, diagnostic tests could be developed and AAAs repaired electively before rupture. Even though our current understanding is that only about 15% of AAAs are visibly genetic, genetic factors could still contribute to the development of apparently sporadic AAA cases in the same way as sporadic breast cancer patients carry mutations in the same genes as patients with heritable forms of the disease.

## ACKNOWLEDGMENTS

The study was supported in part by a grant from NHLBI (HL064310), a grant from the NCHGR (HG01577), and a grant from the NCRR (RR03655). Some of the results were obtained using S.A.G.E., which is also supported by RR03655. We thank Dr. J. Weber and the NHLBI Mammalian Genotyping Service at the Marshfield Medical Research Foundation, Marshfield, WI, for performing the whole genome scan. We gratefully acknowledge the dedicated collaboration of many vascular surgeons, molecular biologists, and geneticists who are shown as coauthors in the original publications listed in the reference section.

## REFERENCES

1. BENGTSSON, H., B. SONESSON & D. BERGQVIST. 1996. Incidence and prevalence of abdominal aortic aneurysms, estimated by necropsy studies and population screening by ultrasound. Ann. N.Y. Acad. Sci. **800:** 1–24.
2. KUIVANIEMI, H. & G. TROMP. 2000. Search for the aneurysm susceptibility gene(s). *In* R.R. Keen & P.B. Dobrin, Eds.: Development of Aneurysms. 219–233. Landes Bioscience. Georgetown.
3. MAJUMDER, P.P. *et al*. 1991. On the inheritance of abdominal aortic aneurysm. Am. J. Hum. Genet. **48:** 164–170.
4. VERLOES, A. *et al*. 1995. Aneurysms of the abdominal aorta: familial and genetic aspects in three hundred thirteen pedigrees. J. Vasc. Surg. **21:** 646–655.
5. KATZ, D.J. *et al*. 1994. Operative mortality rates for intact and ruptured abdominal aortic aneurysms in Michigan: An eleven-year statewide experience. J. Vasc. Surg. **19:** 804–815.
6. KATZ, D.J. *et al*. 1997. Gender differences in abdominal aortic aneurysm prevalence, treatment, and outcome. J. Vasc. Surg. **25:** 561–568.
7. LIMET, R. 1995. Familial risk of abdominal aortic aneurysm and its consequences for organization of selective detection. J. Mal. Vasc. **20:** 285–287.
8. LAMORTE, W.W. *et al*. 1995. Racial differences in the incidence of femoral bypass and abdominal aortic aneurysmectomy in Massachusetts: relationship to cardiovascular risk factors. J. Vasc. Surg. **21:** 422–431.
9. THOMPSON, M.W. *et al*. 1991. Genetics in Medicine. WB Saunders, Harcourt Jovanovich. Philadelphia, PA
10. DARLING, R.C., III *et al*. 1989. Are familial abdominal aortic aneurysms different? J. Vasc. Surg. **10:** 39–43.
11. OLSON, J.M. *et al*. 1999. Genetic mapping of complex traits. Stat. Med. **18:** 2961–2981.

12. NORRGÅRD, O., O. RAIS & K.A. ANGQUIST. 1984. Familial occurrence of abdominal aortic aneurysms. Surgery **95:** 650–656.
13. JOHANSEN, K. & T. KOEPSELL. 1986. Familial tendency for abdominal aortic aneurysms. JAMA **256:** 1934–1936.
14. POWELL, J.T. & R.M. GREENHALGH. 1987. Multifactorial inheritance of abdominal aortic aneurysm. Eur. J. Vasc. Surg. **1:** 29–31.
15. JOHNSTON, K.W. & T.K. SCOBIE. 1988. Multicenter prospective study of nonruptured abdominal aortic aneurysms. I. Population and operative management. J. Vasc. Surg. **7:** 69–81.
16. COLE, C.W. *et al.* 1989. Abdominal aortic aneurysm: consequences of a positive family history. Can. J. Surg. **32:** 117–120.
17. LEDERLE, F.A. *et al.* 1997. Prevalence and associations of abdominal aortic aneurysm detected through screening. Aneurysm Detection and Management (Adam) Veterans Affairs Cooperative Study Group. Ann. Intern. Med. **126:** 441–449.
18. LAWRENCE, P.F. *et al.* 1998. Peripheral aneurysms and arteriomegaly: is there a familial pattern? J. Vasc. Surg. **28:** 599–605.
19. SALKOWSKI, A. *et al.* 1999. Familial incidence of abdominal aortic aneurysms. J. Genet. Couns. **8:** 407.
20. ROSSAAK, J.I. *et al.* 2001. Familial abdominal aortic aneurysms in the Otago region of New Zealand. Cardiovasc. Surg. **9:** 241–248.
21. BENGTSSON, H., O. NORRGARD, *et al.* 1989. Ultrasonographic screening of the abdominal aorta among siblings of patients with abdominal aortic aneurysms. Br. J. Surg. **76:** 589–591.
22. COLLIN, J. & J. WALTON. 1989. Is abdominal aortic aneurysm familial? BMJ **299:** 493.
23. WEBSTER, M.W. *et al.* 1991. Abdominal aortic aneurysm: results of a family study. J. Vasc. Surg. **13:** 366–372.
24. ADAMSON, J. *et al.* 1992. Selection for screening for familial aortic aneurysms. Br. J. Surg. **79:** 897–898.
25. BENGTSSON, H. *et al.* 1992. Prevalence of abdominal aortic aneurysm in the offspring of patients dying from aneurysm rupture. Br. J. Surg. **79:** 1142–1143.
26. VAN DER LUGT, A. *et al.* 1992. Screening for familial occurrence of abdominal aortic aneurysm. Ned. Tijdschr. Geneeskd. **136:** 1910–1913.
27. ADAMS, D.C. *et al.* 1993. Familial abdominal aortic aneurysm: prevalence and implications for screening. Eur. J. Vasc. Surg. **7:** 709–712.
28. MOHER, D. *et al.* 1994. Definition and management of abdominal aortic aneurysms: results from a Canadian survey. Can. J. Surg. **37:** 29–32.
29. FITZGERALD, P. *et al.* 1995. Abdominal aortic aneurysm in the Irish population: a familial screening study. Br. J. Surg. **82:** 483–486.
30. LARCOS, G. *et al.* 1995. Ultrasound screening of families with abdominal aortic aneurysm. Australas. Radiol. **39:** 254–256.
31. BAIRD, P.A. *et al.* 1995. Sibling risks of abdominal aortic aneurysm. Lancet **346:** 601–604.
32. JAAKKOLA, P. *et al.* 1996. Familial abdominal aortic aneurysms: screening of 71 families. Eur. J. Surg. **162:** 611–617.
33. VAN DER GRAAF, Y. *et al.* 1998. Results of aortic screening in the brothers of patients who had elective aortic aneurysm repair. Br. J. Surg. **85:** 778–780.
34. SALO, J.A. *et al.* 1999. Familial occurrence of abdominal aortic aneurysm. Ann. Intern. Med. **130:** 637–642.

35. OGATA, T. *et al*. 2005. The life-time prevalence of abdominal aortic aneurysms among siblings of aneurysm patients is eight-fold higher than among siblings of spouses: an analysis of 187 aneurysm families in Nova Scotia, Canada. J. Vasc. Surg. **42:** 891–897.
36. KUIVANIEMI, H. & H. SHIBAMURA. 2003. Candidate genes for abdominal aortic aneurysms. *In* Diseases of the Aorta. D. Liotta & M. del Rio, Eds.: 89–100. Domingo Liotta Foundation Medical. Buenos Aires, Argentina.
37. SALKOWSKI, A. *et al*. 2001. Web site-based recruitment for research studies on abdominal aortic and intracranial aneurysms. Genet. Test. **5:** 307–310.
38. KUIVANIEMI, H. *et al*. 2003. Familial abdominal aortic aneurysms: collection of 233 multiplex families. J. Vasc. Surg. **37:** 340–345.
39. SHIBAMURA, H. *et al*. 2004. Genome scan for familial abdominal aortic aneurysm using sex and family history as covariates suggests genetic heterogeneity and identifies linkage to chromosome 19q13. Circulation **109:** 2103–2108.
40. BOUCHER, P. *et al*. 2003. LRP: role in vascular wall integrity and protection from atherosclerosis. Science **300:** 329–332.
41. KUIVANIEMI, H. *et al*. 1996. Candidate genes for abdominal aortic aneurysms. Ann. N.Y. Acad. Sci. **800:** 186–197.
42. LENK, G. *et al*. 2006. Global expression profiles in human normal and aneurysmal abdominal aorta based on two distinct whole genome microarray platforms. Ann. N.Y. Acad. Sci. This volume.

# The Candidate Gene Approach to Susceptibility for Abdominal Aortic Aneurysm

## TIMP1, HLA-DR-15, Ferritin Light Chain, and Collagen XI-Alpha-1

M. DAVID TILSON III[a,b] AND CHARLES Y. RO[a]

[a]Department of Surgery, St. Luke's-Roosevelt Hospital Center, Continuum Health Partners, New York, New York, USA

[b]Columbia University in the City of New York, New York, USA

ABSTRACT: There are two approaches to gene discovery for diseases when genetic susceptibility has been implicated by clinical genetic or case-control studies: (1) genome-wide screening and (2) evaluation of candidate genes. Each has specific advantages and disadvantages. The principal advantage of genome-wide screening is that it is impeccably objective in as much as it proceeds without any presuppositions regarding the importance of specific pathobiological features of the disease process. The principal disadvantage is that such a study is expensive and resource intensive. A large population of enrolled patients and multidisciplinary teams of investigators cooperating from several institutions are usually required. The alternative approach of evaluating candidate genes can be pursued by a small independent laboratory with limited funding and resources, a small collection of clinical specimens, and a small number of team players. The disadvantage is that it is by necessity highly subjective in the process of selecting specific candidates among many reasonable possibilities. There is no *a priori* assurance that effort will not be expended on one or more candidates that turn out in the end to be failures. This report reviews efforts in our laboratory to evaluate four genes as candidates. One of these tissue inhibitor of metalloprotease 1(TIMP1) led to the description of a polymorphism, but not a conclusive mutation. The other three (HLA-DR-15, ferritin light chain (FTL), and collagen XI-alpha-1 (COL11A1) are subjects of continuing interest.

Address for correspondence: Martin David Tilson III, M.D., Department of Surgery, St. Luke's-Roosevelt Hospital Center, 1000 Tenth Avenue-Suite 2B, New York, NY 10019. Voice: 212-523-7780; fax: 212-523-6495.

e-mail: mdt1@columbia.edu

Ann. N.Y. Acad. Sci. 1085: 282–290 (2006). © 2006 New York Academy of Sciences.
doi: 10.1196/annals.1383.016

KEYWORDS: abdominal aortic aneurysm; TIMP; HLA-DR; ferritin light chain; collagen XI; COL11A1; susceptibility genes; candidate genes; matrix metalloproteinases; oxidative injury; protease inhibitors; matrix remodeling; autoimmunity; genome-wide screening

## INTRODUCTION

Genome-wide screening is a robust tool for the discovery of susceptibility genes without the need for hypothetical presuppositions based on the state of knowledge in the field of abdominal aortic aneurysm (AAA) pathobiology. Prerequisites include: (1) stable and substantial grant funding to support multiinstitutional and multidisciplinary research groups; (2) access to clinical databases including large numbers of sibling-pairs; (3) high throughput molecular methodology; and (4) computationally intensive data management systems. Notwithstanding all of its advantages, especially absence of bias at the process level for selecting candidate loci, it is unsuitable for a small laboratory with limited resources of grant support, few personnel, and a small specimen inventory. "Candidate genes" may be pursued with modest amounts of money for research support, some "banked" tissue samples obtained from surgical specimens or blood with IRB approval, and cooperation with a CORE institutional facility for primer-synthesis and sequencing work. The "candidate gene" approach requires only: (1) a working knowledge of AAA pathobiology; (2) a collection of tissue samples from AAA patients in formalin or frozen in a refrigerator; (3) inexpensive scientific kits for making cDNA from mRNA or purification of genomic DNA from preserved tissue; (4) a polymerase chain reaction (PCR) machine and an instrument for visualizing gel bands to be harvested and submitted for sequencing; (5) some blind luck from time to time, as promising leads may arise serendipitously in the course of pursuing other endeavors; and (6) some eager volunteer students who want to become involved in a short-term research experience. So this approach may be the most suitable one for a small laboratory with limited resources. This article reports on our experience with four genes that have been approached as candidates during the period from 1988 until 2006. The first, tissue inhibitor of metalloprotease (TIMP1), appeared to be a failure in our hands at the time; but a role for this gene and/or other members of its family has not been ruled out. The other three are in different stages of continuing interest. Since the rationale for approaching each gene as a candidate was different, the following description for each will be captioned for "Background, Methods, Results, and Conclusions."

## TIMP1

*Background.* In an early chart review study (1980), the author found that AAAs were significantly more common in men than in women.[1] However, the ratio of men to women was approximately 50/50 in patients with atherosclerotic occlusive disease of the aorta. Thus, we became interested in the spontaneously aneurysm-prone Blotchy mouse. In this mutation, only males are affected because the causative gene is on the X chromosome. The mutation interferes with cellular copper transport, and we sought evidence to support a role for the Blotchy-locus indirectly by the study of copper levels in tissue from AAA patients and by the study of the lysyl-oxidase-dependent collagen cross-link pyridinoline (Pyr). Our result for tissue copper levels[2] was in conflict with results from two other laboratories, which were also not in agreement with each other. The situation was reviewed by J.F. Blanchard in 1999.[3] The most recent studies of trace metals in AAA do not detect any significant changes in either copper or zinc.[4] Further confounding our hypothesis, the initial results on Pyr[5] were in conflict with our second data set, which was based on a larger number of patients and an improved high-performance liquid chromatography (HPLC) methodology developed in our laboratory.[6] Accordingly, a second paper was written to bring the record up to date.[7] Thereafter, we abandoned copper metabolism as a failed hypothesis, but we retained an interest in the X chromosome as a candidate locus.

TIMP was assigned to the X chromosome, so we turned attention to consider it as a candidate. Only one TIMP was known at the time, although now three members of the family have been described. We studied what is today called TIMP1, and we sequenced the cDNA for this gene from six AAA patients.

*Methods.* mRNA was extracted from six tissue specimens from AAA patients and the cDNAs were sequenced by a collaborator.

*Results.* The sequencing laboratory sent us a preliminary communication that two of the six patients had an identical substitution in the coding sequence. A subsequent message was that the substitution was in the third position of the codon and that the amino acid was unchanged. Consequently, this interesting observation may be trivial.[8] However, our finding of this polymorphism has been confirmed by Wang and coauthors.[9] The transition is a C for T substitution in the third position of codon 101. Wang *et al.* reported that T was more common in both male (51%) and female (73%) controls. However, C was detected in 63% of women with AAA. The difference in the frequency of the transition in the female patients versus the female controls was statistically significant at $P = 0.0019$ by Fisher's exact test.

*Conclusion.* Uncertain. Even if the codon is conserved, it is possible that the transition might have an effect on gene expression. Also, the regulatory sequences have not been thoroughly examined in the AAA context. Accordingly, this gene and other members of the TIMP family remain viable candidates and the question will be unresolved until there are further studies.

## HLA-DR-15

*Background.* In the experiments described above, finding that the Pyr-analog that we measured was high (not low, as predicted), we believed that deoxy-Pyr was an immature cross-link and a sentinel for increased collagen turnover. This interpretation plus other experiments during the early 1990s served to redirect laboratory effort to describing the role of matrix metalloproteinases (MMPs) and plasmin in the destruction of matrix that is a hallmark of AAA pathobiology.[10–11] We began to consider the possibility that the AAA is an autoimmune disease of maturity with features similar to rheumatoid arthritis.[12] Since autoimmune diseases were known to have HLA-DR-DP-DQ susceptibility genes, we submitted a series of specimens from AAA patients for HLA-DR typing at the New York Blood Bank and at the Core Facility at our university.

*Methods and Results.* The results in the aggregate were confusing, so we focused attention on 10 haplotypes from African Americans because AAA in this specific population is uncommon. The results reported at this meeting 10 years ago suggested that DR-2 was among the candidate alleles.[13] DR-2 was subsequently subdivided into molecular subsets DR-15 and DR-16. A former student (H. Hirose, 1995) studied this question again in a larger vascular surgery clinic population in Japan (including control subjects with atherosclerotic occlusive disease of the aorta). He has reported with his coauthors that DR-15 is a susceptibility allele for AAA disease.[14] He also reported that an allele of DQ was a negative risk factor.[15] Another student (T. Jordan, 2001) found that DR-15 cosegregated with aneurysmal diseases (abdominal, thoracic, and cerebral) in an extended kindred of affected persons.[16]

*Conclusion.* HLA DR-15 continues to be a viable candidate allele with a confirmatory report from the group at Mayo Clinic.[17]

## FERRITIN LIGHT CHAIN (FTL)

*Background.* Consideration of FTL as a candidate gene arose serendipitously. We were using "degenerate" primers to try to clone a cDNA for aneurysm-associated-antigenic protein-40 kDa (AAAP-40), and among many uninteresting cDNA sequences that were determined, there was a cDNA for FTL from fibroblasts cultured from a AAA specimen. This finding preempted our attention because there were three substitutions, two of which changed codons.[18] Further studies have been done on genomic DNA from our collection of AAA specimens.

*Methods and Results.* Genomic DNA was extracted from surgical specimens of 19 patients with AAA and primers were designed for the amplification of exons 1 and 2. This work was done by my student C.Y. Ro, coauthor of this article. The candidate substitutions predicted from the cDNA of an AAA fibroblast culture were not detected. The original cell culture could not be recovered to try to confirm the initial finding and the patients could not be traced under IRB requirements for the protection of confidentiality. However, 15 of the 19 new patients were heterozygous for C/T at position number 54,160,889 in a reference build of the UCSD human genome database (chromosome 19q13). Two

Chromosome 19q

Ferritin Light Chain

* Position # 54,160,889 in USCD Genome Build - NO Codon Change
** Position # 54,160,895 in USCD Genome Build - Codon changes from Glu to Lys

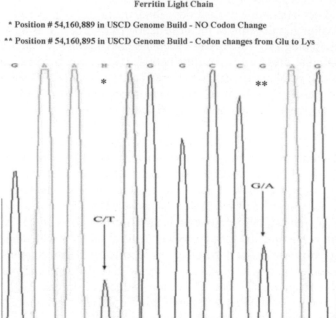

**FIGURE 1.** The two asterisks (**) indicate the nucleotide substitution that results in an altered codon in 2 of 19 patients studied.

patients were heterozygous for A/G at position number 54,160,895, and this substitution changed the codon from a glutamate (normal) to a lysine (possible mutation). A chromatogram from the sequencing analysis from 1 of these 2 patients is shown in FIGURE 1.

*Conclusion.* The A/G substitution may be a mutational event that accounts for susceptibility of a subset of patients with AAA because of possible consequences for protein folding and stability. The FTL locus is of interest because: (1) there is current interest in the roles of inflammatory cytokines and oxidative injury during AAA pathogenesis[19–20] and (2) FTL is at or near a site recently described by Kuivaniemi and coauthors as a susceptibility locus for both cerebral and aortic aneurysmal diseases.[30]

## COLLAGEN XI-ALPHA 1 (COL11A1)

*Background.* With the assistance of T. McCaffrey from the Department of Cardiology at Cornell in New York City at the time, two of my students (D.R. Ewing and J.Y. Gefen, 2000) did a gene chip to evaluate mRNAs that are over- or underexpressed by fibroblasts from aortic adventitia of AAA patients. Among the overexpressed genes, COL11A1 was the outlier (increased 38-fold by comparison to a cell line of putative normal aortic fibroblasts) and further studies showed that antibody against collagen XI was immunoreactive with aortic adventitial microfibrils.[22] A review of the literature informed us that COL11A1 is subject to site-specific expression in aorta versus cartilage. In cartilage there is use of alternative exon 6B and in aorta there is use of 6A. We believed that this situation deserved further study.

*Method 1 (preliminary study).* My student, I.K. Toumpoulis (2004), amplified exon 6A from genomic DNA of 25 AAA patients randomly selected from our collection of surgical specimens. The primers were closely adjacent to the exon of interest.

*Method 2 (repeat study with improved methodology).* Coauthor C.Y. Ro repeated this work in 14 patients with more widely spaced primers that included the flanking introns.

*Result 1 (preliminary study).* The computer report from the sequencing laboratory identified several substitutions detected by its programmatic analysis of the data. Visual inspection of the raw chromatographic data suggested that some of the putative ambiguities were correct and that some were probably incorrect. Molecular biologists were consulted and were helpful in making the best consensus interpretations. However, we became aware of the difficulties that are inherent in the reading of heterozygosities. Accordingly, Ro carried out the second set of experiments in our laboratory.

*Result 2 (expanded study with improved methodology).* More distantly spaced primers resulted in a data set that did not confirm any unambiguous heterozygosities in exon 6A. However, this time there was a consistent heterozygous G for T signal in the upstream intron, 70 bp away from the coding sequence, in all 14 patients. This finding is illustrated in FIGURE 2.

*Conclusion.* This upstream heterozygous substitution may affect the alternative splicing and expression of exon 6A. If one allele produces an abnormal gene product, the whole collagen XI molecule might undergo "protein suicide." Such an event would explain the overexpression of mRNA for COL11A1. Further studies will be required to confirm this hypothesis.

## CONCLUSION

The candidate gene approach lacks the objectivity of genome-wide screening. The candidate gene approach also requires a basic working knowledge

Heterozygous Signal at Position -70 bp (upstream) from Exon 6A
in Fourteen Consecutively Sequenced Patients with AAA

Collagen XI-alpha-1

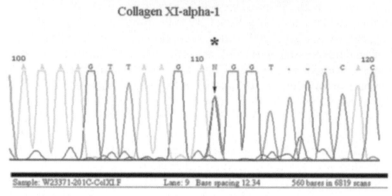

**FIGURE 2.** A heterozygous signal in the intron preceding exon 6A was detected in genomic sequences from 14/19 patients with AAA.

of AAA pathobiology, and the processes of hypothesis formation and subjective judgment are important. Significant findings cannot be guaranteed and encouraging preliminary results must be subjected to further studies. Notwithstanding all of these negative features, this approach may be the best choice for a small laboratory with limited resources. It may lead to candidates with sustained vitality and point the way for future studies on a larger scale, from which conclusions on a higher level of probability may be reached.

## REFERENCES

1. TILSON, M.D. & H.C. STANSEL. 1980. Differences in results for aneurysm vs. occlusive disease after bifurcation grafts: results of 100 elective grafts. Arch. Surg. **115:** 1173–1175.
2. TILSON, M.D. 1982. Decreased hepatic copper levels. A possible chemical marker for the pathogenesis of aortic aneurysms in man. Arch. Surg. **117:** 1212–1213.
3. BLANCHARD, J.F. 1999. Epidemiology of abdominal aortic aneurysms. Epidemiol. Rev. **21:** 207–221.
4. JAAKKOLA, P., M. HIPPELAINEN & M. KANTOLA. 1994. Copper and zinc concentrations of abdominal aorta and liver in patients with infrarenal abdominal aortic aneurysm or aortoiliacal occlusive disease. Ann. Chir. Gynaecol. **83:** 304–308.
5. TILSON, M.D. & G. DAVIS. 1983. Deficiencies of copper and a compound with ion-exchange characteristics of pyridinoline in skin from patients with abdominal aortic aneurysms. Surgery **94:** 134–141.
6. TILSON, M.D., R.N. DREYER, A. HUDSON, *et al.* 1985. Partial characteristics of an analog of pyridinoline isolated from human skin. Biochem. Biophys. Res. Commun. **126:** 1222–1227.

7. TILSON, M.D. 1985. Further studies of a putative cross-linking amino acid (3-deoxypyridinoline) in skin from patients with abdominal aortic aneurysms. Surgery **98:** 888–891.

8. TILSON, M.D., J.M. REILLY, C.M. BROPHY, *et al.* 1993. Expression and sequence of the gene for tissue inhibitor of metalloproteinases in patients with abdominal aortic aneurysms. J. Vasc. Surg. **18:** 266–270.

9. WANG, X., G. TROMP, C.W. COLE, *et al.* 1999. Analysis of coding sequences for tissue inhibitor of metalloproteinases 1 (TIMP1) and 2 (TIMP2) in patients with aneurysms. Matrix Biol. **18:** 121–124.

10. IRIZARRY, E., K.M. NEWMAN, R.H. GANDHI, *et al.* 1993. Demonstration of interstitial collagenase in abdominal aortic aneurysm disease. J. Surg. Res. **54:** 571–574.

11. JEAN-CLAUDE, J., K.M. NEWMAN, H. LI, *et al.* 1994. Possible key role for plasmin in the pathogenesis of abdominal aortic aneurysms. Surgery **116:** 472–478.

12. K.M. NEWMAN, Y. OGATA, A.M. MALON, *et al.* 1994. Identification of matrix metalloproteinases 3 (stromelysin-1) and 9 (gelatinase B) in abdominal aortic aneurysm. Arterioscler. Thromb. **14:** 1315–1320.

13. NEWMAN, K.M., A.M. MALON, R.D. SHIN, *et al.* 1994. Matrix metalloproteinases in abdominal aortic aneurysm: characterization, purification, and their possible sources. Connect. Tissue Res. **30:** 265–276.

14. TILSON, M.D. & K.M. NEWMAN. 1994. Proteolytic mechanisms in the pathogenesis of aortic aneurysms. *In* Aneurysms: new findings and treatments. Yao, J.S. & W.H. Pearce, Eds.: 3–9. Appleton and Lange. Norwalk CT.

15. GREGORY, A.K., N.X. YIN, J. CAPELLA, *et al.* 1996. Features of autoimmunity in the abdominal aortic aneurysm. Arch. Surg. **131:** 85–88.

16. TILSON, M.D., K.J. OZSVATH, H. HIROSE & S. XIA. 1996. A genetic basis for autoimmune manifestations in the abdominal aortic aneurysm resides in the MHC class II locus DR-beta-1. Ann. N.Y.Acad. Sci. **800:** 208–215.

17. HIROSE, H., M. TAKAGI, N. MIYAGAWA, *et al.* 1998. Genetic risk factor for abdominal aortic aneurysm: HLA-DR2(15), a Japanese study. J. Vasc. Surg. **27:** 500–503.

18. HIROSE H. & M.D. TILSON. 1999. Negative genetic risk factor for abdominal aortic aneurysm: HLA-DQ3, a Japanese study. J. Vasc. Surg. **30:** 959–960.

19. JORDAN, T.P. BA, X.G. LI, J.C. OBUNIKE & M.D. TILSON. 2002. Aneurysmal diseases cosegregate in an African-American kindred with HLA class II DR-B1-15. International College of Angiology. New York.

20. RASMUSSEN, T.E., J.W. HALLETT, JR., S. SCHULTE, *et al.* 2001. Genetic similarity in inflammatory and degenerative abdominal aortic aneurysms: a study of human leukocyte antigen class II disease risk genes. J. Vasc. Surg. **34:** 84–89.

21. LI, X., J. OBUNIKE & M.D. TILSON. 2002. Ferritin-like expressed mRNA with two substitutions changing putative expressed protein, from aortic aneurysm adventitial fibroblasts (bases 1-900). *In* GenBank Accession # AY207005.

22. TILSON, M.D. F.C., S.X. XIA, D. SYN, *et al.* 2000. Expression of molecular messages for angiogenesis by fibroblasts from aneurysmal abdominal aorta versus dermal fibroblasts. Int. J. Surg. Invest. **1:** 453–457.

23. PAIK D. & M.D. TILSON. 1996. Neovascularization in the abdominal aortic aneurysm. Endothelial nitric oxide synthase, nitric oxide, and elastolysis. Ann. N. Y. Acad. Sci. **800:** 277.

24. PAIK, D.C., W.G. RAMEY, J. DILLON & M.D. TILSON. 1997. The nitrite/elastin reaction: implications for in vivo degenerative effects. Connect. Tissue Res. **36:** 241–251.

25. MILLER, F.J., JR., W.J. SHARP, X. FANG, *et al*. 2002. Oxidative stress in human abdominal aortic aneurysms: a potential mediator of aneurysmal remodeling. Arterioscler. Thromb. Vasc. Biol. **22:** 560–565.

26. YAJIMA, N., M. MASUDA, M. MIYAZAKI, *et al*. 2002. Oxidative stress is involved in the development of experimental abdominal aortic aneurysm: a study of the transcription profile with complementary DNA microarray. J. Vasc. Surg. **36:** 379–385.

27. SHIBAMURA, H., J.M. OLSON, C. VAN VLIJMEN-VAN KEULEN, *et al*. 2004. Genome scan for familial abdominal aortic aneurysm using sex and family history as covariates suggests genetic heterogeneity and identifies linkage to chromosome 19q13. Circulation **109:** 2103–2108.

28. BHATTI, A. E.D., T.P. JORDAN, T.A. MCCAFFREY, *et al*. 2002. Role of collagen type XI in the pathogenesis of the abdominal aortic aneurysm. J. Am. Coll. Surg. **195** (Suppl):S201.

## ADDITIONAL REFERENCES

29. BELSLEY S.J. & M.D. TILSON. 2003. Two decades of research on etiology and genetic factors in abdominal aortic aneurysm disease. (Review Article) Acta Chir. Belg. **103:** 187–197.

30. KUIVANIEMI H. & T. OGATA. 2006. Highlights of the recent literature on abdominal aortic aneurysm research. (Editorial) Ann. Vasc. Surg. **20:** 1–4.

31. TILSON M.D., III. 2005. The polymorphonuclear leukocyte and the abdominal aortic aneurysm: a neglected cell type and a neglected disease. (Editorial) Circulation **112:** 154–156.

# Aneurysm Outreach Inc., a Nonprofit Organization, Offers Community-Based, Ultrasonography Screening for Abdominal Aortic Aneurysms

SHEILA ARRINGTON,[a] TORU OGATA,[b] P. MICHAEL DAVIS, JR.,[d]
ALBERT D. SAM, II,[e] LARRY H. HOLLIER,[f] GERARD TROMP,[b]
AND HELENA KUIVANIEMI[b,c]

[a]Aneurysm Outreach Inc., Prairieville, LA, USA

[b]The Center for Molecular Medicine and Genetics, Wayne State University School of Medicine, Detroit, Michigan, USA

[c]Department of Surgery, Wayne State University School of Medicine, Detroit, Michigan, USA

[d]CVT Surgical Center, Baton Rouge, LA, USA

[e]Vascular Surgery Associates, Baton Rouge, LA, USA

[f]Department of Surgery, Louisiana State University School of Medicine, New Orleans, LA, USA

ABSTRACT: Aneurysm Outreach Inc. (AOI; www.alink.org) is a nonprofit volunteer organization founded in 1999 whose aim is to (a) raise public awareness about aneurysms; (b) stimulate and fund genetic research through donations; and (c) coordinate a support network for aneurysm patients and their families. Since abdominal ultrasonography examination of an asymptomatic individual is not presently reimbursed by health insurance in the United States, one of the initiatives supported by AOI is to have free ultrasonography screening for abdominal aortic aneurysm (AAA) for those most at risk. One of the initiatives supported by AOI is to have free ultrasonography screening for abdominal aortic aneurysm (AAA). To meet this goal, a free screening program was initiated in September 2001 and by November 2004 approximately 3,000 participants were screened and 61 (2.0%) participants were confirmed to have a dilated aorta and were referred to their primary care physicians or vascular surgeons for further follow-up and treatment, if indicated.

KEYWORDS: aneurysm; aorta; aortic dilation; ultrasonography screening

Address for correspondence: Sheila Arrington, Aneurysm Outreach Inc., 17222 Highway 929, Prairieville, LA 70769, USA. Voice: 225-622-1577, 225-622-2202; fax: 225-622-1502.
e-mail: aoi@alink.org

Ann. N.Y. Acad. Sci. 1085: 291–293 (2006). © 2006 New York Academy of Sciences.
doi: 10.1196/annals.1383.032

We report the results of this screening program and summarize the demographics of those with normal and dilated aortas. Aneurysm Outreach Inc. (AOI) offered free screening for abdominal aortic aneurysm (AAA) to anyone who met the criteria of being (a) over 60 years old; or (b) over 50 years old, male, and with positive family history for AAA; or (c) over 55 years old, female, and with positive family history for AAA. AOI organized 21 events between September 2001 and November 2004 and the number of participants per event varied from 24 to 240. Ultrasonography scans were performed by registered vascular technologists (RVT). The ultrasonography instruments used for the screenings were: (a) ATL HDI 3000$^{TM}$ and ATL HDI 5000$^{TM}$ (PHILIPS, Bothell, WA) donated by Vascular Associates Laboratory (VAL, Baton Rouge, LA); (b) Toshiba 140$^{TM}$ (Toshiba, Tokyo, Japan) and Siemens Antares$^{TM}$ (Siemens, Malvern, PA) donated by CVT surgical center (CVT, Baton Rouge, LA); and (c) SonoSite TITAN$^{TM}$ and SonoSite 180PLUS$^{TM}$, donated by SonoSite, Inc. (Bothell, WA). Altogether 3,088 individuals met the screening criteria; 22 of them were already known to have AAAs. A total of 36 (1.2%) individuals were excluded from the final analysis due to inadequate ultrasonography images. Among the remaining 3,030 individuals, a dilatation of the aorta was detected and confirmed in 61 (2.0%) individuals, in 4.3% of the screened males, and in 0.6% of the screened females. As of January 2005 a total of 13 individuals (0.43%) had their AAAs repaired surgically. The frequencies of males and current smokers were significantly higher in the AAA group than in the group with normal size aortas (male: AAA 83.6% vs. normal 42.0%, $P < 0.0001$; smoker: AAA 54.9% vs. normal 18.1%, $P < 0.0001$). The mean age was significantly higher in the AAA group than in the group with normal size aortas (AAA 71.0 ± 6.2 vs. normal 68.4 ± 7.0, $P = 0.005$). In conclusion, the results of this community-based free ultrasonography screening program are in agreement with randomized controlled screening programs and emphasize the need for systematic screening programs and the importance of finding individuals harboring AAAs before their rupture. Early diagnosis of AAA, prior to rupture, is vital for optimizing patient survival. When ultrasonography screening for AAA becomes a national program covered by health insurance,[1,2] the emphasis of AOI and other similar organizations will shift from both education and providing screening to education and possibly coordinating screening events.

## ACKNOWLEDGMENTS

The research in the Kuivaniemi laboratory is supported by the NHLBI (grant HL064310). Aneurysm Outreach Inc. has received donations from individuals and companies. Full listing of donors is available on the Aneurysm Outreach Inc web site at www.alink.org

# REFERENCES

1. KENT, K.C., R.M. ZWOLAK, M.R. JAFF, *et al.* 2004. Screening for abdominal aortic aneurysm: a consensus statement. J. Vasc. Surg. **39:** 267–269.
2. U.S. PREVENTIVE SERVICES TASK FORCE. 2005. Screening for abdominal aortic aneurysm: recommendation statement. Ann. Intern. Med. **142:** 198–202.

# Diffusion of Alexa Fluor 488-Conjugated Dendrimers in Rat Aortic Tissue

BRENDA S. CHO,[a,b] KAREN J. ROELOFS,[b] ISTVAN J. MAJOROS,[c] JAMES R. BAKER, JR.,[c] JAMES C. STANLEY,[b] PETER K. HENKE,[b] AND GILBERT R. UPCHURCH, JR.[b]

[a]*Department of Biomedical Engineering, University of Michigan, Ann Arbor, MI, USA*

[b]*Department of Surgery, Jobst Vascular Research Laboratories, University of Michigan, Ann Arbor, MI, USA*

[c]*Department of Internal Medicine, University of Michigan, Ann Arbor, MI, USA*

ABSTRACT: In this study, the distribution of labeled dendrimers in native and aneurysmal rat aortic tissue was examined. Adult male rats underwent infrarenal aorta perfusion with generation 5 (G5) acetylated Alexa Fluor 488-conjugated dendrimers for varying lengths of time. In a second set of experiments, rats underwent aortic elastase perfusion followed by aortic dendrimer perfusion 7 days later. Aortic diameters were measured prior to and postelastase perfusion, and again on the day of harvest. Aortas were harvested 0, 12, or 24 h postperfusion, fixed, and mounted. Native aortas were harvested and viewed as negative controls. Aortic cross-sections were viewed and imaged using confocal microscopy. Dendrimers were quantified (counts/high-powered field). Results were evaluated by repeated measures ANOVA and Student's $t$-test. We found that in native aortas, dendrimers penetrated the aortic wall in all groups. For all perfusion times, fewer dendrimers were present as time between dendrimer perfusion and aortic harvest increased. Longer perfusion times resulted in increased diffusion of dendrimers throughout the aortic wall. By 24 h, the majority of the dendrimers were through the wall. Dendrimers in aneurysmal aortas, on day 0 postdendrimer perfusion, diffused farther into the aortic wall than controls. In conclusion, this study documents labeled dendrimers delivered intra-arterially to native rat aortas *in vivo*, and the temporal diffusion of these molecules within the aortic wall. Increasing perfusion time and length of time prior to harvest resulted in continued dendrimer diffusion into the aortic wall. These preliminary data provide a novel mechanism whereby local inhibitory therapy may be delivered locally to aortic tissue.

Address for correspondence: Gilbert R. Upchurch, Jr., M.D., University of Michigan Hospital, 2210 THCC, 1500 East Medical Center Drive, Ann Arbor, MI 48109-0329. Voice: 734-936-5790; fax: 734-647-9867.

e-mail: riversu@umich.edu

Ann. N.Y. Acad. Sci. 1085: 294–305 (2006). © 2006 New York Academy of Sciences.
doi: 10.1196/annals.1383.004

KEYWORDS: aorta; aneurysm; dendrimer; drug delivery; nanotechnology; PAMAM

# BACKGROUND

Local drug delivery has been used to treat many diseases. Local intra-arterial drug delivery is difficult because it may be diluted away from the target site rapidly due to high pressure and flow within the arteries.[1] In one study, extracellular matrix (ECM)-directed local drug delivery was achieved via a polylysine vehicle for treating restenosis in the vessel wall. This was done by maintaining a high concentration of the drug within the target tissue.[2] An alternative drug carrier that has not previously been used to deliver agents to aortic tissue is a poly(amidoamine) (PAMAM) dendrimer. PAMAM dendrimers have been used as carriers for delivering drugs in cancer therapies.[3] PAMAM dendrimers can also be used as imaging agents in humans.[4] Their multifunctional structure makes them appealing for drug delivery applications.[5] In addition, to be useful in biological systems, materials need to be biocompatible and water soluble.[6] Dendrimers are synthetic and very biocompatible with a highly branched structure (FIG. 1).[5] This structure allows for the attachment of multiple agents by covalent linkage or by encapsulation.[4] In this study, dendrimers were acetylated to neutralize some of the primary amine groups and to reduce nonspecific binding. Their shapes and sizes are well defined and uniform, and their surfaces are readily chemically functionalized and modifiable.[5,7]

One potential clinical application for these dendrimers is targeted drug delivery for treating abdominal aortic aneurysms (AAAs). AAAs are the 10th leading cause of death of men and the 14th leading cause of overall death in the United States.[8] Although there are currently no proven effective nonsurgical medical therapies to treat patients with AAAs, doxycycline has been shown to limit the enlargement of experimental AAAs[9–12] and decrease levels of plasma matrix metalloproteinase 9 (MMP-9), an enzyme known to degrade the aortic wall in patients with AAAs.[13] By delivering locally rather than systemically, required doses of compounds such as doxycycline could be reduced, thereby eliminating the risk of unwanted side effects.

In this study, generation 5 (G5) acetylated Alexa Fluor 488-conjugated dendrimers were delivered intra-arterially to native and aneurysmal aortas to examine the diffusion of these labeled dendrimers through the aortic wall.

# METHODS

Adult male Sprague–Dawley rats weighing 190–210 g were obtained from Charles River Laboratories (Wilmington, MA, USA) and were used for all experiments in this study. Surgical procedures and experiments were approved

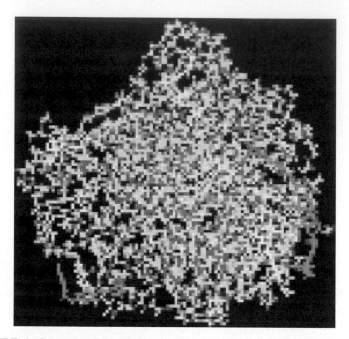

**FIGURE 1.** Structure of dendrimer. Dendrimer synthesis is attained via stepwise additions and reactions; each layer is referred to as a "generation." In this study, generation 5 dendrimers were partially acetylated and conjugated to Alexa Fluor 488 molecules.[3]

by the University of Michigan Universal Committee on the Use and Care of Animals, per Protocol #8833.

### Rodent Elastase Perfusion AAA Model

Rats were anesthetized with 2–3% isoflurane with 100% oxygen. Using sterile techniques, a ventral midline incision was made. The infrarenal abdominal aorta was isolated and perfused with pancreatic porcine elastase as previously described (FIG. 2 A, B).[14] Briefly, the aorta was exposed from the iliac bifurcation (distal) to the level of the left renal vein (proximal), and all side branches within the exposed length of the aorta were tied off with 7–0 silk suture (Ethicon Inc., Somerville, NJ, USA) to ensure pressurization of the aorta. Using 4–0 cotton suture (Genzyme Corp., Fall River, MA, USA) and a vascular clip, temporary distal and proximal aortic control was obtained. A 30-gauge needle was used to make an aortotomy just proximal to the iliac bifurcation. A polyethylene-10 (PE-10) tube was inserted through the aortotomy, and pancreatic porcine elastase (6 units/mL; Lot Number 083K7655; Sigma, St. Louis, MO, USA) was infused into the isolated infrarenal aorta for 30 min. Following perfusion, a 10–0 nylon monofilament suture (Surgical Specialties Corp., Reading, PA, USA) was used to repair the aortotomy in the aorta.

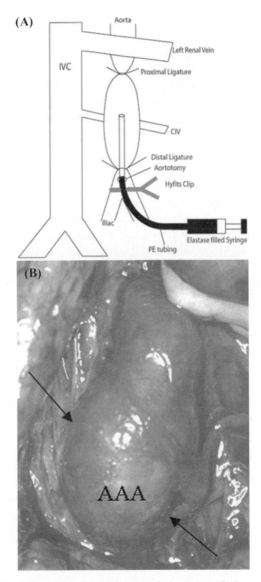

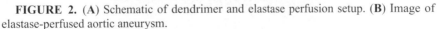

**FIGURE 2.** (**A**) Schematic of dendrimer and elastase perfusion setup. (**B**) Image of elastase-perfused aortic aneurysm.

Images were taken using a Spot Insight Color Optical Camera (Diagnostic Instruments, Sterling Heights, MI, USA) that was attached to the operating microscope (Nikon, Melville, NY, USA), and aortic diameters were measured using Image Pro Express Software (Media Cybernetics Inc., Silver Spring, MD, USA). To close the abdomen, a 3–0 vicryl suture (Ethicon Inc., Somerville, NJ, USA) was used and the rats were allowed to recover.

## Dendrimer Perfusion

The design and synthesis of the G5 acetylated Alexa Fluor 488-conjugated dendrimers (molecular weight of 27,000 g/mol) are described according to Majoros *et al.*[3] To improve water solubility, and decrease aggregation and nonspecific delivery of these dendrimers, the terminal primary amino functionality was acetylated.[15,16] Nonacetylated primary amino groups were used for conjugation of Alexa Fluor 488, an imaging agent.[3,17]

### Experiment 1

Rats were anesthetized as described above for elastase perfusion, and underwent infrarenal aortic perfusion with G5 acetylated Alexa Fluor 488-conjugated dendrimers (200 nM in 1X PBS) at a rate of 2 mL/h for varying lengths of time (10, 30, 60 min; $n = 4$ per perfusion time). Upon dendrimer perfusion, blood was allowed to flush out excess dendrimer solution. Aortas were harvested 0, 12, or 24 h postperfusion ($n = 4$ per time point).

### Experiment 2

Rats were anesthetized and underwent infrarenal aortic elastase perfusion. Seven days following elastase perfusion, rats underwent aortic dendrimer perfusion as described above. Seven and 8 days postelastase perfusion, rats were anesthetized, infrarenal aortas were exposed, and aortic diameters were measured prior to aortic explantation.

For all experiments, upon harvesting, aortic tissue was rinsed with 1X PBS, pH 7.2–7.4, fixed in formalin (10%) for 1 h at room temperature, and mounted in ProLong Gold Antifade Reagent (Molecular Probes, Eugene, OR, USA). Aortic cross-sections were viewed and imaged using confocal microscopy. Dendrimers were quantified within the aortic wall by manually counting them in captured images, and are presented as dendrimers per high-powered field. Native aortas (i.e., not perfused with dendrimers) were harvested and viewed as negative controls.

## RESULTS

### Dendrimer Diffusion in Native Aortas

In native aortas, dendrimers penetrated the aortic wall at all time points. For all perfusion times, fewer dendrimers were present as time between dendrimer perfusion and aortic harvest increased (TABLE 1, FIG. 3). Longer perfusion times resulted in increased diffusion of dendrimers throughout the aortic wall. By 24 h, the majority of the dendrimers were through the wall.

TABLE 1. Dendrimer quantification and location in normal aortic tissue

| Perfusion time (min) | Time before harvest (h) | Average ± SEM number of dendrimers* | Location of dendrimers |
|---|---|---|---|
| 10 | 0 | 99 ± 21 | Media |
| 10 | 24 | 61 ± 4 | Mostly media, some adventitia |
| 30 | 0 | 71 ± 7 | Inner media |
| 30 | 12 | 60 ± 4 | Adventitia |
| 30 | 24 | 35 ± 1 | Adventitia |
| 60 | 0 | 46 ± 2 | Outer media, adventitia |
| 60 | 12 | 34 ± 1 | Adventitia |

*Mean counts from four samples per group.

When native aortas were perfused for 10 min, dendrimers were concentrated in the media (toward lumen) on day 0, and in the media and adventitia 24 h postperfusion. More dendrimers were present on day 0 than 24 h postperfusion. Upon perfusing normal aortas for 30 min with dendrimer, the majority of the dendrimers were in the media on day 0, and in the adventitia 12 h and 24 h postperfusion. There were fewer dendrimers present 12 h postperfusion compared with day 0, and even fewer on 24 h postperfusion. After a 60-min perfusion of normal aortas, the dendrimers were primarily in the media (toward adventitia) and in the adventitia at day 0, and only in the adventitia 12 h postperfusion. Representative images of dendrimer-perfused normal aortas on day 0 are shown in FIGURE 4. Native aortas that were not perfused with dendrimers were harvested and demonstrated no fluorescence.

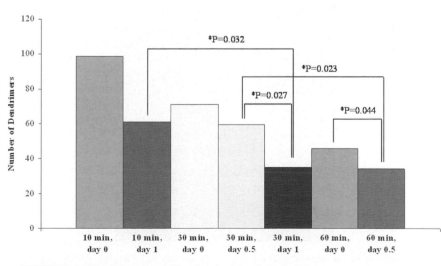

FIGURE 3. Dendrimer quantification in normal aortic tissue.

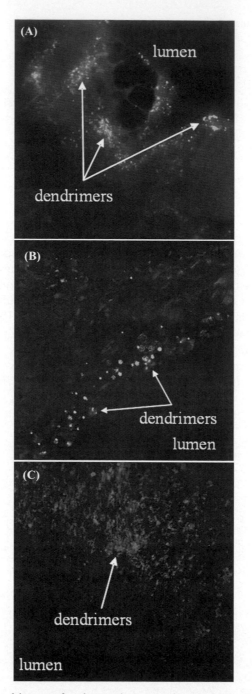

**FIGURE 4.** Dendrimer-perfused normal aorta on day 0, 10 min perfusion (**A**) day 0, 30 min perfusion (**B**) day 0, 60 min perfusion (**C**) 40×.

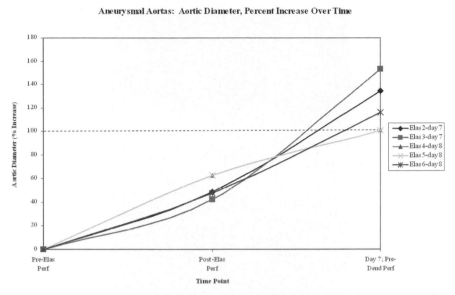

**FIGURE 5.** Percent increase in aortic diameter in elastase-perfused aortas postperfusion and 7 days following perfusion. Each curve represents one animal. All animals formed AAAs (defined as 100% increase in diameter) on postoperative day 7.

## *Experimental AAA Formation*

The mean percentage increase ($\pm$SEM) in aortic diameter in the aneurysmal aortas 7 days following elastase perfusion was $121 \pm 10\%$ (FIG. 5). Each animal formed an aneurysm (defined as 100% increase in aortic diameter) by day 7 postelastase perfusion.

## *Dendrimer Diffusion in Aneurysmal Aortas*

In aneurysmal aortas, dendrimers diffused farther into the aortic wall than in control aortas (30 min perfusion time, day 0 harvest). Fewer dendrimers were present in aortas that were harvested 24 h postdendrimer perfusion than when harvested immediately (FIG. 6). By 24 h, the majority of the dendrimers were through the wall.

Upon perfusing aneurysmal aortas (day 7 postelastase perfusion) for 30 min with dendrimer, the majority of the dendrimers were in the adventitia on both days 7 and 8 (postelastase perfusion). At both time points, dendrimers in aneurysmal tissue diffused farther out than in native tissue (TABLE 2). Representative images of dendrimer-perfused aneurysmal aortas on day 0 are shown in FIGURE 7.

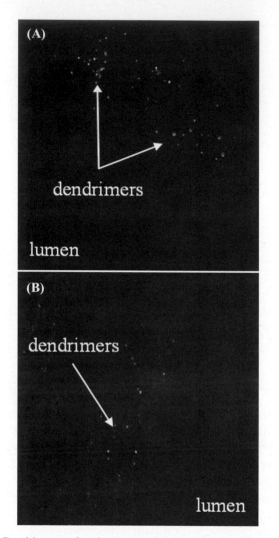

**FIGURE 6.** Dendrimer-perfused aneurysmal aorta on day 7 postelastase perfusion and harvested on day 7, 30 min perfusion (**A**) and day 8, 30 min perfusion (**B**), 40×.

## DISCUSSION

The objective of this study was to determine if dendrimers could be delivered intra-arterially to normal and aneurysmal rat aortas *in vivo*, and to examine the distribution of the labeled dendrimers within the aortic wall. This preliminary study indicates that labeled dendrimers diffuse into the aortic wall from the lumen. These dendrimers are not specific to the aorta, but at early times since they are delivered intra-arterially remain in the aortic wall and do not diffuse

**TABLE 2. Dendrimer quantification and location in aneurysmal aortic tissue**

| Perfusion time (min) | Time before harvest (h) | Average ± SEM number of dendrimers* | Location of dendrimers |
|---|---|---|---|
| 30 | 0 | 50 ± 13 | Adventitia |
| 30 | 24 | 34 ± 9 | Adventitia |

*Mean counts from four samples per group.

out into other tissues. Both normal and aneurysmal aortic tissues are permeable enough to allow for the passage of nanoparticles through the wall. Additionally, varying dendrimer perfusion times, and lengths of time between dendrimer perfusion and explantation affected the concentration gradient-dependent diffusion patterns.

Several factors likely influenced the distribution of the dendrimers, including the pressure within the isolated portion of the aorta during dendrimer perfusion, the resistance of the aortic tissue, and any convective forces present in the aorta. The physical and chemical properties of the dendrimers contribute to their diffusion patterns in the aortic wall. These dendrimers diffuse into the aortic wall because of their small size, and are attractive for local delivery of agents since they are biocompatible and have a highly branched structure, allowing for the attachment of multiple agents.[5] For the present study, dendrimers were acetylated to neutralize some of the primary amine groups. Their shapes and sizes are well defined and uniform, and their surfaces are readily chemically functionalized and modifiable.[5,7] The pressure within the isolated portion of

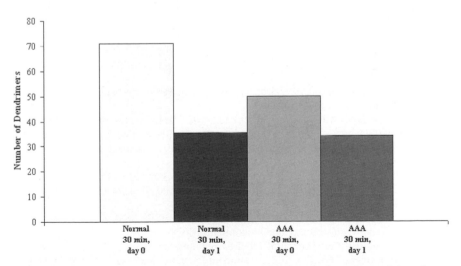

**FIGURE 7.** Dendrimer quantification in aneurysmal aortic tissue (normal data shown for comparison).

the aorta during dendrimer perfusion and any convective forces present in the aorta were similar in the native and aneurysmal aortas.[18] However, due to the remodeling of the aortic ECM during AAA formation, the change in the resistance of the aortic tissue most likely contributed to the different distribution patterns seen in the normal and aneurysmal tissue samples.

These preliminary results warrant further investigation of the use of dendrimers for targeted drug delivery, especially in the area of AAA, where there are no proven effective medical therapies. Because of their biocompatibility and ability to attach these particles to a wide variety of agents, their potential as drug-carrying vehicles is excellent. The size of these dendrimers also makes them good candidates for delivering these agents. In previous studies, liposomes with a mean diameter of approximately 500 nm represented the maximum size that could be used for drug delivery.[19]

Future experiments may include binding agents to dendrimers, and delivering them intra-arterially to experimental AAAs during development and following formation of small AAAs. Candidate agents include: (1) doxycycline, which has been shown to inhibit formation of experimental AAAs[9–12] and slow the growth of small AAAs in humans[13] and (2) 17-beta estradiol, which has been shown to inhibit the development of experimental AAAs.[20]

## ACKNOWLEDGMENTS

This study was supported by NIH KO8 (HL67885–02) (GRU), VonLeibig Award-Lifeline Foundation (GRU), NIH Cellular Biotechnology Training Program (BSC), Surgery Research Advisory Committee Grant (BSC), and the Jobst Foundation.

## REFERENCES

1. BRIEGER, D. & E. TOPOL. 1997. Local delivery systems and prevention of restenosis. Cardiovasc. Res. **35:** 405–413.
2. SAKHAROV, D.V., A.F. JIE, M.E. BEKKERS, et al. 2001. Polylysine as a vehicle for extracellular matrix-targeted local drug delivery, providing high accumulation and long-term retention within the vascular wall. Arterioscler. Thromb. Vasc. Biol. **21:** 943–948.
3. MAJOROS, I.J., T.P. THOMAS, C.B. MEHTA & J.R. BAKER. 2005. Poly(amidoamine) dendrimer-based multifunctional engineered nanodevice for cancer therapy. J. Med. Chem. **48:** 5892–5899.
4. MALIK, N., R. WIWATTANAPATAPEE, R. KLOPSCH, et al. 2000. Dendrimers: relationship between structure and biocompatibility in vitro, and preliminary studies on the biodistribution of 125I-labelled polyamidoamine dendrimers in vivo. J. Control Release. **65:** 133–148. Erratum in: J. Control Release 2000. **68:** 299–302.
5. PATRI, A.K., I.J. MAJOROS & J.R. BAKER. 2002. Dendritic polymer macromolecular carriers for drug delivery. Curr. Opin. Chem. Biol. **6:** 466–471.

6. LESNIAK, W., A.U. BIELINSKA, K. SUN, *et al.* 2005. Silver/dendrimer nanocomposites as biomarkers: fabrication, characterization, *in vitro* toxicity, and intracellular detection. Nano. Lett. **5:** 2123–2130.
7. BOSMAN, A.W., H.M. JANSSEN & E.W. MEIJER. 1999. About dendrimers: structure, physical properties, and applications. Chem. Rev. **99:** 1665–1688.
8. AILAWADI, G., J.L. ELIASON & G.R. UPCHURCH JR. 2003. Current concepts in the pathogenesis of abdominal aortic aneurysm. J. Vasc. Surg. **38:** 584–588.
9. PETRINEC, D., S. LIAO, D.R. HOLMES, *et al.* 1996. Doxycycline inhibition of aneurysmal degeneration in an elastase-induced rat model of abdominal aortic aneurysm: preservation of aortic elastin associated with suppressed production of 92-kD gelatinase. J. Vasc. Surg. **23:** 336–346.
10. SHO, E., J. CHU, M. SHO, *et al.* 2004. Continuous periaortic infusion improves doxycycline efficacy in experimental aortic aneurysms. J. Vasc. Surg. **39:** 1312–1321.
11. THOMPSON, R.W., S. LIAO & J.A. CURCI. 1998. Therapeutic potential of tetracycline derivatives to suppress the growth of abdominal aortic aneurysms. Adv. Dent. Res. **12:** 159–165.
12. CURCI, J.A., D. PETRINEC, S. LIAO, *et al.* 1998. Pharmacologic suppression of experimental abdominal aortic aneurysms: a comparison of doxycycline and four chemically modified tetracyclines. J. Vasc. Surg. **28:** 1082–1093.
13. BAXTER, B.T., W.H. PEARCE, E.A. WALTKE, *et al.* 2002. Prolonged administration of doxycycline in patients with small asymptomatic abdominal aortic aneurysms: report of a prospective (phase II) multicenter study. J. Vasc. Surg. **36:** 1–12.
14. ANIDJAR, S., J.L. SALZMANN, D. GENTRIC, *et al.* 1990. Elastase-induced experimental aneurysms in rats. Circulation **82:** 973–981.
15. PATRI, A.K., J.F. KUKOWSKA-LATALLO & J.R. BAKER. 2005. Targeted drug delivery with dendrimers: comparison of the release kinetics of covalently conjugated drug and non-covalent drug inclusion complex. Adv. Drug Deliv. Rev. **57:** 2203–2214.
16. QUINTANA, A., E. RACZKA, L. PIEHLER, *et al.* 2002. Design and function of a dendrimer-based therapeutic nanodevice targeted to tumor cells through the folate receptor. Pharm. Res. **19:** 1310–1316.
17. PANCHUK-VOLOSHINA, N., R.P. HAUGLAND, J. BISHOP-STEWART, *et al.* 1999. Alexa dyes, a series of new fluorescent dyes that yield exceptionally bright, photostable conjugates. J. Histochem. Cytochem. **47:** 1179–1188.
18. LOVICH, M.A. & E.R. EDELMAN. 1995. Mechanisms of transmural heparin transport in the rat abdominal aorta after local vascular delivery. Circ. Res. **77:** 1143–1150.
19. PRICE, R.J., D.M. SKYBA, S. KAUL & T.C. SKALAK. 1998. Delivery of colloidal particles and red blood cells to tissue through microvessel ruptures created by targeted microbubble destruction with ultrasound. Circulation **98:** 1264–1267.
20. AILAWADI, G., J.L. ELIASON, K.J. ROELOFS, *et al.* 2004. Gender differences in experimental aortic aneurysm formation. Arterioscler. Thromb. Vasc. Biol. **24:** 2116–2122.

# Hypoxia at the Site of Abdominal Aortic Aneurysm Rupture Is Not Associated with Increased Lactate

EDWARD CHOKE, GILLIAN W. COCKERILL, JOSEPH DAWSON, YUEN-LI CHUNG, JOHN GRIFFITHS, RICHARD W. WILSON, IAN M. LOFTUS, AND MATTHEW M. THOMPSON

*Department of Cardiovascular Sciences, Academic Vascular Surgery Unit, St. George's, University of London, UK*

ABSTRACT: The mechanisms of hypoxia-mediated aneurysm wall weakening and rupture are unknown. During hypoxia, strategies to maintain cellular ATP levels include increasing glycolysis (glycolytic strategy) or decreasing ATP consumption (metabolic depression). This study demonstrated that compared to anterior aneurysm sac, rupture edge overexpressed hypoxia-inducible factor-1-$\alpha$ (marker of hypoxia) and showed no significant difference in levels of combined ADP and ATP or lactate (glycolytic end product). Further studies are needed to confirm whether hypoxic AAA cells adapt through metabolic depression rather than glycolysis. The downregulation of protein synthesis during such metabolic depression may be a factor in hypoxia-mediated wall weakening.

KEYWORDS: hypoxia; glycolysis; lactate; protein synthesis; abdominal aortic aneurysm; rupture

## INTRODUCTION

Localized hypoxia is a potential cause of focal aneurysm wall weakening.[1] However, the mechanisms of hypoxia-mediated wall degeneration are not well understood. During hypoxia, several strategies exist for cells to maintain their ATP levels. The first strategy is to increase the rate of glycolysis (glycolytic strategy) and the second is to depress the rate of ATP consumption (metabolic depression strategy). There are trade-offs with both strategies leading to undesirable consequences on the structural integrity of the hypoxic segment of aneurysm wall. The drawback with glycolytic strategy is the accumulation of anaerobic end products (lactate). On the other hand, protein synthesis, which

Address for correspondence: Prof. M.M. Thompson, Department of Vascular Surgery, 4th Floor St. James Wing, St George's Hospital, Blackshaw Rd., London SW17 0QT. Voice: 44-208-725-3205; fax: 44-208-725-3495.

e-mail: Matt.Thompson@stgeorges.nhs.uk

Ann. N.Y. Acad. Sci. 1085: 306–310 (2006). © 2006 New York Academy of Sciences.
doi: 10.1196/annals.1383.005

accounts for a significant portion of energy consumption, is likely to be down-regulated to conserve ATP levels during metabolic depression and may be a mechanism by which hypoxia leads to a physically compromised aortic wall and eventual rupture. An understanding of the metabolic response adopted by hypoxic aneurysmal segments may open new avenues for therapy against aneurysm rupture. This study assessed the transcript and protein levels of a marker of hypoxia (hypoxia-inducible factor (HIF)-1-$\alpha$) at the aneurysm rupture edge in relation to their paired anterior aneurysm wall and evaluated the metabolite profiles at these two sites.

## METHODS

Paired samples of aneurysm rupture edge and anterior aneurysm wall (2 cm distal to left renal vein) obtained during emergency open repair for ruptured AAAs ($n = 12$) were analyzed. Immunohistochemistry (IHC) was performed with a labeled streptavidin-biotin method using antibodies to HIF-1-$\alpha$ (Clone ESEE122 diluted 1:500, Novus Biologicals, CO, USA) and CD31 (Clone JC70A diluted 1:50, DAKO, UK). The percentage area of HIF-1-$\alpha$ immunostaining was quantified following IHC. Molecular analyses involved the extraction of total RNA (RNeasy® Fibrous Tissue RNA extraction kit, Qiagen, UK), reverse transcription into cDNA (high-capacity cDNA archive kit, Applied Biosystems, UK) and quantification of HIF-1-$\alpha$ gene expression by QRT-PCR (TaqMan® Gene Expression Assays, Applied Biosystems, UK). Metabolomic studies involved the extraction of water soluble metabolites using 6% perchloric acid (PCA) followed by the generation of $^1$H nuclear magnetic resonance (NMR) spectra using a Bruker 600MHz spectrometer. All data were reported as mean $\pm$ SEM. The distributions of mRNA levels of HIF-1-$\alpha$ were skewed and logarithmic transformation was used for normalization. Differences in HIF-1-$\alpha$ expression and levels of metabolites between rupture site and anterior sac were determined using paired two-tailed Student's $t$ test. A value of $P < 0.05$ was considered significant.

## RESULTS

### HIF-1-$\alpha$

Compared to anterior sac, aneurysm rupture edge demonstrated increased protein expression of HIF-1-$\alpha$ (percentage area fraction of HIF-1-$\alpha$ staining): rAAA anterior sac, 3.36 $\pm$ 0.81% versus rAAA rupture edge, 5.92 $\pm$ 1.15% ($P = 0.021$) and upregulated gene expression of HIF-1-$\alpha$ (arbitrary units normalized to 18s rRNA): rAAA anterior sac, 2.85 $\pm$ 0.13 versus rAAA rupture edge, $3.18 \pm 0.15$ ($P = 0.013$, 95% CI 0.084 to 0.576). The upregulation of HIF-1-$\alpha$ protein and mRNA expression supported the presence of hypoxia at the rupture edge relative to anterior sac.

## Metabolomic Analysis

A total of 20 metabolites were quantified using high-resolution NMR spectroscopy. The quantitative data for these metabolites are detailed in TABLE 1. Eighteen of 20 metabolites profiled were not significantly different between the rupture edge and anterior sac. Interestingly, rupture edge demonstrated similar levels of combined ADP and ATP (energy levels) compared to anterior sac ($P = 0.67$). Although faced with an environment of relative hypoxia, rupture edge specimens demonstrated no metabolic evidence for increased anaerobic metabolism to maintain ADP/ATP at a similar level to anterior aneurysm sac. Specifically, no difference in lactate levels (glycolytic end product) was found ($P = 0.14$) between rupture edge and anterior sac biopsies. Glutamine ($P = 0.0007$) and succinate ($P = 0.04$) were the only metabolites significantly increased at the rupture edge.

**TABLE 1. Metabolite profiles of anterior aneurysm sac and aneurysm rupture edge**

|  | Anterior sac | Rupture edge | $P$ value |
|---|---|---|---|
| Combined ADP and ATP | 0.007772 ($\pm$0.0027) | 0.007194 ($\pm$0.0016) | 0.667 |
| Lactate | 0.368224 ($\pm$0.0464) | 0.435732 ($\pm$0.0392) | 0.143 |
| Leucine | 0.01521 ($\pm$0.0024) | 0.017004 ($\pm$0.0023) | 0.371 |
| Iso-leucine | 0.005747 ($\pm$0.0009) | 0.006548 ($\pm$0.0009) | 0.418 |
| Valine | 0.013412 ($\pm$0.0018) | 0.0149 ($\pm$0.0013) | 0.397 |
| $\beta$-hydroxybutyrate | 0.012493 ($\pm$0.0021) | 0.02098 ($\pm$0.0069) | 0.231 |
| Alanine | 0.036311 ($\pm$0.0030) | 0.038689 ($\pm$0.0054) | 0.625 |
| Acetate | 0.282182 ($\pm$0.1391) | 0.429914 ($\pm$0.2118) | 0.637 |
| Glutamate | 0.066556 ($\pm$0.0126) | 0.071631 ($\pm$0.0103) | 0.575 |
| Succinate | 0.013581 ($\pm$0.0019) | 0.021088 ($\pm$0.0033) | 0.041* |
| Glutamine | 0.024643 ($\pm$0.0048) | 0.051559 ($\pm$0.0066) | 0.0007* |
| Aspartate | 0.016288 ($\pm$0.0060) | 0.02265 ($\pm$0.0113) | 0.401 |
| Choline | 0.008227($\pm$0.0013) | 0.009276 ($\pm$0.0014) | 0.507 |
| Phosphocholine | 0.047677 ($\pm$0.0112) | 0.03594 ($\pm$0.0052) | 0.256 |
| Myoinositol | 0.093168 ($\pm$0.0174) | 0.084955 ($\pm$0.0131) | 0.548 |
| Glycine | 0.047472 ($\pm$0.0073) | 0.042202 ($\pm$0.0058) | 0.717 |
| Creatine | 0.026471 ($\pm$0.0042) | 0.030561 ($\pm$0.0047) | 0.566 |
| Glucose | 0.062202 ($\pm$0.0114) | 0.072166 ($\pm$0.0125) | 0.430 |
| Tyrosine | 0.004804 ($\pm$0.0008) | 0.007181 ($\pm$0.0012) | 0.076 |
| Phenylalanine | 0.008074 ($\pm$0.0011) | 0.00963 ($\pm$0.0011) | 0.186 |
| Formate | 0.061083 ($\pm$0.0236) | 0.069742 ($\pm$0.0259) | 0.814 |

Data presented are given in $\mu$mol/g wet weight (mean $\pm$ SE). $P$-values for differences were derived from paired Student's $t$-test.
*Significant.

## DISCUSSION

The HIF transcriptional system is a key component of cellular response to hypoxia.[2] HIF-1-α is degraded under normoxic conditions, but stable under hypoxic conditions, and appears within minutes of cells becoming hypoxic. Immunohistochemical staining of tissues for HIF-1-α therefore provides a guide to the activity of the system. The localized overexpression of HIF-1-α indicated that hypoxic conditions were present at the aneurysm rupture edge.

Despite evidence for relative hypoxia at the rupture edge compared with anterior sac, there was no difference in combined ADP and ATP levels at both sites. Therefore, mechanisms must exist to compensate for the downregulation of aerobic ATP production at the hypoxic rupture edge. In the absence of any evidence of increased anaerobic component (unaltered lactate levels) at the rupture edge, there are many processes that could be downregulated to conserve energy during metabolic depression, and probably are. In cancer research, the data on downregulation of protein synthesis, which account for a significant portion (20–30%) of the energy consumption, are the most consistent.[3] If hypoxic aneurysm cells exhibit similar adaptations, the impact of such protein synthesis downregulation on tissue repair, maintenance of aneurysm wall strength, and propensity to rupture are likely to be significant. A recent study demonstrated the importance of c-Jun N-terminal-kinase (JNK) pathway and abnormal protein synthesis in the pathogenesis of AAA.[4] However, the subject of protein synthesis in aneurysm research is still a neglected area compared to extracellular matrix degradation.

The overexpression of HIF-1-α supported the presence of hypoxic conditions at the aneurysm rupture edge. The maintenance of ATP levels in the absence of increased lactate production suggested that glycolysis was not a strategy used by hypoxic aneurysm segments. Further studies are needed to confirm whether hypoxic AAA cells adapt through an alternative strategy, namely metabolic depression, and if such metabolic depression plays a role in hypoxia-mediated wall weakening and eventual rupture.

## ACKNOWLEDGMENTS

This work was supported by a research fellowship from the Royal College of Surgeons of England. We are grateful to Mr. Robert McFarland, Mr. Thomas Loosemore, and Mr. Josh Derodra for assistance with collecting the tissue specimens, and to Dr. Jan Poloniecki for expert help with statistical analysis.

## REFERENCES

1. VORP, D.A. *et al*. 2005. Biomechanical determinants of abdominal aortic aneurysm rupture. Arterioscler. Thromb. Vasc. Biol. **25:** 1558–1566.
2. PUGH, C.W. *et al*. 2003. Regulation of angiogenesis by hypoxia: role of the HIF system. Nat. Med. **9:** 677–684.
3. GUPPY, M. *et al*. 2005. Metabolic depression: a response of cancer cells to hypoxia? Comp Biochem. Physiol. B. Biochem. Mol. Biol. **140:** 233–239.
4. YOSHIMURA, K. *et al*. 2005. Regression of abdominal aortic aneurysm by inhibition of c-Jun N-terminal kinase. Nat. Med. **11:** 1330–1338.

# Gene Expression Profile of Abdominal Aortic Aneurysm Rupture

EDWARD CHOKE, MATTHEW M. THOMPSON, ALUN JONES,
EVELYN TORSNEY, JOSEPH DAWSON, KENNETH LAING,
HOSAAM NASR, IAN M. LOFTUS, AND GILLIAN W. COCKERILL

*Department of Cardiovascular Sciences, Academic Vascular Surgery Unit,
St. George's, University of London, UK*

ABSTRACT: To search for novel transcriptional pathways that are activated in abdominal aortic aneurysm rupture, cDNA microarrays were
used to compare global mRNA expression at the aneurysm rupture edge
to anterior sac, and selected results were confirmed using quantitative
real-time-polymerase chain reaction (QRT-PCR). This study identified
apoptosis, angiogenesis, and inflammation as potentially important participants during the process of aneurysm rupture.

KEYWORDS: abdominal aortic aneurysm; rupture; genes; microarray

## INTRODUCTION

It is increasingly recognized that abdominal aortic aneurysm (AAA) rupture
is a multifaceted biological process involving biochemical, cellular, and proteolytic influences in addition to biomechanical factors.[1] An understanding of
such biological processes is crucial if pharmacological inhibition of aneurysm
rupture is to be made possible. Transcriptional profiling using high-density microarrays provides unique data about regulatory pathways and gene function in
diseases by comparing the level of mRNA transcribed in cells in a given pathologic state versus a control. This study used this technology to provide insight
into the pathophysiologic processes involved in AAA rupture by comparing
the gene expression of aneurysm rupture edge to anterior aneurysm sac. These
findings could in turn provide a reference framework for the development of
protective strategies specifically targeted at preventing rupture.

## METHODS

Paired samples of aneurysm rupture edge and anterior aneurysm wall
(2 cm distal to left renal vein) obtained during emergency open repair for

Address for correspondence: Dr. Gillian W. Cockerill, St. George's University of London, Cranmer
Terrace, London SW17 0RE, UK. Voice: 00-44-208-725-5582; fax: 00-44-208-725-5582.
e-mail: gcockeri@sgul.ac.uk

Ann. N.Y. Acad. Sci. 1085: 311–314 (2006). © 2006 New York Academy of Sciences.
doi: 10.1196/annals.1383.006

ruptured AAAs were analyzed. Pooled samples from 12 patients were subjected to cDNA microarray processing in triplicates. Affymetrix chip processing was performed at the John Innes Centre Genome Laboratory (Norwich, UK) using the Affymetrix Human Genome U133A Plus 2.0 microarray (Affymetrix, Santa Clara, CA, USA). The U133A Plus 2.0 microarray is an oligonucleotide microarray that allows detection of up to 60,000 transcripts. Data were normalized using GeneSpring software (Agilent Technologies, West Lothian, UK) and a threshold level of significance was set at $P < 0.015$.

Immunohistochemistry (IHC) was performed with a labeled streptavidin-biotin method using antibodies to GADD45-$\gamma$ (Clone C-16, diluted 1:500) and IEX-1 (Clone C-20, diluted 1:50) (Santa Cruz Biotechnology, CA, USA). Validation of selected differentially expressed genes was performed using quantitative real-time-polymerase chain reaction (QRT-PCR). This involved the extraction of total RNA (RNeasy® Fibrous Tissue RNA Extraction Kit, Qiagen, UK), reverse transcription into cDNA (high-capacity cDNA Archive Kit, Applied Biosystems, UK), and quantification of gene expression using TaqMan® Gene Expression Assays (Applied Biosystems).

## RESULTS

Following normalization of the 54,675 transcripts on each array, 624 (1.14%) were differentially expressed with a $P$ value of $< 0.015$. Of these, genes regarded as candidate effectors for aneurysm rupture were analyzed in more detail (TABLE 1). These genes are involved in the following cellular pathways: (1) apoptosis, (2) angiogenesis, and (3) inflammation. Immediate early response-3 (IER-3), GADD45G, and vascular endothelial growth factor (VEGF) differential expression were selected for validation with QRT-PCR. In all three cases, the direction of the fold change by microarray and QRT-PCR was the same (TABLE 2). Immunostaining for IER-3 showed more numerous nuclei staining per high power field (HPF) within aneurysm rupture edge specimens. GADD45-$\gamma$ also showed more cell nuclei staining at aneurysm rupture edge and was expressed by endothelial cells and smooth muscle cells (SMC).

## DISCUSSION

To search for novel transcriptional pathways that are activated in aneurysm rupture, cDNA microarrays were used to compare global mRNA expression at the aneurysm rupture edge to anterior aneurysm wall. This study identified the following cellular pathways—apoptosis, angiogenesis, and inflammation—as potentially important participants during the process of aneurysm rupture.

A number of studies previously suggested that depletion of medial SMC through apoptosis plays an important role in aneurysm formation by

TABLE 1. cDNA microarray analysis of differentially expressed genes in aneurysm rupture edge

| Gene accession no. | Gene name | Fold change Rupture edge/Anterior sac | Transcript function |
|---|---|---|---|
| A1935096 | Nuclear receptor 4A2 | 6.4 | Apoptosis |
| NM-003897 | IER-3 | 2.6 | Apoptosis |
| NM-006705 | GADD45G | 2.5 | Apoptosis |
| NM-003811 | TNF SF9 | 3.5 | Apoptosis |
| BC 031280 | RAD21 | 1.4 | Apoptosis |
| AF098518 | Four and a half Lim 1 | 2.8 | Angiogenesis |
| M27281 | VEGF | 2.9 | Angiogenesis |
| AF182069 | PROK 2 | 7.1 | Angiogenesis |
| NM-001430 | IL-8 | 5.8 | Angiogenesis |
| NM-000450 | E-selectin | 27.7 | Inflammation |
| BC010943 | Oncostatin M Receptor | 2.4 | Inflammation |
| BF304996 | Regulated G-protein S16 | 6.1 | Inflammation |

($P < 0.015$).

eradicating a cell population capable of accomplishing connective tissue repair.[2–5] While the importance of SMC apoptosis in aneurysm development has previously been demonstrated, this is the first report to associate apoptosis with aneurysm rupture and provide a number of potential target genes for future studies investigating how apoptosis might trigger aneurysm rupture. This study also supports previous work from our laboratory that demonstrated an association between aneurysm rupture with increased angiogenesis and overexpression of key proangiogenic cytokines, including VEGF. These data provide additional and potentially important starting points for further investigations on the cellular and molecular mechanisms underlying aneurysm rupture.

## ACKNOWLEDGMENTS

This work was supported by a research fellowship from the Royal College of Surgeons of England. We are grateful to Mr. Robert McFarland, Mr. Thomas Looscmore, and Mr. Josh Derodra for assistance with collecting the tissue specimens, and to Dr. Jan Poloniecki for expert help with statistical analysis.

TABLE 2. Quantification of mRNA expression by QRT-PCR

| Gene name | Anterior sac | Rupture edge | $P$ value |
|---|---|---|---|
| IER-3 | $1.050 \pm 0.157$ | $1.700 \pm 0.107$ | 0.030 |
| GADD45G | $1.124 \pm 0.071$ | $1.723 \pm 0.118$ | 0.003 |
| VEGF | $1.69 \pm 0.25$ | $2.22 \pm 0.21$ | 0.004 |

# REFERENCES

1. CHOKE, E. *et al.* 2005. A review of biological factors implicated in abdominal aortic aneurysm rupture. Eur. J. Vasc. Endovasc. Surg. **30:** 227–244.
2. HOLMES, D.R. *et al.* 1996. Smooth muscle cell apoptosis and p53 expression in human abdominal aortic aneurysms. Ann. N. Y. Acad. Sci. **800:** 286–287.
3. LIAO, S. *et al.* 2000. Accelerated replicative senescence of medial smooth muscle cells derived from abdominal aortic aneurysms compared to the adjacent inferior mesenteric artery. J. Surg. Res. **92:** 85–95.
4. LOPEZ-CANDALES, A. *et al.* 1997. Decreased vascular smooth muscle cell density in medial degeneration of human abdominal aortic aneurysms. Am. J. Pathol. **150:** 993–1007.
5. THOMPSON, R.W. *et al.* 1997. Vascular smooth muscle cell apoptosis in abdominal aortic aneurysms. Coron. Artery Dis. **8:** 623–631.

# Increased Angiogenesis at the Site of Abdominal Aortic Aneurysm Rupture

EDWARD CHOKE, GILLIAN W. COCKERILL, JOSEPH DAWSON, RICHARD W. WILSON, ALUN JONES, IAN M. LOFTUS, AND MATTHEW M. THOMPSON

*Department of Cardiovascular Sciences, Academic Vascular Surgery Unit, St. George's, University of London, UK*

ABSTRACT: Abdominal aortic aneurysm (AAA) rupture is associated with elevated levels of matrix metalloproteinase (MMP). Medial neovascularization is a known characteristic of established AAAs and involves proteolytic degradation of extracellular matrix by MMPs to facilitate endothelial cell proliferation and migration. This study evaluated the extent of neovascularization in abdominal aortic aneurysm rupture. Results indicated upregulation of proangiogenic cytokines and increased medial neovascularization at the aneurysm rupture edge compared with paired aneurysm anterior sac. Further investigations into the role of angiogenesis in aneurysm rupture may open novel therapeutic avenues to prevent aneurysm rupture.

KEYWORDS: aneurysm; rupture; angiogenesis; metalloproteinases; neovascularization

## INTRODUCTION

Matrix metalloproteinases (MMPs) have been implicated in aneurysm wall weakening and rupture.[1–3] The MMP family is closely involved in the process of neovascularization[4] and plays key proangiogenic roles.[5–7] Neoangiogenesis of the medial layer is a known feature of established abdominal aortic aneurysm (AAA),[8] however, the role of this pathological angiogenic response in aneurysm rupture is not known.[9,10] Immunolocalization studies have indicated that MMPs produced in aneurysms were associated with proliferative microvessels,[8] therefore the expression of MMPs during such angiogenic response may lead to proteolytic disruption and degradation of aortic media. In view of these considerations, this study assessed the hypothesis that increased medial neovascularization is associated with aneurysm rupture.

Address for correspondence: Prof. M.M. Thompson, Department of Vascular Surgery, 4th Floor St. James Wing, St. George's Hospital, Blackshaw Rd., London SW17 0QT. Voice: 44-208-725-3205; fax: 44-208-725-3495.

e-mail: Matt.Thompson@stgeorges.nhs.uk

Ann. N.Y. Acad. Sci. 1085: 315–319 (2006). © 2006 New York Academy of Sciences.
doi: 10.1196/annals.1383.007

# METHODS

## Sample Collection

During emergency open repair for ruptured AAAs ($n = 12$), strips of aortic wall from the aneurysm rupture site, and anterior aneurysm wall (2 cm distal to left renal vein) were carefully excised. From these biopsies, tissues from (1) rupture edge, (2) level of rupture at least 3 cm away from the rupture edge, and (3) anterior sac were analyzed. Anterior aneurysm sac biopsies (also 2 cm distal to the left renal vein) were similarly obtained during elective open repair of nonruptured AAAs (nrAAAs) ($n = 10$). These nrAAA control tissues were used for IHC only.

## Immunohistochemistry (IHC)

IHC was performed with a labeled streptavidin-biotin method using antibodies to CD31, CD68, α-actin smooth muscle (α-SMA) (DAKO, UK), and $α_v$-integrin (R&D Systems, UK).

## Morphometric Analysis

Following IHC, quantification was performed for medial neovascularization (CD31+microvessels per HPF as adapted[11] from previous published studies),[12] microvessel diameter, inflammatory infiltrate (% area inflammatory cells), and vessel maturity index (% microvessels with outer smooth muscle coat).

## Quantitative Real-Time-Polymerase Chain Reaction (QRT-PCR)

Total RNA was extracted (RNeasy® Fibrous Tissue RNA extraction kit, Qiagen, UK) and reverse transcribed into cDNA (high-capacity cDNA Archive Kit, Applied Biosystems, UK). Gene expressions of candidate angiogenic mediators were determined by QRT-PCR using TaqMan® Gene Expression Assays (Assays-on-Demand™ Gene Expression Products, Applied Biosystems, Foster City, CA, USA).

# RESULTS

## Morphometric Analysis

TABLE 1 details the results for morphometric analysis. Compared with nrAAA and rAAA anterior sac, rAAA rupture edge showed increased mean

**TABLE 1. Morphometric analysis of medial neovascularization**

|  | nrAAA anterior sac | rAAA anterior sac | rAAA rupture edge | *P value |
|---|---|---|---|---|
| Medial neovascularization (microvessels per HPF) | 4.0 ± 0.4 | 3.7 ± 0.3 | 11.4 ± 1.5 | <0.001 |
| Diameter (μm) | 37.3 ± 3.3 | 41.8 ± 4.8 | 17.3 ± 2.2 | <0.001 |
| Inflammatory infiltrate (% area inflammatory cells) | 8.3 ± 2.8 | 4.9 ± 0.8 | 5.8 ± 1.1 | 0.35 |
| Maturity index (% mature microvessels) |  | 83.3 ± 2.3 | 47.6 ± 5.4 | <0.001 |

*Paired Student's *t*-test.

microvessel density in the medial layer ($P < 0.001$), smaller mean diameter of medial microvessels ($P < 0.001$), and lower maturity index ($P < 0.001$). There was a close spatial correlation between medial neovascularization and inflammatory infiltration. However, the extent of inflammatory infiltrate in areas of medial neovascularization was not significantly different in all representative samples ($P = 0.35$).

## Proangiogenic Cytokines

Normalized values for expression of angiogenic mediators in the rupture edge, aneurysm wall at the level of rupture, and anterior sac are summarized in TABLE 2. The genes for $\alpha_V$-integrin, vascular endothelial growth factor (VEGF), VE-Cadherin, monocyte chemoattractant protein-1 (MCP-1), and Vimentin were significantly upregulated at the rupture edge. Of the various proangiogenic mediators upregulated at the mRNA level, $\alpha_V$-integrin was selected for quantitative assessment of protein expression. The percentage area fraction of $\alpha_V$-integrin IHC staining was significantly higher at the rupture edge ($P = 0.034$).

## DISCUSSION

This study has demonstrated that there were focal areas of increased medial neovascularization localized to aneurysm rupture edge with a concomitant increase in gene expression of key angiogenic factors ($\alpha_V$-integrin, VEGF, Ve-Cadherin, MCP-1, and Vimentin) and protein expression of $\alpha_V$-integrin. The presence of small lumen and immature microvessels supports the notion of an ongoing active angiogenic environment at the rupture edge. It is not known if the increased angiogenesis was a causative factor in aneurysm rupture or simply a consequence of the disease process. Ongoing work includes investigations into whether VEGF-induced angiogenesis has any influence on aneurysm

**TABLE 2.** Summary of gene expressions (arbitrary units normalized to 18S rRNA) of candidate angiogenic mediators and protein expression (% area IHC staining) of $\alpha_v$-integrin

| | rAAA anterior sac | rAAA level of rupture | rAAA rupture edge | $P$ value |
|---|---|---|---|---|
| mRNA expression* | | | | |
| $\alpha_v$-integrin | $3.08 \pm 0.18$ | $2.77 \pm 0.05$ | $3.32 \pm 0.23$ | **0.0354** |
| VEGF | $1.69 \pm 0.25$ | $0.77 \pm 0.17$ | $2.22 \pm 0.21$ | **<0.0001** |
| VE-Cadherin | $2.49 \pm 0.15$ | $2.00 \pm 0.05$ | $2.58 \pm 0.18$ | **0.005** |
| MCP-1 | $2.60 \pm 0.25$ | $2.18 \pm 0.14$ | $2.96 \pm 0.18$ | **0.015** |
| Vimentin | $4.76 \pm 0.18$ | $4.40 \pm 0.09$ | $4.88 \pm 0.16$ | **0.039** |
| TGF-$\beta$-1 | $2.87 \pm 0.13$ | $3.06 \pm 0.10$ | $3.20 \pm 0.15$ | 0.106 |
| Basic FGF | $1.51 \pm 0.14$ | $1.85 \pm 0.14$ | $1.85 \pm 0.22$ | 0.110 |
| HGF | $1.13 \pm 0.12$ | $1.27 \pm 0.09$ | $1.09 \pm 0.15$ | 0.504 |
| VEGFR2 | $2.50 \pm 0.17$ | $2.05 \pm 0.12$ | $2.48 \pm 0.20$ | 0.059 |
| CD68 | $3.11 \pm 0.13$ | $2.95 \pm 0.11$ | $3.18 \pm 0.15$ | 0.429 |
| Protein expression** | | | | |
| $\alpha_v$-integrin | $2.39 \pm 0.53$ | – | $5.57 \pm 1.2$ | **0.012** |

Data are in mean ± SEM. Comparison used *repeated measures ANOVA.
**Paired Student's $t$-test. Significant values in bold.

rupture in angiotensin II-induced aneurysms in apoE-/-hyperlipidemic mice. Insights obtained from these experiments may open novel therapeutic avenues to prevent AAA rupture.

## ACKNOWLEDGMENTS

This work was supported by a research fellowship from the Royal College of Surgeons of England. We are grateful to Mr. Robert McFarland, Mr. Thomas Loosemore, and Mr. Josh Derodra for assistance with collecting the tissue specimens, and to Dr. Jan Poloniecki for expert help with statistical analysis.

## REFERENCES

1. ALLAIRE, E. *et al*. 1998. Local overexpression of TIMP-1 prevents aortic aneurysm degeneration and rupture in a rat model. J. Clin. Invest. **102:** 1413–1420.
2. ALLAIRE, E. *et al*. 1998. Prevention of aneurysm development and rupture by local overexpression of plasminogen activator inhibitor-1. Circulation **98:** 249–255.
3. WILSON, R.W. *et al*. 2006. Matrix metalloproteinase-8 and -9 are increased at the site of abdominal aortic aneurysm rupture. Circulation **113:** 438–445.
4. COCKERILL, G.W. *et al*. 1995. Angiogenesis: models and modulators. Int. Rev. Cytol. **159:** 113–160.
5. HERRON, G.S. *et al*. 1986. Secretion of metalloproteinases by stimulated capillary endothelial cells. I. Production of procollagenase and prostromelysin exceeds expression of proteolytic activity. J. Biol. Chem. **261:** 2810–2813.

6. KALLURI, R. *et al.* 2003. Basement membranes: structure, assembly and role in tumour angiogenesis. Nat. Rev. Cancer **3:** 422–433.
7. RUNDHAUG, J.E. *et al.* 2005. Matrix metalloproteinases and angiogenesis. J. Cell. Mol. Med. **9:** 267–285.
8. HERRON, G.S. *et al.* 1991. Connective tissue proteinases and inhibitors in abdominal aortic aneurysms. Involvement of the vasa vasorum in the pathogenesis of aortic aneurysms. Arterioscler. Thromb. **11:** 1667–1677.
9. THOMPSON, M.M. *et al.* 1996. Angiogenesis in abdominal aortic aneurysms. Eur. J. Vasc. Endovasc. Surg. **11:** 464–469.
10. HOLMES, D.R. *et al.* 1995. Medial neovascularization in abdominal aortic aneurysms: a histopathologic marker of aneurysmal degeneration with pathophysiologic implications. J. Vasc. Surg. **21:** 761–771.
11. VACCA, A. *et al.* 1993. Melanocyte tumor progression is associated with changes in angiogenesis and expression of the 67-kilodalton laminin receptor. Cancer **72:** 455–461.
12. WEIDNER, N. *et al.* 1992. Tumor angiogenesis: a new significant and independent prognostic indicator in early-stage breast carcinoma. J. Natl. Cancer Inst. **84:** 1875–1887.

# Aortic Aneurysms as a Source of Circulating Interleukin-6

JOE DAWSON, GILLIAN COCKERILL, EDWARD CHOKE, IAN LOFTUS, AND MATT M. THOMPSON

*Department of Vascular Surgery, St. George's Hospital and St. George's, University of London, London, UK*

ABSTRACT: In keeping with the inflammatory paradigm of abdominal aortic aneurysm (AAA) pathophysiology, *in vitro* studies suggest that aneurysms secrete the proinflammatory cytokine interleukin-6 (IL-6). Circulating IL-6 levels are higher in patients with AAA with elevated circulating IL-6 an independent risk factor for cardiovascular mortality. To investigate whether aneurysms secrete IL-6 into the circulation, arterial IL-6 was measured from within the aorta in three groups of patients undergoing endovascular procedures; 27 AAA, 10 thoracic aneurysms (TA), and 15 controls. Overall, IL-6 was higher in the aneurysm groups ($P < 0.0008$) with significant rises corresponding to positions downstream to the aneurysm in both AAA and TA. There were no significant differences in IL-6 with aortic position in the control group. These data support the hypothesis that aneurysms secrete IL-6 into the circulation and may account for the high cardiovascular mortality observed in patients with aneurysms.

KEYWORDS: abdominal aortic aneurysm; interleukin-6; inflammation; cytokines; cardiovascular mortality

## INTRODUCTION

The multifunctional cytokine interleukin-6 (IL-6) has been consistently implicated in abdominal aortic aneurysm (AAA) pathophysiology. Venous plasma concentrations are higher in patients with AAA compared controls[1,2] and *in vitro* tissue culture models demonstrate that aneurysms actively secrete IL-6.[3,4] This suggests that AAAs may secrete IL-6 into the circulation. As elevated circulating IL-6 is an independent risk factor for future MI, cardiovascular, and all-cause mortality,[5,6] this may account for the fact that 67% of AAA patients die from cardiovascular causes unrelated to their aneurysm.[7]

Address for correspondence: Matt M. Thompson, Department of Vascular Surgery, St. George's Hospital, Blackshaw Road, Tooting, London, SW17 ORE, UK. Voice: 44-208-725-3205; fax: 44-208-725-3495.

e-mail: matt.thompson@stgeorges.nhs.uk

Ann. N.Y. Acad. Sci. 1085: 320–323 (2006). © 2006 New York Academy of Sciences.
doi: 10.1196/annals.1383.009

Circumstantial evidence from the UK Small Aneurysm Trial would support this as patients who underwent early surgery had a 7.2% survival advantage over those under surveillance. It was suggested that this could be due to reduced temporal exposure to IL-6 from the aneurysm.[7] The purpose of this study was to measure plasma IL-6 from several points within the aorta in patients with aneurysms to test the hypothesis that IL-6 is secreted by the aneurysm.

## METHODS

Twenty-seven patients with AAA and 10 patients with thoracic aortic aneurysms (TA) undergoing endovascular aneurysm repair were recruited. In addition, 15 patients without aneurysms undergoing angiography comprised a control group. Prior to stent insertion or intervention, a catheter was used to sample blood at five sequential points within the aorta; ascending aorta (TA only), arch of aorta or TA , descending aorta, proximal abdominal aorta (AAA and controls only), distal abdominal aorta, and common iliac artery. Plasma IL-6 was determined by enzyme-linked immunosorbent assay (ELISA). In addition, C-reactive protein (CRP) was measured in the AAA and control groups.

## RESULTS

Overall mean IL-6 was significantly higher in the aneurysm groups than controls (10.81 pg/mL ± 3.32 vs. 4.94 pg/mL ± 0.48 vs 2.65 pg/mL ± 0.51,

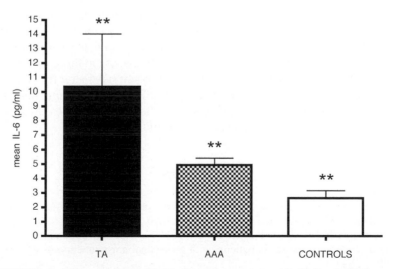

**FIGURE 1.** Mean circulating IL-6 in TA, AAA, and controls. ** $P = 0.0008$, one-way analysis of variance (ANOVA).

**TABLE 1.** Variation in circulating IL-6 with aortic location in patients with TA, AAA, and controls

| | IL-6 (pg/mL) | | |
|---|---|---|---|
| Aorta position | TA ($n = 10$) | AAA ($n = 27$) | Control ($n = 15$) |
| Ascending | $10.37 \pm 3.26$ | – | – |
| Arch or TA | $10.35 \pm 3.16$ | $4.70 \pm 0.47$ | $2.45 \pm 0.50$ |
| Descending | $11.64 \pm 3.55$ | $4.73 \pm 0.48$ | $2.65 \pm 0.54$ |
| Proximal abdo | – | $5.00 \pm 0.51$ | $2.82 \pm 0.59$ |
| Distal abdo | $10.82 \pm 3.44$ | $5.09 \pm 0.50$ | $2.80 \pm 0.59$ |
| Iliac artery | $10.88 \pm 3.27$ | $5.17 \pm 0.46$ | $2.54 \pm 0.47$ |
| $P$-value | $0.02^*$ | $0.002^*$ | $0.26^+$ |
| Overall mean IL-6 | $10.81 \pm 3.32$ | $4.94 \pm 0.48$ | $2.65 \pm 0.51$ |
| $P$-value | | $0.0008^\ddagger$ | |

*Repeated measures and $\ddagger$ one-way ANOVA, $+$ Friedman repeated measures test. Results expressed as mean $\pm$ SEM.

$P = 0.0008$, FIG. 1). Within the AAA and TA groups, IL-6 significantly differed with aorta position ($P = 0.002$ and $P = 0.02$, respectively) with levels rising downstream to the aneurysm (TABLE 1). However, there were no significant differences in IL-6 with position in the control group ($P = 0.24$) or CRP in either group ($P = 0.35$).

## CONCLUSIONS

As IL-6 levels correspond to aneurysm position with no differences in CRP, these data suggest the aneurysm as a source of circulating IL-6 rather than merely reflecting systemic inflammation. The higher levels seen in the thoracic aneurysm group may reflect more extensive disease in these patients. As circulating IL-6 has been identified as an independent risk factor for mortality, it is reasonable to suggest that the biological effect of aneurysms may have more far reaching and insidious effects upon cardiovascular health than the well-documented mortality associated with rupture and repair.

## REFERENCES

1. TRESKA, V., O. TOPOLCAN & L. PECEN. 2000. Cytokines as plasma markers of abdominal aortic aneurysm. Clin. Chem. Lab. Med. **38:** 1161–1164.
2. JUVONEN, J., H-M. SURCEL, J. SATTA, et al. 1997. Elevated circulating levels of inflammatory cytokines in patients with abdominal aortic aneurysm. ATVB **17:** 2843–2847.
3. WALTON, L.J., I.J. FRANKLIN, T. BAYSTON, et al. 1999. Inhibition of prostaglandin E2 synthesis in abdominal aortic aneurysms: implications for smooth muscle cell

viability, inflammatory processes, and expansion of abdominal aortic aneurysms. Circulation **100:** 48–54.

4. SZEKANECZ, Z., M.R. SHAH, W.H. PEARCE, *et al.* 1994. Human atherosclerotic abdominal aortic aneurysms produce interleukin (IL)-6 and interferon-gamma but not IL-2 and IL-4: the possible role for IL-6 and interferon-gamma in vascular inflammation. Agents Actions **42:** 159–162.

5. RIDKER, P.M., N. Rifai, M.J. Stampfer, *et al.* 2000. Plasma concentrations of interleukin-6 and the risk of future myocardial infarction among apparently healthy men. Circulation **101:** 1767–1772.

6. JONES, K.G., D.J. BRULL, L.C. BROWN, *et al.* 2001. Interleukin-6 (IL-6) and the prognosis of abdominal aortic aneurysms. Circulation **103:** 2260–2265.

7. PARTICIPANTS UK SMALL ANEURYSM TRIAL. 1998. Mortality results for randomised controlled trial of early elective surgery or ultrasonographic surveillance for small abdominal aortic aneurysms. Lancet **352:** 1649–1655.

# Circulating Cytokines in Patients with Abdominal Aortic Aneurysms

JOE DAWSON, GILLIAN COCKERILL, EDWARD CHOKE, IAN LOFTUS, AND MATT M. THOMPSON

*Department of Vascular Surgery, St. George's Hospital and St. George's, University of London, London, UK*

ABSTRACT: Studies suggest that aneurysm-derived cytokines perpetuate the cycle of inflammation and proteolysis that is the pathological hallmark of abdominal aortic aneurysms (AAA). As interleukin (IL)-6 is an independent risk factor for cardiovascular mortality, such cytokines may also have important systemic effects. The purpose of this study was to investigate the effect of aneurysm repair on circulating levels of cytokines. Inflammatory cytokines were measured in 99 patients with AAA and 100 patients who had undergone AAA repair in the past. There was a significant reduction in IL-10 in the postoperative group, and a nonsignificant trend toward reduction in IL-6 and CRP in the postoperative group. Subgroup analysis of the postoperative group revealed significantly lower levels of IL-6 and CRP in the open group compared to endovascular aneurysm repair (EVAR). These results suggest that aneurysm repair may have an effect upon chronic levels of circulating inflammatory cytokines, and that the type of repair may exert some influence.

KEYWORDS: abdominal aortic aneurysm; interleukin-6; inflammation; cytokines; cardiovascular mortality

## INTRODUCTION

The emergence of inflammation as a key process in the pathogenesis of abdominal aortic aneurysms[1] (AAAs) has encouraged elucidation of the role of inflammatory cytokines in aneurysm disease. Several studies have suggested that aneurysms secrete increased amounts of inflammatory cytokines *in vitro*,[2] and elevated circulating concentrations are present in patients with aneurysms.[3] Among these, interleukin (IL)-6 has been found to be higher in AAA patients compared to normal controls and those with coronary heart disease. This may be clinically relevant considering elevated circulating IL-6 is an independent risk factor for cardiovascular mortality,[4] and two-thirds of patients with AAA die from cardiovascular causes unrelated to their aneurysm.

Address for correspondence: Prof. M.M. Thompson, St. George's Hospital, Blackshaw Rd., Tooting, London, SW17 ORE, UK. Voice: 44-208-725-3205; fax: 44-208-725-3495.
e-mail: Matt.Thompson@stgeorges.nhs.uk

Ann. N.Y. Acad. Sci. 1085: 324–326 (2006). © 2006 New York Academy of Sciences.
doi: 10.1196/annals.1383.010

**TABLE 1.** Circulating cytokine profile in pre- and postoperative abdominal aortic aneurysm patients

| Cytokine | Preop | Postop | $P$ value* |
|---|---|---|---|
| IFN-γ (pg/mL) | undetectable | undetectable | – |
| TNF-α (pg/mL) | 8.4 (5.4–9.9) | 8.4 (4.9–10.3) | 0.86 |
| IL-1β (pg/mL) | 2.5 (1.5–3.0) | 2.7 (1.4–3.2) | 0.46 |
| IL-6 (pg/mL) | 5.52 (3.8–7.6) | 5.48 (3.0–6.6) | 0.28 |
| IL-8 (pg/mL) | 28.7(12.5–39.6) | 33.9(11.1–49.3) | 0.24 |
| IL-10 (pg/mL) | 2.0 (1.2–2.5) | 1.8 (1.1–2.2) | 0.03 |
| hs-CRP (mg/L) | 4.5 (1.8–8.0) | 4.1 (2.2–6.8) | 0.6 |

Results expressed as median + interquartile range.
*Mann–Whitney test.

Furthermore, UK Small Aneurysm Trial patients who underwent early surgery displayed a 7.2% survival advantage over those under surveillance. Although it was suggested that this may be due to lifestyle changes in the surgery group, it was also postulated that this was possibly due to reduced temporal exposure to aneurysm-derived IL-6.[5] The purpose of this study, therefore, was to determine whether excluding the aneurysm from the circulation by means of aneurysm repair reduced long-term circulating cytokine concentrations.

## METHODS

Venous blood was collected from 199 patients: 99 patients with aneurysms (50 small (< 5.5 cm) and 49 large (> 5.5 cm)) and 100 patients who had undergone aneurysm repair in the past (66 endovascular aneurysm repair (EVAR) and 34 open repair). IL-6 and associated inflammatory mediators were analyzed; interferon-gamma, (IFN-γ), tumor necrosis factor-alpha (TNF-α), interleukins-1-beta (IL-1-β), IL-6, IL-8, IL-10, and high-sensitivity C-reactive protein (hs-CRP). Cytokines were determined using the Luminex system (Luminex Corp. Austin, TX, USA), hs-CRP by rate turbidemetry immunoassay (Synchron LX® System, Beckman Coulter, Inc. Fullerton, CA, USA). In a separate experiment, paired pre- and postoperative plasma samples were compared from 28 patients who underwent AAA repair. In both experiments, samples in the postoperative cohort were obtained at least 6 weeks after surgery, avoiding the period of transient increase in inflammatory cytokines associated with surgical trauma.

## RESULTS

IL-10 was significantly lower in postoperative group ($P = 0.03$), whereas there were no statistically significant differences in IFN-γ, TNF-α, IL-1-β, and

**TABLE 2. Paired IL-6 concentrations pre- and postabdominal aortic aneurysm repair**

| Paired | Preop | Postop | $^{+}P$ value |
|---|---|---|---|
| IL-6 (pg/mL) | $11.1 \pm 2.8$ | $9.1 \pm 1.6$ | 0.47 |

Results expressed as mean $\pm$ SE.
$^{+}$Paired $t$-test.

IL-8 (TABLE 1). There was a nonsignificant trend toward lower postoperative levels of IL-6 and CRP (TABLES 1 and 2). However, subgroup analysis of the postoperative group revealed significantly lower levels of IL-6 (5.9 pg/mL (3.7–6.8) vs. 4.2 pg/mL (2.2–6.1), $P = 0.03$) and CRP (4.5 pg/mL (2.5–7.3) vs. 2.6 pg/mL (1.1–4.3), $P = 0.04$) in the open group compared to EVAR.

## CONCLUSIONS

These results suggest that aneurysm repair may have an effect upon circulating inflammatory cytokines, and that the type of repair may influence aneurysm biology. The influence of these subtle differences in circulating cytokines on long-term cardiovascular mortality remains to be seen.

## REFERENCES

1. BROPHY, C.M., J.M. REILLY, G.L. SMITH, et al. 1991. The role of inflammation in nonspecific abdominal aortic aneurysm disease. Ann. Vasc. Surg. **5:** 229–233.
2. NEWMAN, K.M., J. JEAN-CLAUDE, H. LI, et al. 1994. Cytokines that activate proteolysis are increased in abdominal aortic aneurysms. Circulation **90:** 224–227.
3. TRESKA, V., O. TOPOLCAN & L. PECEN. 2000. Cytokines as plasma markers of abdominal aortic aneurysm. Clin. Chem. Lab. Med. **38:** 1161–1164.
4. RIDKER, P.M., N. RIFAI, M.J. STAMPFER, et al. 2000. Plasma concentrations of interleukin-6 and the risk of future myocardial infarction among apparently healthy men. Circulation **101:** 1767–1772.
5. PARTICIPANTS UK SMALL ANEURYSM TRIAL. 1998. Mortality results for randomised controlled trial of early elective surgery or ultrasonographic surveillance for small abdominal aortic aneurysms. Lancet **352:** 1649–1655.

# Endothelial Progenitor Cells and Abdominal Aortic Aneurysms

JOE DAWSON,[a] JENNY TOOZE,[b] GILLIAN COCKERILL,[a] EDWARD CHOKE,[a] IAN LOFTUS,[a] AND MATT M. THOMPSON[a]

[a]*Department of Vascular Surgery, St. George's Hospital and St. George's, University of London, London, UK*

[b]*Department of Haematology, St. George's Hospital and St. George's, University of London, London, UK*

ABSTRACT: Endothelial progenitor cells (EPCs) are a population of circulating stem cells that hone in to sites of vascular injury where they undergo differentiation to become incorporated into damaged tissue. The aim of this study was to enumerate EPCs in patients with abdominal aortic aneurysms (AAA). CD133$^+$ peripheral blood mononuclear cells were immunomagnetically selected and CD34/CD133 was used as a marker of EPCs. EPCs were detected using flow cytometry. AAA patients had significantly higher levels of circulating EPCs than age-matched controls (2.43% vs. 1.25% of all events, $P = 0.008$). The role and function of EPCs in AAA remain to be determined, but their implication with angiogenesis may represent one plausible mechanism.

KEYWORDS: abdominal aortic aneurysm; endothelial progenitor cells; stem cells; EPCs

## INTRODUCTION

Abdominal aortic aneurysms (AAAs) develop as the result of an imbalance between destructive and restorative processes. We currently have limited knowledge regarding potential reparative mechanisms. However, a population of circulating stem cells known as endothelial progenitor cells (EPCs) have recently emerged as playing an important role in vascular repair and may modulate disease resistance. EPCs reside in the bone marrow and mobilization occurs following stimulation by a growing number of identified factors including vascular injury.[1] EPCs then hone in to areas of vascular damage where they differentiate and appear to engraft into damaged tissue including experimental aneurysms.[2] The use of EPC therapy in animals has shown promise

Address for correspondence: Prof. Matt M. Thompson, Department of Vascular Surgery, St. George's Hospital, Blackshaw Road, Tooting, London, SW17 0RE, UK. Voice: 44-208-725-3205; fax: 44-208-725-3495.

e-mail: matt.thompson@stgeorges.nhs.uk

Ann. N.Y. Acad. Sci. 1085: 327–330 (2006). © 2006 New York Academy of Sciences.
doi: 10.1196/annals.1383.011

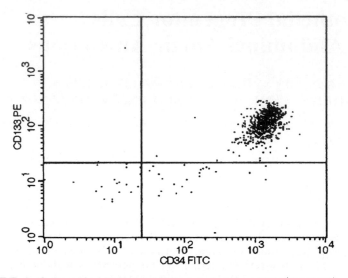

**FIGURE 1.** Cytometric data demonstrating a dual-stained CD34$^+$/CD133$^+$ progenitor cell population following CD133 immunomagnetic separation.

with transplantation of EPCs limiting the evolution of experimental atherosclerosis.[3] In addition, recent studies have suggested that a reduction in the number of circulating EPCs correlated with an increased risk of cardiovascular events and death from cardiovascular causes.[4] The aim of this study was to investigate the number of circulating EPCs in patients with AAA.

## METHODS

### Collection of Blood and Isolation of Peripheral Blood Mononuclear Cells

Venous blood was drawn from 25 patients with AAA and 18 age-matched controls. Peripheral blood mononuclear cells (PBMNs) were isolated using density gradient centrifugation.

### Immunomagnetic Cell Separation and Fluorochrome Staining

The combination of CD34 (a hematopoietic stem and EPC marker) and CD133 (a more specific progenitor marker) acts as putative markers to represent a population of circulating EPCs. To facilitate identification of this extremely rare population of cells, PBMNs were CD133 enriched using immunomagnetic cell separation. These cells were then incubated with CD133-PE and CD34-FITC-conjugated fluorochromes for 30 min prior to flow cytometric analysis.

**TABLE 1. Cell numbers expressing EPC cell surface markers expressed as % of total events (mean ± SE)**

| Cell surface marker | AAA | Controls | *P*-value* |
|---|---|---|---|
| CD133+ | 2.45 ± 0.36 | 1.25 ± 0.14 | 0.01 |
| CD34+ | 2.63 ± 0.36 | 1.41 ± 0.16 | 0.008 |
| CD133+ / CD34+ | 2.43 ± 0.34 | 1.25 ± 0.14 | 0.008 |

*Student's *t*-test.

## *Flow Cytometry*

Gates were set on the forward and side scatter plot corresponding to known morphology of progenitor cells. To correct for nonspecific antibody binding, positive cells were compared to negative mouse isotype controls. Results were expressed as a percentage of total events.

## RESULTS

Cell purities were similar in both groups following magnetic separation and a discrete population of CD34+/CD133+ cells was identified by flow cytometry (FIG. 1). We found significantly more CD133+/CD34+ cells in the AAA group compared to controls (2.43 vs. 1.25, *P* = 0.008, TABLE 1 and FIG. 2).

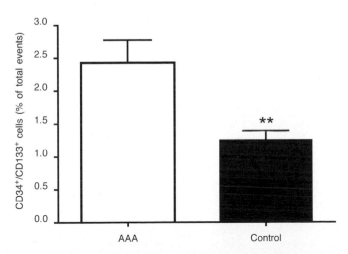

**FIGURE 2.** Percentage of circulating CD133-isolated cells expressing CD34+ /CD133+ cells in patients with abdominal aortic aneurysms compared to age-matched controls. **\*\***P = 0.008, Student's *t*-test.

## CONCLUSIONS

These preliminary data suggest that EPCs are mobilized in patients with AAA, perhaps as an ongoing attempt at repair. EPCs have been shown to be mobilized by angiogenic factors such as hypoxia and vascular endothelial growth factor (VEGF)[5]—factors also identified in aneurysms. As such, EPCs may be required for the neovascularization identified in aneurysms.[6] The role and functional capacity of EPCs in this population remain to be determined, but they may well represent a novel method of disease modification and warrant further study.

## REFERENCES

1. GILL, M., K. DIAS, M.L. HATTORI, et al. 2001. Vascular trauma induces rapid but transient mobilization of VEGFR2(+) AC133(+) endothelial precursor cells. Circ. Res. **88:** 167–174.
2. SHO, E., M. SHO, H. NANJO, et al. 2004. Hemodynamic regulation of CD34+ cell localisation and differentiation in experimental aneurysms. Arterioscler. Thromb. Vac. Biol. **24:** 1916–1921.
3. RAUSCHER, F.M., P.J. GOLDSCHMIDT-CLERMONT, B.H. DAVIS, et al. 2003. Aging, progenitor cell exhaustion, and atherosclerosis. Circulation **108:** 457–463.
4. WERNER, N., S. KOSIOL, T. SCHIEGL, et al. 2005. Circulating endothelial progenitor cells and cardiovascular outcomes. N. Engl. J. Med. **353:** 999–1007.
5. TAKAHASHI, T., C. KALKA, H. MASUDA, et al. 1999. Ischemia and cytokine-induced mobilization of bone marrow-derived endothelial progenitor cells for neovascularization. Nat. Med. **5:** 434–438.
6. THOMPSON, M.M., L. JONES, A. NASIM, et al. 1996. Angiogenesis in abdominal aortic aneurysms. Eur. J. Vasc. Endovasc. Surg. **11:** 464–469.

# Increasing Evidence for Immune-Mediated Processes and New Therapeutic Approaches in Abdominal Aortic Aneurysms—A Review

CHRISTINA DUFTNER,[a,c] RÜDIGER SEILER,[b] CHRISTIAN DEJACO,[a,c] GUSTAV FRAEDRICH,[b] AND MICHAEL SCHIRMER[a,c]

[a]*Department of Internal Medicine, Clinical Division of General Internal Medicine, Innsbruck Medical University, Innsbruck, Austria*

[b]*Department of Surgery, Division of Vascular Surgery, Innsbruck Medical University, Innsbruck, Austria*

[c]*Department of Internal Medicine, General Hospital of the Elisabethinen, Klagenfurt, Austria*

ABSTRACT: Animal models for abdominal aortic aneurysms (AAAs), immunogenetical and pathophysiological studies support the importance of immune-mediated processes in the pathogenesis of AAA disease. Neutrophils, natural killer (NK) cells, monocytes/macrophages, and proinflammatory cytokines are involved in the complex and dynamic tissue remodeling of the AAA vessel wall. Our group showed an increased prevalence of circulating interferon-$\gamma$ (IFN-$\gamma$) producing CD28$^-$ T cells especially in smaller AAAs, thus supporting the concept of a T cell-mediated pathophysiology of AAAs, especially during the early development of AAAs. Further research should now assess the possible benefit of anti-inflammatory therapeutic approaches in AAA patients, especially with small AAAs.

KEYWORDS: abdominal aortic aneurysms; inflammation; lymphocytes; interferon-$\gamma$; costimulatory molecule

## INTRODUCTION

The pathophysiology of abdominal aortic aneurysms (AAAs) has not been totally clarified. Previously, inflammatory AAAs (IAAAs) were defined by the presence of a thickened aneurysm wall, marked perianeurysmal and retroperitoneal fibrosis, and dense adhesions of adjacent abdominal organs. These

Address for correspondence: Michael Schirmer, M.D., Department of Internal Medicine, General Hospital of the Elisabethinen, Völkermarkterstrasse 15–19, A-9020 Klagenfurt, Austria. Voice: +43-650-5830-161; fax: +43-463-5830-159.
e-mail: michael.schirmer@ekh.at

Ann. N.Y. Acad. Sci. 1085: 331–338 (2006). © 2006 New York Academy of Sciences.
doi: 10.1196/annals.1383.036

IAAAs represent 4–9% of all AAAs.[1] Presently, an underlying immune-mediated inflammatory process is supported for the majority of AAAs. In 1981 Rose and Dent noted that no sharp histological distinction existed between non-IAAAs, including the "usual atherosclerotic aneurysms," and IAAAs, and proposed that the IAAA was the extreme end of an inflammatory process responsible for both IAAAs and nonspecific AAAs.[2] This concept of a common immune-mediated pathogenesis was supported by the demonstration of identical HLA alleles functioning in both IAAAs and degenerative non-IAAAs.[3]

## IMMUNOGENETICAL STUDIES SUPPORT ROLE OF HLA MOLECULES

A specific immunogenetic background has been examined and has documented that approximately 15% of patients with AAAs, but without any recognizable connective tissue disorder like Ehlers-Danlos or Marfan syndrome, have a positive family history.[4] Two segregation studies from the early 1990s favored a genetic model and suggested the presence of a major gene effect.[5,6] Recently, genetic heterogeneity and the presence of susceptibility loci for familial AAA were also described on chromosomes 19q13 and 4q31.[7] Interestingly, there are several plausible candidate genes in the two regions with the highest LOD scores described on chromosome 19 such as interleukin (IL-)15, GRB2-associated binding protein 1, or PDCD5 (protein for programmed cell death 5) involved in inflammation and cellular growth arrest and apoptosis. Rasmussen et al. detected HLA-DRB1*15 and B1*0404 alleles as genetic risk factors for IAAA in a White American population,[8] and a Japanese research group found HLA-DRB1*02 to be a genetic risk factor and HLA-DQB1*03 a protective factor for nonspecific infrarenal AAAs.[9] More detailed studies then revealed genetic similarities between degenerative and IAAAs, and in a North American, Caucasian cohort, both HLA-DRB1*02 and B1*04 alleles were associated with risk for both degenerative (odds ratio [OR] 2.2 and 2.0) and IAAAs (OR 3.7 and OR 2.5, respectively).[3]

## CELLULAR ASPECTS OF IMMUNOLOGICAL BACKGROUND

During the last years, more and more studies have confirmed the presence of extensive inflammatory infiltrates in the media and adventitia leading to increased expression of proinflammatory cytokines and C-reactive protein in aneurysmal tissue.[10,11] The inflammatory cells enter the media and adventitia via neovessels with medial thinning and activation of monocytes, thus triggering the production of matrix metalloproteinases (MMPs) and apoptosis of medial smooth muscle cells.[12,13] Inflammatory cells accumulate in AAA lesions with a predominance of CD4$^+$ T cells (3- to 20-fold increase in comparison to CD8$^+$ T cells) and to a lesser extent B cells and macrophages.[14] B cells rarely exist in occlusive atherosclerotic aortas,[14,15] whereas AAAs often display local deposition of immunoglobulin,[16,17] potentially reflecting humoral immune responses. Besides, also NK cells and significant proportions of NKT cells that express T cell receptor (TCR) $\alpha\beta$, CD4, and the NK markers CD56 and CD161 were found in AAA lesions. Thus a type 1 CD4$^+$ T and CD4$^+$CD161$^+$ NKT cells medicated regulation of vascular smooth muscle cell proliferation and apoptosis was implicated.[18] Increased circulating levels of NK cells were described in AAA patients with increased NK cytotoxicitiy possibly involved in the potentiation and generation of inflammation in patients with AAAs.[19] The reduced prevalence of immunorcgulatory CD31$^+$ T cells may additionally promote the development of AAAs.[20]

The pivotal role of interferon-$\gamma$ (IFN-$\gamma$) producing CD4$^+$ T cells in orchestrating matrix remodeling in AAA has now been demonstrated in an AAA mouse CD4$^{-/-}$ knockout model. Whereas CD4$^{-/-}$ mice were resistant to aneurysm induction, intraperitoneal application of IFN-$\gamma$ could partially reconstitute the development of aneurysms. Furthermore, mice with targeted deletion of IFN-$\gamma$ showed attenuation of MMP expression and inhibition of aneurysm development and aneurysms in IFN-$\gamma^{-/-}$ knockout mice were reconstituted by infusion of competent splenocytes from the corresponding wild-type mice.[21] CD4$^+$ T cells isolated from ancurysmal tissue specimens were also shown to produce large amounts of IFN-$\gamma$, but not IL-4. In aneurysm tissue, overexpression of the transcriptional factor Tbet, involved in the regulation of proinflammatory immune responses and IFN-$\gamma$ itself, has been described.[22] Thus, both the mouse model and human studies favor the concept of a T cell-mediated and IFN-$\gamma$ triggered pathophysiological process in AAAs.

Our own studies showed an increased prevalence of circulating CD4$^+$ and CD8$^+$CD28$^-$ T cells in AAA patients without a history of neoplasm, recent acute infection, or history of any other immune-mediated chronic disease.[23] In the peripheral blood percentages of CD28$^-$ out of the CD3$^+$CD4$^+$ and the CD3$^+$CD8$^+$ cells were enriched to 7.8 $\pm$ 8.8% and 41.9 $\pm$ 15.7% in AAA patients compared to healthy controls with 2.2 $\pm$ 6.1% and 24.9 $\pm$ 15.5%, respectively ($P = 0.002$ and $P \leq 0.001$, after adjustment for age and sex). This subgroup of proinflammatory IFN-$\gamma$ producing T cells, which lack the costimulatory molecule CD28 on their surface, has already been identified in patients with immune-mediated disorders, including rheumatoid arthritis, ankylosing spondylitis, multiple sclerosis, Wegener's granulomatosis, and unstable angina,[24–28] and are considered markers for chronic inflammation and early aging. Functionally, these T cells are capable of releasing large amounts of IFN-$\gamma$, perforin, and granzyme B, providing them with the ability to lyse target cells.[29] Phenotypically, CD4$^+$ and CD8$^+$CD28$^-$ T cells mostly lack the expression of the lymphocyte marker CD7, but highly express the NK cell marker CD57. A marker for naïve T cells, CD45RA, was expressed on

$53.4 \pm 26.4\%$ of CD4$^+$CD28$^-$ T cells and $72.7 \pm 14.8\%$ of CD8$^+$CD28$^-$ T cells in comparison to $19.7 \pm 10.4\%$ of CD4$^+$CD28$^+$ T cells and $20.8 \pm 16.4\%$ on CD8$^+$CD28$^+$ T cells ($P = 0.010$ and $P < 0.001$, respectively). Thus, CD28$^-$ T cells from AAA patients reveal an end-differentiated memory-effector phenotype with reconversion of CD45RA.[30,31] From the functional perspective, both CD4$^+$ and CD8$^+$CD28$^-$ T cells produce large amounts of IFN-$\gamma$ and perforin, but lack the production of IL-4. Interestingly, in this study patients with small AAAs ($<4$ cm) showed higher peripheral levels of CD4$^+$CD28$^-$ T cells ($11.7 \pm 9.0\%$) than those patients with intermediate ($4$–$6$ cm, $6.6 \pm 7.7\%$, $P = 0.025$) and large AAAs ($\geq 6$ cm, $6.7 \pm 5.6\%$, $P = 0.065$). No correlation was detected between the peripheral levels of CD8$^+$CD28$^-$ T cells and maximal AAA diameter.

Besides the necessity of specific T cells for the development of AAAs, depletion of polymorphonuclear (PMN) cells in C57BL6 mice by pretreatment with anti-PMN antibodies not only induced neutropenia, but resulted in AAA resistance in the Anidjar/Dobrin mouse model and showed the role for PMNs in AAA disease.[32] Besides, L-selectin knockout mice were significantly more resistant to AAA development than wild-type controls.[33] Fewer macrophages and neutrophils were recruited to the aorta and the formation of AAAs was either prevented or delayed, supporting the important role of L-selectin-mediated recruitment of inflammatory cells in the development of AAAs.

The role of macrophage-derived leukotrienes was recently analyzed in apolipoprotein E-deficient mice fed with a high cholesterol diet.[34] The 5-lipoxygenase (5-LO), a key enzyme in the formation of proinflammatory leukotrienes, was found to be upregulated in the macrophages solely on the outer layer of the aorta and promoted aneurysm formation with stimulated expression of MIP-1$\alpha$ in macrophages and MIP-2 in endothelial cells. These data now link the 5-LO pathway to hyperlipidemia-dependent inflammation of the arterial wall and to pathogenesis of aortic aneurysms.

## SEROLOGICAL MARKERS OF INFLAMMATION

An elevated erythrocyte sedimentation rate (ESR) is present in only 40-88% of IAAA patients, but even less frequent in patients with unspecific AAA as first described in Walker's original paper and confirmed in subsequent reports.[35] The results of studies on C-reactive protein (CRP) are still controversial. CRP has been described as elevated in patients who present with symptoms or ruptured AAAs.[36] Increased levels of high sensitivity CRP (hsCRP) were recently shown to be associated with an increased risk of AAA.[37] In a small study with 39 AAA patients, serum levels of hsCRP correlated with aneurysm size,[11] but a larger study showed AAA disease progression to be independent of serum CRP levels.[38] Direct proof of CRP mRNA in 4 out of 16 AAA tissues examined by reverse transcription polymerase chain reaction (RT-PCR) suggest that production of CRP occurs in the aneurysmal aortic tissue itself.[11] Previous studies already reported elevated serum levels of IL-1β, TNF-α, and IL-6 in AAA patients.[39] In AAA tissue samples, TNF-α levels were found to be higher in small-sized AAAs compared to large-sized AAAs, and may be related to infiltration of macrophages.[12] In addition, TNF-α and TNF-α converting enzyme (TACE) mRNA levels were highest in the media and adventitia of the transition zone compared to mid-portions of AAAs.[40]

## ANTI-INFLAMMATORY THERAPIES IN AAA

Until today, several animal studies showed promising results in stabilizing preexisting AAAs and preventing rupture by immuno-modulating therapy. The effect of rapamycin as an immunosuppressive agent has been demonstrated in elastase-treated rats.[41] Treatment with simvastatin suppresses the development of experimental AAAs in both normal C57Bl/6 wild-type and hypercholesterolemic apoE-deficient mice, and the mechanisms of this effect are independent of lipid-lowering and include preservation of medial elastin and smooth muscle cells as well as altered aortic wall expression of MMPs and their inhibitors.[42] In addition, gene array analysis provided evidence that several mediators of inflammation, matrix remodeling and oxidative stress are downregulated by simvastatin treatment. Kalyanasundaram *et al.* suggested that simvastatin may be useful as an adjuvant therapy to suppress the growth of small aneurysms.[44] Treatment with nonsteroidal anti-inflammatory drugs, such as indomethacin proved succesful in the prevention of AAAs in animal models. The overexpression of TGF-ß1, a multipotent cytokine with anti-inflammatory effects, by endovascular gene therapy stabilized AAAs already injured by inflammation and proteolysis.[45]

So far little is known about anti-inflammatory approaches in humans. However recently, it was demonstrated in a retrospective analysis of 150 AAA patients that the use of statins was associated with attenuation of AAA growth.[46]

## CONCLUSIONS

Recent studies provide more details on immune-mediated mechanisms in the pathogenesis of AAA. Animal and human tissue studies suggest a role for IFN-γ producing T cells in the development of AAAs. These immune-mediated processes in AAAs offer many opportunities for promising new therapeutic approaches, especially for small AAAs.

## ACKNOWLEDGMENTS

We thank the Research Fund of the Austrian National Bank (OeNB, projects # 8835 and # 9715), the Verein zur Förderung der Hämatologie, Onkologie und Immunologie (Innsbruck), the Medical Research Fund of the Innsbruck

Medical University (MFF), and the Tyrolean Research Fund (project # 0404/121) for their financial support of this work.

## REFERENCES

1. VAGLIO, A. & C. BUZIO. 2005. Chronic periaortitis: a spectrum of diseases. Curr. Opin. Rheumatol. **17:** 34–40.
2. ROSE, A.G. & D.M. DENT. 1981. Inflammatory variant of abdominal atherosclerotic aneurysm. Arch. Pathol. Lab. Med. **105:** 409–413.
3. RASMUSSEN, T.E., J.W. HALLETT JR, S. SCHULTE S, *et al.* 2001. Genetic similarity in inflammatory and degenerative abdominal aortic aneurysms: a study of human leukocyte antigen class II disease risk genes. J. Vasc. Surg. **34:** 84–89.
4. NITECKI, S.S., J.W. HALLETT JR, A.W. STANSON, *et al.* 1996. Inflammatory abdominal aortic aneurysms: a case-control study. J. Vasc. Surg. **23:** 860–868.
5. MAJUMDER, P.P., P.L. ST JEAN, R.E. FERRELL, *et al.* 1991. On the inheritance of abdominal aortic aneurysm. Am. J. Hum. Genet. **48:** 164–170.
6. VERLOES, A., N. SAKALIHASAN, L. KOULISCHER, *et al.* 1995. Aneurysms of the abdominal aorta: familial and genetic aspects in three hundred thirteen pedigrees. J. Vasc. Surg. **21:** 646–655.
7. SHIBAMURA, H., J.M. OLSON, C. VAN VLIJMEN-VAN KEULEN, *et al.* 2004. Genome scan for familial abdominal aortic aneurysm using sex and family history as covariates suggests genetic heterogeneity and identifies linkage to chromosome 19q13. Circulation **109:** 2103–2108.
8. RASMUSSEN, T.E., J.W. HALLETT JR, H.D. TAZELAAR, *et al.* 2002. Human leukocyte antigen class II immune response genes, female gender, and cigarette smoking as risk and modulating factors in abdominal aortic aneurysms. J. Vasc. Surg. **35:** 988–993.
9. HIROSE, H., M. TAKAGI, N. MIYAGAWA, *et al.* 1998. Genetic risk factor for abdominal aortic aneurysm: HLA-DR2(15), a Japanese study. J. Vasc. Surg. **27:** 500–503.
10. RASMUSSEN, T.E., J.W. HALLETT JR, S. SCHULTE, *et al.* 2001. Genetic similarity in inflammatory and degenerative abdominal aortic aneurysms: a study of human leukocyte antigen class II disease risk genes. J. Vasc. Surg. **34:** 84–89.
11. VAINAS, T., T. LUBBERS, F.R. STASSEN, *et al.* 2003. Serum C-reactive protein level is associated with abdominal aortic aneurysm size and may be produced by aneurysmal tissue. Circulation **107:** 1103–1105.
12. HAMANO, K., T.S. LI, M. TAKAHASHI, *et al.* 2003. Enhanced tumor necrosis factor-alpha expression in small sized abdominal aortic aneurysms. World J. Surg. **27:** 476–480.
13. KEELING, W.B., P.A. ARMSTRONG, P.A. STONE, *et al.* 2005. An overview of matrix metalloproteinases in the pathogenesis and treatment of abdominal aortic aneurysms. Vasc. Endovasc. Surg. **39:** 457–464.
14. HENDERSON, E.L., Y.J. GENG, G.K. SUKHOVA, *et al.* 1999. Death of smooth muscle cells and expression of mediators of apoptosis by T lymphocytes in human abdominal aortic aneurysms. Circulation **99:** 96–104.
15. KOCH, A.E., G.K. HAINES, R.J. RIZZO, *et al.* 1990. Human abdominal aortic aneurysms. Immunophenotypic analysis suggesting an immune-mediated response. Am. J. Pathol. **137:** 1199–1213.

16. HANSSON, G.K., L. JONASSON, P.S. SEIFERT, *et al.* 1989. Immune mechanisms in atherosclerosis. Arteriosclerosis **9:** 567–578.

17. BROPHY, C.M., J.M. REILLY, G.J. SMITH, *et al.* 1991. The role of inflammation in nonspecific abdominal aortic aneurysm disease. Ann. Vasc. Surg. **5:** 229–233.

18. CHEW, D.K., J. KNOETGEN, S. XIA, *et al.* 2003. The role of a putative microfibrillar protein (80 kDa) in abdominal aortic aneurysm disease. J. Surg. Res. **114:** 25–29.

19. CHAN, W.L., N. PEJNOVIC, H. HAMILTON, *et al.* 2005. Atherosclerotic abdominal aortic aneurysm and the interaction between autologous human plaque-derived vascular smooth muscle cells, type 1 NKT, and helper T cells. Circ. Res. **96:** 675–683.

20. FORESTER, N.D., S.M. CRUICKSHANK, D.J. SCOTT, *et al.* 2006. Increased natural killer cell activity in patients with an abdominal aortic aneurysm. Br. J. Surg. **93:** 46–54.

21. CALIGIURI, G., P. ROSSIGNOL, P. JULIA, *et al.* 2006. Reduced immunoregulatory CD31+ T cells in patients with atherosclerotic abdominal aortic aneurysm. Arterioscler. Thromb. Vasc. Biol. **26:** 618–623.

22. XIONG, W., Y. ZHAO, A. PRALL, *et al.* 2004. Key roles of CD4+ T cells and IFN-gamma in the development of abdominal aortic aneurysms in a murine model. J. Immunol. **172:** 2607–2612.

23. GALLE, C., L. SCHANDENE, P. STORDEUR P, *et al.* 2005. Predominance of type 1 CD4+ T cells in human abdominal aortic aneurysm. Clin. Exp. Immunol. **142:** 519–527.

24. DUFTNER, C., R. SEILER, P. KLEIN-WEIGEL, *et al.* 2005. High prevalence of circulating CD4+CD28- T-cells in patients with small abdominal aortic aneurysms. Arterioscler. Thromb. Vasc. Biol. **25:** 1347–1352.

25. MARTENS, P.B., J.J. GORONZY, D. SCHAID, *et al.* 1997. Expansion of unusual CD4+ T cells in severe rheumatoid arthritis. Arthritis Rheum. **40:** 1106–1114.

26. DUFTNER, C., C. GOLDBERGER, A. FALKENBACH, *et al.* 2003. Prevalence, clinical relevance and characterization of circulating cytotoxic CD4+CD28- T cells in ankylosing spondylitis. Arthritis Res. Ther. **5:** R292–300.

27. MARKOVIC-PLESE, S., I. CORTESE, K.P. WANDINGER, *et al.* 2001. CD4+CD28- costimulation-independent T cells in multiple sclerosis. J. Clin. Invest. **108:** 1185–1194.

28. LAMPRECHT, P., F. MOOSIG, E. CSERNOK, *et al.* 2001. CD28 negative T cells are enriched in granulomatous lesions of the respiratory tract in Wegener's granulomatosis. Thorax **56:** 751–757.

29. LIUZZO, G., S.L. KOPECKY, R.L. FRYE, *et al.* 1999. Perturbation of the T-cell repertoire in patients with unstable angina. Circulation **100:** 2135–2139.

30. NAKAJIMA, T., S. SCHULTE, K.J. WARRINGTON, *et al.* 2002. T-cell-mediated lysis of endothelial cells in acute coronary syndromes. Circulation **105:** 570–575.

31. HAMANN, D., P.A. BAARS, M.H. REP, *et al.* 1997. Phenotypic and functional separation of memory and effector human CD8+ T cells. J. Exp. Med. **186:** 1407–1418.

32. ARLETTAZ, L., C. BARBEY, F. DUMONT-GIRARD, *et al.* 1999. CD45 isoform phenotypes of human T cells: CD4(+)CD45RA(−)RO(+) memory T cells re-acquire CD45RA without losing CD45RO. Eur. J. Immunol. **29:** 3987–3994.

33. ELIASON, J.L., K.K. HANNAWA, G. AILAWADI, *et al.* 2005. Neutrophil depletion inhibits experimental abdominal aortic aneurysm formation. Circulation **112:** 232–240.

34. HANNAWA, K.K., J.L. ELIASON, D.T. WOODRUM, et al. 2005. L-selectin-mediated neutrophil recruitment in experimental rodent aneurysm formation. Circulation 112: 241–247.
35. ZHAO, L., M.P. MOOS, R. GRABNER, et al. 2004. The 5-lipoxygenase pathway promotes pathogenesis of hyperlipidemia-dependent aortic aneurysm. Nat. Med. 10: 966–973.
36. TANG, T., J.R. BOYLE, A.K. DIXON, et al. 2005. Inflammatory abdominal aortic aneurysms. Eur. J. Vasc. Endovasc. Surg. 29: 353–362.
37. DOMANOVITS, H., M. SCHILLINGER, M. MULLNER, et al. 2002. Acute phase reactants in patients with abdominal aortic aneurysm. Atherosclerosis 163: 297–302.
38. WANHAINEN, A., D. BERGQVIST, K. BOMAN, et al. 2005. Risk factors associated with abdominal aortic aneurysm: a population-based study with historical and current data. J. Vasc. Surg. 41: 390–396.
39. NORMAN, P., C.A. SPENCER, M.M. LAWRENCE-BROWN, et al. 2004. C-reactive protein levels and the expansion of screen-detected abdominal aortic aneurysms in men. Circulation 110: 862–866.
40. ROHDE, L.E., L.H. ARROYO, N. RIFAI, et al. 1999. Plasma concentrations of interleukin-6 and abdominal aortic diameter among subjects without aortic dilatation. Arterioscler. Thromb. Vasc. Biol. 19: 1695–1699.
41. SATOH, H., M. NAKAMURA, M. SATOH, et al. 2004. Expression and localization of tumour necrosis factor-alpha and its converting enzyme in human abdominal aortic aneurysm. Clin. Sci. (Lond) 106: 301–306.
42. LAWRENCE, D.M., R.S. SINGH, D.P. FRANKLIN, et al. 2004. Rapamycin suppresses experimental aortic aneurysm growth. J. Vasc. Surg. 40: 334–338.
43. STEINMETZ, E.F., C. BUCKLEY, M.L. SHAMES, et al. 2005. Treatment with simvastatin suppresses the development of experimental abdominal aortic aneurysms in normal and hypercholesterolemic mice. Ann. Surg. 241: 92–101.
44. KALYANASUNDARAM, A., J.R. ELMORE, J.R. MANAZER, et al. 2006. Simvastatin suppresses experimental aortic aneurysm expansion. J. Vasc. Surg. 43: 117–124.
45. HOLMES, D.R., D. PETRINEC, W. WESTER, et al. 1996. Indomethacin prevents elastase-induced abdominal aortic aneurysms in the rat. J. Surg. Res. 63: 305–309.
46. DAI, J., F. LOSY, A.M. GUINAULT, et al. 2005. Overexpression of transforming growth factor-beta1 stabilizes already-formed aortic aneurysms: a first approach to induction of functional healing by endovascular gene therapy. Circulation 112: 1008–1015.
47. SCHOUTEN, O., J.H. VAN LAANEN, E. BOERSMA, et al. 2006. Statins are associated with a reduced infrarenal abdominal aortic aneurysm growth. Eur. J. Vasc. Endovasc. Surg. 32(1): 21–26.

# Pathogenesis of Thoracic and Abdominal Aortic Aneurysms

DONG-CHUAN GUO,[a] CHRISTINA L. PAPKE,[a] RUMIN HE,[b]
AND DIANNA M. MILEWICZ[a]

[a]*Department of Internal Medicine, The University of Texas Medical School,
Houston, Texas, USA*

[b]*Ruijin Hospital, The Medical College of Shanghai Jiaotong University, China*

ABSTRACT: The major disease processes affecting the aorta are aortic
aneurysms and dissections. Aneurysms are usually described in terms of
their anatomic location, with thoracic aortic aneurysms (TAAs) involving
the ascending and descending aorta in the thoracic cavity and abdominal
aortic aneurysms (AAAs) involving the infrarenal abdominal aorta. Both
thoracic and abdominal aortas are elastic arteries, and share similarities
in their physical structures and cellular components. However, thoracic
and abdominal aortas differ in their biochemical properties and the origin of their vascular smooth muscle cells (VSMCs). These similarities
and differences between thoracic and abdominal aortas provide the basis for the various pathologic mechanisms observed in this disease. This
review focuses on the comparison of the pathologic mechanisms involved
in TAA and AAA.

KEYWORDS: abdominal aortic aneurysm; thoracic aortic aneurysm;
apoptosis; inflammation; pathogenesis

## INTRODUCTION

The major disease processes affecting the aorta are aortic aneurysms and dissections, and these diseases account for nearly 16,000 deaths annually. Aortic
aneurysms tend to expand asymptomatically until a catastrophic event occurs
such as aortic rupture or dissection, which is associated with a high degree
of morbidity, mortality, and medical expenditure. The most common location for aneurysms is the infrarenal abdominal aorta, followed by the ascending thoracic aorta. The histopathologic abnormality underlying thoracic aortic
aneurysms (TAAs) is medial degeneration, traditionally termed *cystic medial
necrosis*, which is characterized by the triad of loss of smooth muscle cells

Address for correspondence: Dong-chuan Guo, Ph.D., Department of Internal Medicine, University
of Texas Medical School, Houston, 6431 Fannin, MSB 6.039, Houston, TX 77030. Voice: 713-500-
6849; fax: 713-500-0693.
  e-mail: Dongchuan.Guo@uth.tmc.edu

Ann. N.Y. Acad. Sci. 1085: 339–352 (2006). © 2006 New York Academy of Sciences.
doi: 10.1196/annals.1383.013

(SMCs), fragmented and diminished number of elastic fibers, and increased accumulation of proteoglycans. In contrast, AAAs are primarily associated with atherosclerosis. TAAs and AAAs share some similar pathological phenotypes including the loss of vascular smooth muscle cells (VSMCs) and destruction of matrix elastic fibers; however, TAAs and AAAs also display some important differences in pathology associated with these two types of aneurysms (TABLE 1). The involvement of inflammation in the pathogenesis of AAAs has been recognized and characterized over decades, while cystic medial necrosis in TAA aortas was previously described as a noninflammatory lesion. However, recent studies indicate that infiltration of inflammatory cells into the thoracic aorta contribute to the formation and development of TAAs. In the past decade, significant progress has been made toward understanding the pathology, molecular biology, and genetics of aortic aneurysms.

## Pathology of Atherosclerosis, AAA, and TAA

AAAs are primarily associated with atherosclerosis, and some evidence suggests that AAAs progress from occlusive disease.[1] However, only 9% to 16% of patients with atherosclerotic abdominal aortas develop AAAs,[2,3] which suggests that chronic atherosclerosis may be a prerequisite for AAA formation. The pathology of atherosclerosis in a variety of arteries has been extensively investigated and involves major changes in the aortic intima when it occurs in abdominal aorta. During formation of atheroma in abdominal aorta, mechanical or chemical insults including hypertension, smoking metabolites, and oxidized lipids may initially damage the endothelial surface. As a result, endothelial cells increase expression of vascular cell adhesion molecule-1 (VCAM-1) and intercellular adhesion molecule-1 (ICAM-1), and reduce nitric oxide synthesis.[4] Increased expression of adhesion molecules, especially VCAM-1, is considered to play a major role in recruitment of monocytes to the site of injury. Endothelial cells and VSMCs can express monocyte chemoattractant proteins in response to oxidized low-density lipoprotein (LDL) stimulation.[5] These cells as well as macrophages residing in the intima express chemoattractant proteins that promote migration of monocytes through the endothelium, recruitment of more monocytes into the intima, and formation of nascent atheroma.[6] Macrophages and T lymphocytes also express growth factors, cytokines, and matrix metalloproteinases (MMPs) that induce migration and proliferation of VSMCs into the intima and formation of atherosclerotic plaques. The plaques contain a thin VSMC-rich fibrous cap and a lipid core with accumulated foam cells. Apoptosis of inflammatory cells and VSMCs in the plaques contributes to the development of atherosclerotic lesions. The majority of cells undergoing apoptosis in atherosclerotic plaques are macrophage foam cells in the lipid core.[7,8] Apoptosis of macrophages contributes to the formation and enlargement of the lipid core.[9] Apoptosis of VSMCs occurs in

TABLE 1. Comparison of the pathogenesis of thoracic and abdominal aneurysms

| | AAA | TAA |
|---|---|---|
| Risk factors | Hypertension, smoking, high cholesterol, and obesity[49] | Hypertension, smoking[55] |
| Gender (Male: Female) | 2–5:1[49,50] | 1.7:1[56] |
| Average age of patients at the time of diagnosis | 65–70 years old[49] | 60–65 years old |
| Pathology | Associated with atherosclerosis[51] | Associated with medial degeneration[57] |
| Apoptosis of VSMCs | Yes[16] | Yes[29–32] |
| Destruction of elastic fibers | Yes[16] | Yes[31] |
| Proteinases that may be involved | MMP-1, MMP-2, MMP-3, MMP-9, MMP-12, Plasminogen activator,Cystatin C[30,52–54] | MMP-2, MMP-9[29,58] |
| Inflammation | Th2-predominant immune response or NK and NKT cells involvement[38,42] | Th1-predominant immune response[48] |
| Cytokine levels elevated | IL-4, IL-5, and IL-10 significantly increase and INF-$\gamma$, IL-12, and IL-18 detectable[38] | INF-$\gamma$ [48] |
| Genetic predisposition | 19q13 and 4q31[33] | TAAD1, TAAD2, FAA1, TAAD/PDA[32,34–36] |

the shoulder regions of plaques and affects the stability of the plaques.[10,11] VSMC-derived apoptotic bodies are also able to concentrate and crystallize calcium that initiates vascular calcification.[12,13]

AAAs demonstrate extensive structural remodeling, which is characterized by degeneration of extracellular matrix, destruction of elastic lamina, and reduction of VSMCs,[14,15] and these changes are associated with progressive weakening of the aortic wall. In end-stage AAA aortas, $\alpha$-actin immunostaining showed a decrease in the numbers of VSMCs in some areas and fragmentation of some remaining VSMCs in others.[16] Compared to a normal aorta, elastin concentration is significantly reduced, collagen concentration is slightly increased, and the aortic media is significantly thinner in the AAA aorta.[17,18] MMPs may play an important role in extracellular matrix remodeling, especially elastin and collagen turnover.[16,19–21] Histological studies have demonstrated that AAA tissue contains an excess of MMP-1, MMP-2, MMP-3, and MMP-9 compared with normal aortic tissue.[22–24] MMP-2 and MMP-9 can degrade a variety of substrates, including both collagen and elastin. Genetically engineered mice lacking either MMP-2 or MMP-9 demonstrate resistance to $CaCl_2$-induced AAA formation,[25,26] which suggests that these molecules contribute to weakening of the aortic wall and aneurysm formation. Another proposed mechanism for weakening of the aortic wall is the apoptosis of VSMCs. Henderson *et al.* demonstrated that apoptosis of VSMCs and macrophages is present in the media of AAA aortas using TUNEL staining and antibodies directed against $\alpha$-actin and CD68. Elevated levels of Fas in both VSMCs and leukocytes and co-localization of perforin with activated T cells in the AAA media suggest that immune cells play an important role in the apoptosis of VSMCs and macrophages in AAA aortas.[16]

The ascending aorta differs from the abdominal aorta in structure, biochemistry, and cell biology. The ascending aorta has a thinner intima, thicker media, and more medial lamellar units compared to the abdominal aorta. Compared to the abdominal aorta, the thoracic aorta has significantly higher elastin and collagen content and a lower collagen-to-elastin ratio.[18] VSMCs in the ascending aorta originate from the neural crest, while those in the descending and abdominal aortas originate from mesoderm and endothelial cells.[27,28] The differences in the physical structure of thoracic and abdominal aortas may contribute to the differences observed in the pathogenesis of TAAs and AAAs. In contrast with the abdominal aorta, atherosclerosis rarely presents in the ascending aorta. The medial degeneration associated with TAAs is observed in the thoracic aorta with aging, but this degeneration is qualitatively and quantitatively much greater in patients with TAAs. Medial degeneration in the TAA aorta is most commonly associated with loss of VSMCs and destruction of the medial elastic fibers. The intima and adventitia are thicker, and the media is thinner in TAA aorta compared with control aortas.[29] However, because of aortic dilation, TAA aorta has a greater medial area compared to control aortas. Sirius red and elastin van Gieson staining results indicate that collagen and

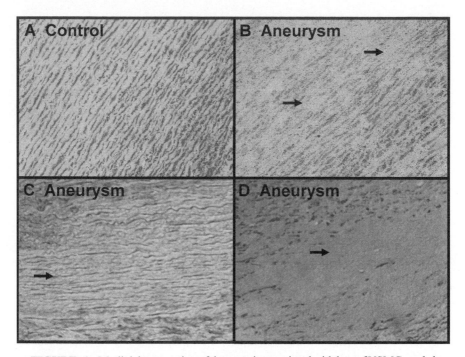

**FIGURE 1.** Medial degeneration of the aorta is associated with loss of VSMCs and elastic fibers. Immunohistochemical staining was performed on human control and aneurysm aortic tissue using a monoclonal antibody directed against SMC-α-actin. **(A)** The control aortas showed an orderly array of VSMCs and elastic fibers in the media. **(B–D)** The aortas of the patients with ascending aortic aneurysms showed regions with primarily loss of SMCs or regions with primarily loss of elastic fibers, or both. Magnification 100x for panels A and B and magnification 400x for panels C and D. (Panels C and D from He *et al.*[31] reproduced by permission).

elastin are significantly reduced in TAA aortas compared to control aortas.[29] MMP-2 and MMP-9 immunoreactivity was increased at the edges of areas of medial degeneration in aortas from patients with sporadic TAA,[30] and MMPs are suggested to play a role in the destruction of extracellular matrix in TAA.

The results of studies to determine whether medial degeneration is associated with decreased density of VSMC in aortic media and apoptosis of VSMCs are contradictory. Tang *et al.* and Lesauskaite *et al.* reported that VSMC density is not reduced in TAA.[29,30] However, He *et al.* reported that VSMC density in the aortic media was significantly reduced in TAA.[31] Since loss of VSMC in TAA aortic media is observed in focal areas (FIG. 1), the number of VSMCs counted in a few high magnification fields may not truly reflect the VSMC density in a large area of aortic media. He *et al.* used an image tool to trace and quantify areas of positive α-actin staining, and found that normal aortas contained significantly more α-actin-positive staining than aortas affected by aneurysm or dissection.[31] It is interesting to note that reduction of VSMC density has also been observed in aortic media of patients with familial form of TAA who have mutations in the smooth muscle myosin heavy chain gene, *MYH11*.[32]

Significantly increased transferase-mediated dUTP nick end labeling-(TUNEL-) positive staining in TAA aortas compared to controls was observed by all three groups. He *et al.* used double staining with a combination of TUNEL and immunohistochemistry to confirm the co-localization of TUNEL-positive cells with VSMCs, T lymphocytes, and macrophages, and concluded that apoptosis of VSMCs presented in the TAA aortic media.[31] However, Lesauskaite *et al.* suggested that TUNEL-positive staining might not be due to apoptosis of VSMCs because they did not observe degraded apoptotic DNA ladder in electrophoresis gel assay.[30] Tang *et al.* came to a similar conclusion that apoptosis in TAA aortas was not significant, and they suggested that cells undergoing apoptosis in TAA aortas were infiltrating leukocytes due to lack of a significant change observed in VSMC density.[29] Therefore, both the questions of decreased VSMCs and whether VSMCs undergo apoptosis remain to be definitively answered. The increased knowledge of the genes predisposing individuals to these diseases has highlighted the significant number and heterogeneity of defective genes leading to TAAs, and the different genes may lead to differences in VSMC density and apoptosis.

Familial aggregation studies have indicated that approximately 15% of patients with AAA who do not have any recognizable connective tissue disorder have a positive family history for AAA. One recent study has shown that markers at two chromosomal loci, 19q13 and 4q31, are linked to familial AAA, providing genetic evidence that inheritance of altered genes at these chromosomal loci may predispose individuals to AAAs.[33] A genetic predisposition to thoracic aneurysms, like abdominal aneurysms, has been linked to several putative loci on chromosomes; however, important structural and cellular differences between the thoracic and abdominal aorta provide an explanation for the different pathological mechanisms observed in AAA and TAA. Familial aggregation studies have indicated that up to 20% of patients with TAA have a first-degree relative with the disease. Four chromosomal loci have been identified for familial TAA including TAAD1, TAAD2, FAA1, and TAD/PDA.[32,34-36] About 5% of patients who have a family histroy of TAAs develop AAAs. The different genes predisposing individuals to TAAs and AAAs further suggest that differences in pathogenesis exist between TAAs and AAAs.

## Inflammation in TAAs and AAAs

Studies on inflammatory infiltrates associated with atherosclerosis in coronary arteries indicate that macrophages are the predominant inflammatory cells in atheromas and the inflammatory cell infiltration is primarily confined to the diseased intima. A Th1-predominant immune response causes aortic wall remodeling and exacerbates formation of atherosclerotic lesions.[37] Western blot assays using proteins extracted from atheromas showed significant elevation of Th1-promoting cytokines IFN-$\gamma$, IL-2, IL-12, and IL-18 compared to control and AAA aortas. Th2-promoting cytokines IL-4, IL-5, and IL-10 were undetectable in atheromas.[38] Increased expression of IFN-$\gamma$ receptor (IDN-$\gamma$R-$\alpha$) and IL-18 receptor (IL-18R-$\alpha$) further support the hypothesis that a Th1-predominant immune response is involved in pathogenesis of atherosclerosis.

Compared to atherosclerosis, inflammatory response in AAAs is usually transmural in distribution and inflammatory cells infiltrated primarily focus on the outer media and adventitia.[15] Inflammatory cells infiltrate AAA aortas either through the vasa vasorum in the adventitia or through the intima into the media.[15,39,40] Inflammatory cells in aortic media and adventitia are involved in the destruction of extracellular matrix and apoptosis of VSMCs, and are proposed to play a major role in the formation of AAAs. The majority of inflammatory cells recovered from AAA tissues are CD4-positive lymphocytes or T cells, followed by B lymphocytes. Several studies have suggested that a Th2-predominant immune response plays an important role in AAA formation.[25,41] Expression of Th2-promoting cytokines IL-4, IL-5, and IL-10 is significantly increased in AAA aortas compared to both normal and atheroma aortas. Expression of Th1-promoting cytokines IL-2 and IL-15 were undetectable in AAA aortas, and expression of INF-$\gamma$, IL-12, and IL-18 were significantly lower in AAA aortas compared to atheromas.[38] Shimizu *et al.* suggested that the factors triggering an immune response switch from Th1- to Th2-dominant determined which individuals would develop AAA.[41] However, Chan *et al.* observed that natural killer (NK) and natural killer T (NKT) cells are present in the media and adventitia of AAA aortas.[42] Since NKT and NK cells have a Th0 cytokine profile and can produce Th2, as well as Th1 cytokines, Chan *et al.* suggested that NK and NKT may play important roles in pathogenesis of AAA rather than Th2-specific cells.[42]

Hirose and Tilson hypothesized that an autoimmune mechanism is involved in AAA formation.[43] A 40-kDa autoimmune abdominal aortic protein has been identified, and Western blot analysis demonstrated that this protein reacts with immunoglobulin G isolated from human AAA tissue.[44] An association study of HLA genotypes with Japanese AAA population suggests that HLA A-2 and HLA B-61 are important genetic risk factors for the development of AAA among the Japanese population.[45] These data further support the hypothesis that an autoimmune mechanism may be involved in the pathogenesis of AAA. Analysis of the T cell receptor (TCR) V$\beta$ repertoire using competitive RT-PCR indicates that TCR usage in T lymphocytes infiltrated in AAA aortic tissue is not restricted.[46] However, the result of another group showed that the oligoclonal populations of $\gamma\delta$ TCR+ T cells were present in AAA lesions. This result provides evidence that AAA is a specific antigen-driven T cell disease.[47]

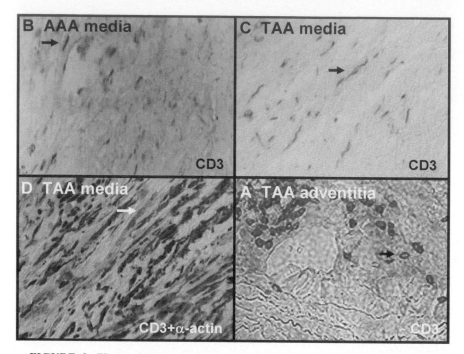

**FIGURE 2.** Flattened T lymphocytes are present in the aortic media of patients with TAA and AAA. Immunohistochemical staining was performed on a cross-section of aortas of patients with TAA and AAA with a monoclonal antibody directed against CD3. Immuno-histochemical staining demonstrated that flattened T lymphocytes presented in the media of patients with AAA (**A**) and TAA (**B**). (**C**) Double immunostaining using antibodies against CD3 and α-actin revealed that the cells positive for SMC-α-actin (*brown*) were distinct from those staining for CD3 (*red*). (**D**) Immunohistochemical staining showed the presence of round T lymphocytes in the adventitia of a patient with TAA. Magnification 400x. (Panel B from Henderson *et al.*[16] reproduced by permission). Shown in color in online version.

The pathology associated with TAAs, termed cystic medial necrosis, was historically described as a noninflammatory lesion. Involvement of inflammatory cells in the pathogenesis of TAAs has only recently been investigated. Immunohistochemical staining using monoclonal antibodies against CD3+ indicated that the numbers of T lymphocytes were significantly increased in TAA aortas compared to control aortas. Some of the CD3+ cells appear flattened in the aortic media when they reside between the SMC layers (FIG. 2).[17,31] To confirm the flattened shape of the T lymphocytes, double immunostaining was performed using antibodies against CD3 and α-actin, and the results revealed that the cells positive for SMC- α-actin were distinct from those staining for CD3. Quantitative RT-PCR assay failed to detect CD3-α mRNA isolated from VSMC cultures explanted from patients' aortas, providing further evidence that the SMCs are not expressing CD3-$\alpha$.[31] Flattened T lymphocytes in the media appear similar to VSMCs in shape under H and E staining. This similarity of cell shape between T lymphocytes and VSMCs may partially explain why infiltration of T lymphocytes in TAA aortas was not recognized for decades.

Immunohistochemical staining showed that T lymphocytes were the predominant inflammatory cells infiltrated in the aortas of patients with sporadic TAA, followed by macrophages.[31,48] Large numbers of T lymphocytes present around vasa vasorum suggest that infiltration of T lymphocytes into TAA aortas occurs through the vasa vasorum.[31] Quantitative RT-PCR assay on cytokines suggests that Th1-type immune responses predominate in TAA aortas.[48] The mRNA levels of the Th1-promoting cytokine IFN-$\gamma$ and the IFN-$\gamma$-inducible chemokines IP-10 and Mig are significantly increased in TAA aortas compared to control aortas, while mRNA levels of Th2-promoting cytokines are undetectable in TAA aortas.[48] Our recent case-control association study on the association of HLA genotypes with sporadic TAA identified one HLA class I haplotype and two HLA class II haplotypes significantly associated with sporadic TAA (unpublished data). We have also observed restricted usage of TCR V-$\beta$ in the T lymphocytes infiltrated in TAA aortas (unpublished data).

## CONCLUSION

Formation of TAAs and AAAs is a complex and chronic process that results from the interaction of genetic and environmental factors. Overlaps in pathogenesis and histological phenotypes have been observed in TAAs and AAAs. Extensive structural remodeling of the extracellular matrix is observed in all aortic aneurysms, including loss of VSMCs and degradation of elastic matrix. Inflammation presents in the aortic wall and plays an important role in the pathogenesis of these aneurysms. However, aneurysms caused by different disease processes show different susceptibility to some genetic and environmental risk factors, and differences in pathological phenotypes and pathogenesis. Different HLA genotypes associated with AAAs and TAAs suggest that different autoimmune antigens may be involved in the formation of these aneurysms. Differences in the pathogenesis of TAAs and AAAs may result from differences in aortic structures, biochemical properties, and origin of VSMCs. Shimizu *et al.* have proposed a two-step model of pathogenesis of AAAs,[41] and this model may also apply to the pathogenesis of TAAs (FIG. 3). The first step involves environmental or genetic factors that produce initial damage to the aortic wall. In abdominal aorta, an exaggerated Th1-predominant inflammatory response may initiate atherosclerotic lesion, while in ascending aorta, the initial damage may result in medial degeneration. In familial TAAs and AAAs,

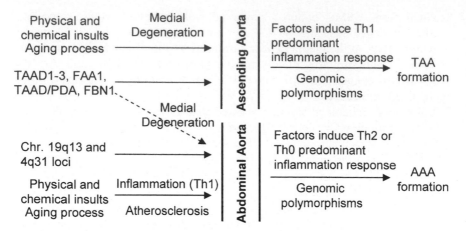

**FIGURE 3.** A two-step procedure is involved in the pathogenesis of TAAs and AAAs, and this procedure may also apply to the pathogenesis of TAAs. The first step involves environmental or genetic factors that produce initial damages to the aortic wall and endothelial cells. VSMCs respond to these damages and attempt to eliminate the injuring agents. When an exaggerated inflammatory or cellular response occurs, it may initiate atherosclerotic lesion or medial degeneration in aortas. Genetic study of familial aortic aneurysms indicates that genes' responses to familial TAA are different from those of AAA. However, some overlap exists, and about 5% of affected individuals carrying defective genes for familial TAA develop AAA. The second step involves environmental factors, which aggravate the aortic damages and inflammation responses. Genomic polymorphisms predispose certain individuals to formation of aortic aneurysms.

mutations in genes may initiate the medial degeneration in aortas. Genetic heterogeneity of defective genes predisposing individuals to familial TAAs and AAAs may initiate medial degeneration through either apoptosis of VSMCs or destruction of extracellular matrix. The second step involves environmental factors that aggravate existing damages. Inflammatory responses and genetically determined cellular responses determine individuals who will develop aortic aneurysms. Mutations in *MYH11* result in the loss of VSMCs in ascending aorta and lead to the development of familial TAAs. Mutations in *TGFBR2* result in familial TAAs and indicate that TGF-β signaling is required for maintaining homeostasis within the aortic wall. Knowledge of environmental and genetic factors that contribute to the formation of aortic aneurysms is still poorly understood. Association of genomic polymorphisms with these diseases suggests that cellular responses may be involved in the development of aortic aneurysms, and may also determine the age onset of disease in the individuals with familial TAAs and AAAs. Further study is necessary to better characterize the nature and causes of the inflammatory response observed in TAAs and AAAs.

# ACKNOWLEDGMENTS

This work was supported by MO1RR02558 (General Clinical Research Center), RO1 HL62594 (D.M.M.), and Doris Duke Foundation.

# REFERENCES

1. KOCH, A.E., G.K. HAINES, R.J. RIZZO, *et al.* 1990. Human abdominal aortic aneurysms. Immunophenotypic analysis suggesting an immune-mediated response. Am. J. Pathol. **137:** 1199–1213.
2. JAFFER, F.A., C.J. O'DONNELL, M.G. LARSON, *et al.* 2002. Age and sex distribution of subclinical aortic atherosclerosis: a magnetic resonance imaging examination of the Framingham Heart Study. Arterioscler. Thromb. Vasc. Biol. **22:** 849–854.
3. SCOTT, R.A., K.A. VARDULAKI, N.M. WALKER, *et al.* 2001. The long-term benefits of a single scan for abdominal aortic aneurysm (AAA) at age 65. Eur. J. Vasc. Endovasc. Surg. **21:** 535–540.
4. ROSS, R. 1993. The pathogenesis of atherosclerosis: a perspective for the 1990s. Nature **362:** 801–809.
5. CUSHING, S.D., J.A. BERLINER, A.J. VALENTE, *et al.* 1990. Minimally modified low density lipoprotein induces monocyte chemotactic protein 1 in human endothelial cells and smooth muscle cells. Proc. Natl. Acad. Sci. USA **87:** 5134–5138.
6. YLA-HERTTUALA, S., B.A. LIPTON, M.E. ROSENFELD, *et al.* 1991. Expression of monocyte chemoattractant protein 1 in macrophage-rich areas of human and rabbit atherosclerotic lesions. Proc. Natl. Acad. Sci. USA **88:** 5252–5256.
7. BJORKERUD, S. & B. BJORKERUD. 1996. Apoptosis is abundant in human atherosclerotic lesions, especially in inflammatory cells (macrophages and T cells), and may contribute to the accumulation of gruel and plaque instability. Am. J. Pathol. **149:** 367–380.
8. HEGYI, L., J.N. SKEPPER, N.R. CARY & M.J. MITCHINSON. 1996. Foam cell apoptosis and the development of the lipid core of human atherosclerosis. J. Pathol. **180:** 423–429.
9. BALL, R.Y., E.C. STOWERS, J.H. BURTON, *et al.* 1995. Evidence that the death of macrophage foam cells contributes to the lipid core of atheroma. Atherosclerosis **114:** 45–54.
10. GENG, Y.J. & P. LIBBY. 1995. Evidence for apoptosis in advanced human atheroma. Colocalization with interleukin-1 beta-converting enzyme. Am. J. Pathol. **147:** 251–266.
11. BENNETT, M.R. 1999. Apoptosis of vascular smooth muscle cells in vascular remodelling and atherosclerotic plaque rupture. Cardiovasc. Res. **41:** 361–368.
12. TRION, A. & L.A. VAN DER. 2004. Vascular smooth muscle cells and calcification in atherosclerosis. Am. Heart J. **147:** 808–814.
13. PROUDFOOT, D., J.N. SKEPPER, L. HEGYI, *et al.* 2000. Apoptosis regulates human vascular calcification in vitro: evidence for initiation of vascular calcification by apoptotic bodies. Circ. Res. **87:** 1055–1062.
14. THOMPSON, R.W., S. LIAO & J.A. CURCI. 1997. Vascular smooth muscle cell apoptosis in abdominal aortic aneurysms. Coron. Artery Dis. **8:** 623–631.

15. THOMPSON, R.W., P.J. GERAGHTY & J.K. LEE. 2002. Abdominal aortic aneurysms: basic mechanisms and clinical implications. Curr. Probl. Surg. **39:** 110–230.

16. HENDERSON, E.L., Y.J. GENG, G.K. SUKHOVA, *et al.* 1999. Death of smooth muscle cells and expression of mediators of apoptosis by T lymphocytes in human abdominal aortic aneurysms. Circulation **99:** 96–104.

17. LIMET, R., B. NUSGENS, A. VERLOES & N. SAKALIHASAN. 1998. Pathogenesis of abdominal aortic aneurysm (AAA) formation. Acta. Chir. Belg. **98:** 195–198.

18. GHORPADE, A. & B.T. BAXTER. 1996. Biochemistry and molecular regulation of matrix macromolecules in abdominal aortic aneurysms. Ann. N. Y. Acad. Sci. **800:** 138–150.

19. SATTA, J., T. JUVONEN, K. HAUKIPURO, *et al.* 1995. Increased turnover of collagen in abdominal aortic aneurysms, demonstrated by measuring the concentration of the aminoterminal propeptide of type III procollagen in peripheral and aortal blood samples. J. Vasc. Surg. **22:** 155–160.

20. SATTA, J., K. HAUKIPURO, M.I. KAIRALUOMA & T. JUVONEN. 1997. Aminoterminal propeptide of type III procollagen in the follow-up of patients with abdominal aortic aneurysms. J. Vasc. Surg. **25:** 909–915.

21. CAMPA, J.S., R.M. GREENHALGH & J.T. POWELL. 1987. Elastin degradation in abdominal aortic aneurysms. Atherosclerosis **65:** 13–21.

22. SANGIORGI, G., R. D'AVERIO, A. MAURIELLO, *et al.* 2001. Plasma levels of metalloproteinases-3 and -9 as markers of successful abdominal aortic aneurysm exclusion after endovascular graft treatment. Circulation **104:** I288–I295.

23. SILENCE, J., F. LUPU, D. COLLEN & H.R. LIJNEN. 2001. Persistence of atherosclerotic plaque but reduced aneurysm formation in mice with stromelysin-1 (MMP-3) gene inactivation. Arterioscler. Thromb. Vasc. Biol. **21:** 1440–1445.

24. THOMPSON, R.W. & W.C. PARKS. 1996. Role of matrix metalloproteinases in abdominal aortic aneurysms. Ann. N. Y. Acad. Sci. **800:** 157–174.

25. LONGO, G.M., W. XIONG, T.C. GREINER, *et al.* 2002. Matrix metalloproteinases 2 and 9 work in concert to produce aortic aneurysms. J. Clin. Invest **110:** 625–632.

26. IKONOMIDIS, J.S., J.R. BARBOUR, Z. AMANI, *et al.* 2005. Effects of deletion of the matrix metalloproteinase 9 gene on development of murine thoracic aortic aneurysms. Circulation **112:** I242–I248.

27. GITTENBERGER-DE GROOT, A.C., M.C. DERUITER, M. BERGWERFF & R.E. POELMANN. 1999. Smooth muscle cell origin and its relation to heterogeneity in development and disease. Arterioscler. Thromb. Vasc. Biol. **19:** 1589–1594.

28. BERGWERFF, M., M.E. VERBERNE, M.C. DERUITER, *et al.* 1998. Neural crest cell contribution to the developing circulatory system: implications for vascular morphology. Circ. Res. **82:** 221–231.

29. TANG, P.C., M.A. COADY, C. LOVOULOS, *et al.* 2005. Hyperplastic cellular remodeling of the media in ascending thoracic aortic aneurysms. Circulation **112:** 1098–1105.

30. LESAUSKAITE, V., P. TANGANELLI, C. SASSI, *et al.* 2001. Smooth muscle cells of the media in the dilatative pathology of ascending thoracic aorta: morphology, immunoreactivity for osteopontin, matrix metalloproteinases, and their inhibitors. Hum. Pathol. **32:** 1003–1011.

31. HE, R., D.C. GUO, A.L. ESTRERA, *et al.* 2006. Characterization of the inflammatory and apoptotic cells in the aortas of patients with ascending thoracic aortic aneurysms and dissections. J. Thorac. Cardiovasc. Surg. **131:** 671–678.

32. ZHU, L., R. VRANCKX, P.K. VAN KIEN, *et al.* 2006. Mutations in myosin heavy chain 11 cause a syndrome associating thoracic aortic aneurysm/aortic dissection and patent ductus arteriosus. Nat. Genet. **38(3):** 343–349.

33. SHIBAMURA, H., J.M. OLSON, C. VLIJMEN-VAN KEULEN, *et al.* 2004. Genome scan for familial abdominal aortic aneurysm using sex and family history as covariates suggests genetic heterogeneity and identifies linkage to chromosome 19q13. Circulation **109:** 2103 2108.

34. GUO, D., S. HASHAM, S.Q. KUANG, *et al.* 2001. Familial thoracic aortic aneurysms and dissections: genetic heterogeneity with a major locus mapping to 5q13-14. Circulation **103:** 2461–2468.

35. HASHAM, S.N., M.C. WILLING, D.C. GUO, *et al.* 2003. Mapping a locus for familial thoracic aortic aneurysms and dissections (TAAD2) to 3p24-25. Circulation **107:** 3184–3190.

36. VAUGHAN, C.J., M. CASEY, J.E.M. VEUGELERS, *et al.* 2001. Familial aortic aneurysms are genetically heterogeneous: identification of a novel genetic locus on chromosome 11q23. Circulation **103:** 2469–2475.

37. LIBBY, P. 2002. Inflammation in atherosclerosis. Nature **420:** 868–874.

38. SCHONBECK, U., G.K. SUKHOVA, N. GERDES & P. LIBBY. 2002. T(H)2 predominant immune responses prevail in human abdominal aortic aneurysm. Am. J. Pathol. **161:** 499–506.

39. NUMANO, F. 2000. Vasa vasoritis, vasculitis and atherosclerosis. Int. J. Cardiol. **75**(Suppl 1): S1–S8.

40. HERRON, G.S., E. UNEMORI, M. WONG, *et al.* 1991. Connective tissue proteinases and inhibitors in abdominal aortic aneurysms. Involvement of the vasa vasorum in the pathogenesis of aortic aneurysms. Arterioscler. Thromb. **11:** 1667–1677.

41. SHIMIZU, K., R.N. MITCHELL & P. LIBBY. 2006. Inflammation and cellular immune responses in abdominal aortic aneurysms. Arterioscler. Thromb. Vasc. Biol. **26(5):** 987–994.

42. CHAN, W.L., N. PEJNOVIC, T.V. LIEW & H. HAMILTON. 2005. Predominance of Th2 response in human abdominal aortic aneurysm: mistaken identity for IL-4-producing NK and NKT cells. Cell. Immunol. **233:** 109–114.

43. HIROSE, H. & M.D. TILSON. 2001. Abdominal aortic aneurysm as an autoimmune disease. Ann. N. Y. Acad. Sci. **947:** 416–418.

44. XIA, S., K. OZSVATH, H. HIROSE & M.D. TILSON. 1996. Partial amino acid sequence of a novel 40-kDa human aortic protein, with vitronectin-like, fibrinogen-like, and calcium binding domains: aortic aneurysm-associated protein-40 (AAAP-40) [human MAGP-3, proposed]. Biochem. Biophys. Res. Commun. **219:** 36–39.

45. SUGIMOTO, T., M. SADA, T. MIYAMOTO & H. YAO. 2003. Genetic analysis on HLA loci in Japanese patients with abdominal aortic aneurysm. Eur. J. Vasc. Endovasc. Surg. **26:** 215–218.

46. YEN, H.C., F.Y. LEE & L.Y. CHAU. 1997. Analysis of the T cell receptor V beta repertoire in human aortic aneurysms. Atherosclerosis **135:** 29–36.

47. PLATSOUCAS, C.D., S. LU, I. NWANESHIUDU, *et al.* 2006. Abdominal aortic aneurysms (AAA) is a specific antigen-driven T-cell. Disease 125–127.

48. TANG, P.C., A.O. YAKIMOV, M.A. TEESDALE, *et al.* 2005. Transmural inflammation by interferon-gamma-producing T cells correlates with outward vascular remodeling and intimal expansion of ascending thoracic aortic aneurysms. FASEB J. **19:** 1528–1530.

49. BLANCHARD, J.F. 1999. Epidemiology of abdominal aortic aneurysms. Epidemiol. Rev. **21:** 207–221.
50. BENGTSSON, H., B. SONESSON & D. BERGQVIST. 1996. Incidence and prevalence of abdominal aortic aneurysms, estimated by necropsy studies and population screening by ultrasound. Ann. N. Y. Acad. Sci. **800:** 1–24.
51. GRANGE, J.J., V. DAVIS & B.T. BAXTER. 1997. Pathogenesis of abdominal aortic aneurysm: an update and look toward the future. Cardiovasc. Surg. **5:** 256–265.
52. DAVIS, V., R. PERSIDSKAIA, L. BACA-REGEN, *et al*. 1998. Matrix metalloproteinase-2 production and its binding to the matrix are increased in abdominal aortic aneurysms. Arterioscler. Thromb. Vasc. Biol. **18:** 1625–1633.
53. YOON, S., G. TROMP, S. VONGPUNSAWAD, *et al*. 1999. Genetic analysis of MMP3, MMP9, and PAI-1 in Finnish patients with abdominal aortic or intracranial aneurysms. Biochem. Biophys. Res. Commun. **265:** 563–568.
54. SHI, G.P., G.K. SUKHOVA, A. GRUBB, *et al*. 1999. Cystatin C deficiency in human atherosclerosis and aortic aneurysms. J. Clin. Invest **104:** 1191–1197.
55. DAPUNT, O.E., J.D. GALLA, A.M. SADEGHI, *et al*. 1994. The natural history of thoracic aortic aneurysms. J. Thorac. Cardiovasc. Surg. **107:** 1323–1332.
56. BICKERSTAFF, L.K., P.C. PAIROLERO, L.H. HOLLIER, *et al*. 1982. Thoracic aortic aneurysms: a population-based study. Surgery **92:** 1103–1108.
57. ERDHEIM, J. 1930. Medionecrosis aortae idiopathica cystica Virchows. Arch. Path. Anat. **276:** 187–192.
58. NATAATMADJA, M., M. WEST, J. WEST, *et al*. 2003. Abnormal extracellular matrix protein transport associated with increased apoptosis of vascular smooth muscle cells in marfan syndrome and bicuspid aortic valve thoracic aortic aneurysm. Circulation **108**(Suppl 1): II329–II334.

# Attenuation of Experimental Aortic Aneurysm Formation in P-Selectin Knockout Mice

KEVIN K. HANNAWA, BRENDA S. CHO, INDRANIL SINHA,
KAREN J. ROELOFS, DANIEL D. MYERS, THOMAS J.
WAKEFIELD, JAMES C. STANLEY, PETER K. HENKE,
AND GILBERT R. UPCHURCH, JR.

*Jobst Vascular Research Laboratories, Section of Vascular Surgery,
Department of Surgery, University of Michigan, Ann Arbor, Michigan, USA*

ABSTRACT: The aim of this study was to determine the role of P-selectin, an adhesion molecule found on the surface of activated platelets and endothelial cells during experimental aortic aneurysm formation. Infrarenal abdominal aortas of C57 black wild-type (WT) mice and P-selectin knockout (PKO) mice were measured *in situ* and then perfused with porcine pancreatic elastase (0.332 U/mL). Whole blood was drawn from the tail artery on day 2 pre-perfusion to determine total and differential white blood cell (WBC) counts. On day 14 postperfusion, aortic diameters (AD) of WT mice ($N = 19$) and PKO mice ($N = 9$) were measured. An aortic aneurysm was defined as a 100% or greater increase in AD from pre-perfusion measurement. Immunohistochemistry, including H&E, trichrome and von Gieson staining, was performed on harvested aortic tissue. Statistical analysis was performed by $t$-test and Fisher's exact test. There were no significant differences in peripheral leukocyte counts at baseline between the two groups. WT mice had significantly larger AD compared to PKO mice at day 14 postperfusion (116 % vs. 38 %, $P < 0.001$). Aortic aneurysm penetrance was 52% in WT mice, while 0% ($P = 0.01$) of PKO mice formed aneurysms. On histologic examination, WT mouse aortas were associated with a significant inflammatory response and degradation of elastin and collagen fibers, while PKO mouse aortas lacked signs of inflammation or vessel wall injury. P-selectin deficiency attenuates aneurysm formation in the elastase aortic perfusion model. This was associated with a blunting of the inflammatory response and preserved vessel wall intergrity following elastase perfusion in the P-selectin knockout mice. Further investigation to elucidate the independent contributions of endothelial cell and platelet P-selectin in experimental aortic aneurysm formation is required.

Address for correspondence: Gilbert R. Upchurch, Jr., M.D., University of Michigan Hospital, 2210 THCC, 1500 East Medical Center Drive, Ann Arbor, MI 48109-0329. Voice: 734-936-5790; fax: 734-647-9867.
e-mail: riversu@umich.edu

Ann. N.Y. Acad. Sci. 1085: 353–359 (2006). © 2006 New York Academy of Sciences.
doi: 10.1196/annals.1383.014

KEYWORDS: AAAs; inflammation; adhesion; selectin

## BACKGROUND

Abdominal aortic aneurysms (AAAs) affect 3% to 9% of the United States population and are the 14th leading cause of death.[1] Currently, AAA formation is seen as a multifactorial process characterized by infiltration of inflammatory cells (e.g., neutrophils and monocytes) into the aortic wall followed by destruction of structural proteins such as elastin and collagen by extracellular matrix-degrading enzymes.[2]

The role of adhesion molecules during early inflammatory cell recruitment prior to AAA formation has not been well investigated. Recently, Hannawa *et al.* demonstrated the importance of a specific adhesion molecule, L-selectin, on the recruitment of neutrophils during the initial stages of AAA pathogenesis following elastase aortic perfusion in mice.[3] The objective of this study was to further investigate the role of another member of the selectin family, P-selectin, found on the surface of endothelial cells and platelets during AAA formation.

## METHODS

### Elastase Perfusion

C57Bl/6 wild-type (WT) mice and P-selectin KO (PKO) mice were anesthetized under 2% isoflurane inhalation on day 2 pre-perfusion and approximately 0.25 mL of blood was drawn from a prewarmed ventral tail artery by laceration and analyzed using a HEMAVET® 1500FS multispecies hematology instrument (CDC Technologies, Oxford, CT, USA). On the day of perfusion, baseline digital images of the aorta were obtained and aortic diameter (AD) was measured using Image Pro Express. Temporary control of the aorta was obtained and an aortotomy was made near the bifurcation using a 30-gauge needle. The aorta was then cannulated with PE-10 tubing and perfused with 0.332 units/mL of elastase in 1mL of saline for 5 min.[3] WT (N = 19) and PKO (N = 9) mouse aortas were measured and harvested at 14 days postperfusion. Aneurysmal aortas were defined as greater than a 100% increase from baseline.

### Histology/Immunohistochemistry

Harvested aortas were fixed in fresh, cold 4% paraformaldehyde. Aortas were then paraffin embedded, cut into 4 mm sections, and mounted onto slides. Aortic sections were stained with hematoxlin/eosin, Masson's trichrome, and

Verhoff's von Gieson stain for qualitative analysis of aortic wall structure, collagen staining, and elastin staining, respectively.

## RESULTS

There were no significant differences in circulating white blood cell (WBC) counts at baseline between WT and PKO mice ($8.64 \times 10^3$ WBC/$\mu$L vs. $10.58 \times 10^3$ WBC/$\mu$L, $P = 0.078$, respectively). WT mice had significantly larger AD compared to PKO mice 14 days following elastase perfusion (116% vs. 38% increase from pre-perfusion diameter, $P < 0.001$, FIG. 1). In addition, 52% of WT mice formed an AAA, while none of the PKO mice formed AAAs ($P = 0.01$).

Representative abdominal aortic tissue sections of WT mice documented increased inflammatory response and destruction of aortic wall structure. (FIG. 2A) More specifically, trichrome (FIG. 2B) and von Gieson staining (FIG. 2C) demonstrated medial and adventitial collagen degradation (*arrows*) and loss of medial elastin (*arrows*), respectively. In contrast, aortic sections from PKO mice demonstrated preserved aortic wall structure (FIG. 2D) as well as intact collagen (FIG. 2E, *arrows*) and elastin fibers (FIG. 2F, *arrows*).

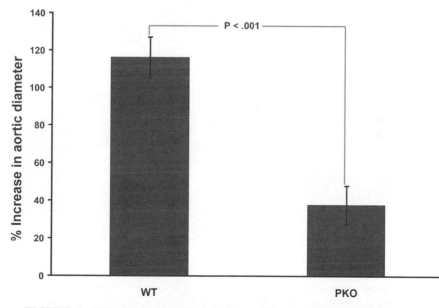

**FIGURE 1.** WT mice had significantly larger AD compared to PKO mice at day 14 postelastase perfusion (116% vs. 38%, $P < 0.001$). In addition, more WT mice (52%) than PKO mice (0%; $P = 0.01$) had aneurysms. An aortic aneurysm was defined as a 100% or greater increase in AD from pre-perfusion measurement (*dashed line*).

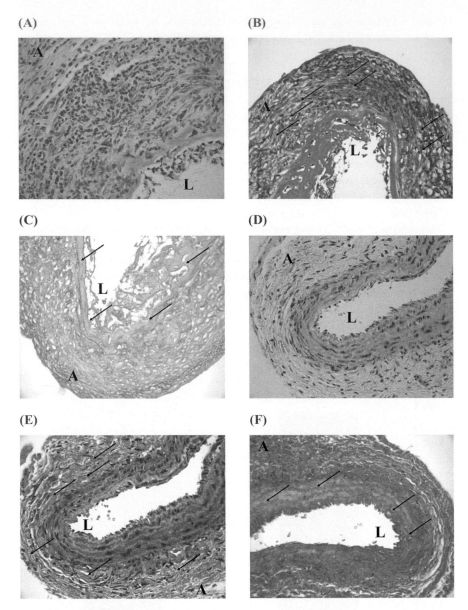

**FIGURE 2.** Representative abdominal aortic tissue sections (40× magnification) at 14 days postelastase perfusion of aortas in WT and PKO mice. Aortic sections from WT mice (**A**) show an increased inflammatory response and destruction of aortic wall structure. More specifically, trichrome staining (**B**) and von Gieson's stain (**C**) demonstrate adventitial collagen degradation (*arrows*) and loss of medial elastin (*arrows*), respectively. In contrast, PKO mouse aortic sections demonstrated preserved aortic wall structure (**D**), collagen staining (**E**, *arrows*), and elastin fibers (**F**, *arrows*). **A** = adventitia; **L** = lumen.

## DISCUSSION

In this study, AAA formation in PKO mice was attenuated suggesting a critical role for P-selectin. This inhibition of AAA development in PKO mice was associated with diminished aortic wall degradation and preserved elastin and collagen.

AAA pathogenesis is a multifactorial process[2,4] that may be initiated by some unknown injury to the aortic wall. Following this event, which serves as a catalyst for the inflammatory response, enhanced chemokine and cytokine production further promotes leukocyte recruitment into the aortic wall. Ultimately, secretion of proteolytic enzymes such as matrix metalloproteinases by leukocytes and smooth muscle cells results in aortic wall extracellular matrix destruction and aneurysm formation.

A better understanding of the initial events associated with recruitment of inflammatory cells into the aortic wall is needed as most studies of AAA disease have focused on understanding the enzymology associated with vessel wall degradation and repair. A study by Ricci *et al.*[5] focusing on events initiating inflammatory cell recruitment demonstrated that inhibiting leukocyte recruitment diminished AAA formation in an experimental model. Using antibody blockade of CD18, a subunit of the integrin adhesion molecule found on leukocytes, which promotes firm adhesion to the endothelial surface, AAA size and macrophage recruitment were inhibited following rodent aortic elastase perfusion.

This study sought to clarify the role of the selectins, specifically P-selectin, during AAA formation. The selectins are a family of three adhesion molecules: E-selectin on the surface of endothelial cells, P-selectin on the surface of endothelial cells and activated platelets, and L-selectin that is constitutively expressed on the surface of most leukocytes.[6,7] The primary function of selectins is to promote leukocyte capture to sites of inflammation. Without selectins, inflammatory cell recruitment, an early and critical event during AAA formation, is significantly diminished.[8–12] While the role of P-selectin during AAA formation prior to this study has not been investigated, a study by Hannawa and colleagues documented the critical nature of L-selectin, found only on leukocytes, during AAA formation.[3] After documenting early upregulation of L-selectin in the rat elastase AAA model, L-selectin knockout mice were studied and found to have attenuated AAA formation associated with diminished aortic wall neutrophils and macrophages.

P-selectin in particular appears to be an attractive target for pharmacologic therapy to inhibit leukocytes in the inflammatory influx. Myers and others, in a model of deep venous thrombosis, using an oral, novel P-selectin inhibitor documented decrease in thrombus weights associated with increased vessel wall leukocytes.[13] In this same model, Thanaporn and colleagues documented that a P-selectin receptor antagonist was associated with decreased perithrombotic inflammation and increased thrombus dissolution.[14] These strategies may also be attractive for inhibition of AAAs in the elastase AAA model.

Limitations of this study include the observation that the cell of origin was not determined. To differentiate whether endothelial cell P-selectin, platelet P-selectin, or both are necessary for aneurysm formation, a set of experiments involving either bone marrow transplant or aortic transplant between WT and PKO mice should be undertaken. Despite this limitation, we have identified another critical component, P-selectin, of the inflammatory cascade that contributes to the formation of experimental AAAs.

## ACKNOWLEDGMENT

This work was supported by NIH KO8 (HL67885-02) (GRU), von Liebig Award–Lifeline Foundation (GRU), the Lifeline Medical Student Research Award (KH, IS), the Griswold and Margery H. Ruth Alpha Omega Alpha Medical Student Research Fellowship (IS), and the Jobst Foundation.

## REFERENCES

1. ANDERSON, R.N. 2002. Deaths: leading causes for. National Center for Health Statistics. National Vital Statistics Reports **50:** 1–86.
2. WASSEF, M., B.T. BAXTER, R.L. CHISHOLM, *et al.* 2001. Pathogenesis of abdominal aortic aneurysms: a multidisciplinary research program supported by the National Heart, Lung, and Blood Institute. J. Vasc. Surg. **34:** 730–738.
3. HANNAWA, K.K., J.L. ELIASON, D.T. WOODRUM, *et al.* 2005. L-selectin mediated neutrophil recruitment in experimental rodent aneurysm formation. Circulation **112:** 241–247.
4. AILAWADI, G., J.L. ELIASON & G.R. UPCHURCH, JR. 2003. Current concepts in the pathogenesis of abdominal aortic aneurysm. J. Vasc. Surg. **38:** 584–588.
5. RICCI, M.A., G. STRINDBERG, J.M. SLAIBY, *et al.* 1996. Anti-CD 18 monoclonal antibody slows experimental aortic aneurysm expansion. J. Vasc. Surg. **23:** 301–317.
6. LEY, K. 1997. The selectins as rolling receptors. *In* The Selectins. D. Vestweber, Ed.: 63–104. Harwood Amsterdam.
7. VESTWEBER, D. & J.E. BLANKS. 1999. Mechanisms that regulate the function of the selectins and their ligands. Physiol. Rev. **79:** 181–213.
8. ARBONES, M.L., D.C. ORD, K. LEY, *et al.* 1994. Lymphocyte homing and leukocyte rolling and migration are impaired in L-selectin-deficient mice. Immunity **1:** 247–260.
9. BULLARD, D.C., L. QIN, I. LORENZO, *et al.* 1995. P-selectin/ICAM-1 double mutant mice: acute emigration of neutrophils into the peritoneum is completely absent but is normal into pulmonary alveoli. J. Clin. Invest. **95:** 1782–1788.
10. BULLARD, D.C., E.J. KUNKEL, H. KUBO, *et al.* 1996. Infectious susceptibility and severe deficiency of leukocyte rolling and recruitment in E-selectin and P-selectin double mutant mice. J. Exp. Med. **183:** 2329–2336.

11.  JOHNSON, R.C., T.N. MAYADAS, P.S. FRENETTE, *et al.*1995. Blood cell dynamics in P-selectin-deficient mice. Blood **86:** 1106–1114.
12.  TEDDER, T.F., D.A. STEEBER & P. PIZCUETA. 1995. L-selectin-deficient mice have impaired leukocyte recruitment into inflammatory sites. J. Exp. Med. **181:** 2259–2264.
13.  MYERS, D.D. JR, J.E. RECTENWALD, P.W. BEDARD, *et al.* 2005. Decreased venous thrombosis with an oral inhibitor of P selectin. **42:** 329–336.
14.  THANAPORN, P., D.D. MYERS, S.K. WROBLESKI, *et al.* 2003. P-selectin inhibition decreases post-thrombotic vein wall fibrosis in a rat model. Surgery **134:** 365–371.

# Global Expression Profiles in Human Normal and Aneurysmal Abdominal Aorta Based on Two Distinct Whole Genome Microarray Platforms

GUY M. LENK,[a] GERARD TROMP,[a] MAGDALENA SKUNCA,[a]
ZORAN GATALICA,[c] RAMON BERGUER,[d]
AND HELENA KUIVANIEMI[a,b]

[a]Center for Molecular Medicine and Genetics, Wayne State University School
of Medicine, Detroit, MI, USA

[b]Department of Surgery, Wayne State University School of Medicine, Detroit,
MI, USA

[c]Department of Pathology, Creighton University School of Medicine, Omaha,
NE, USA

[d]Department of Surgery, University of Michigan, Ann Arbor, MI, USA

ABSTRACT: Abdominal aortic aneurysms (AAA) are the thirteenth cause
of death in the United States. The etiology of the disease is yet largely unknown, although several environmental risk factors (e.g., smoking) have
been identified and the search for finding genetic risk factors has been
initiated. The purpose of our study was to gain insight into the pathobiology of AAA by determining which genes are expressed in the abdominal
aorta under either the diseased or normal states, thereby generating the
whole-genome-wide expression profiles for these conditions.

KEYWORDS: abdominal aortic aneurysm; gene expression; genomics;
pathway analysis; gene ontology

We used two distinct microarray platforms to generate global gene expression profiles to analyze the transcriptome of both aneurysmal[1-3] and nonaneurysmal abdominal aorta. Aortic tissue samples were collected from patients from the following four groups: (a) male abdominal aortic aneurysm
(AAA) patients ($n = 4$); (b) male autopsy controls ($n = 4$); (c) female AAA
patients ($n = 3$); and (d) female autopsy controls ($n = 3$). Case and control

Address for correspondence: Helena Kuivaniemi, M.D., Ph.D., Center for Molecular Medicine and
Genetics, Wayne State University School of Medicine, 3317 Gordon H. Scott Hall of Basic Medical
Sciences, 540 E. Canfield Ave., Detroit, MI 48201, USA. Voice: 313-577-8733; fax: 313-577-5218.
e-mail: kuivan@sanger.med.wayne.edu

Ann. N.Y. Acad. Sci. 1085: 360–362 (2006). © 2006 New York Academy of Sciences.
doi: 10.1196/annals.1383.041

groups were matched for age and ethnicity. RNA was isolated from abdominal aortic tissues, labeled, and hybridized to two different whole genome microarray platforms (Affymetrix and Illumina). The samples were run as pools (both platforms) and also as individual samples (Illumina only). The results were analyzed using the statistical program R (version 2.0; Bioconductor package), GeneSpring (version 7.2), and BeadStudio (version 1.5.0.34). Cluster (version 3.0) was used for hierarchical clustering of genes with expression differences between the cases and controls and visualized with TreeView (version 1.0.12). The online database PANTHER was used to annotate the genes into ontological categories.[4]

The number of unique genes shared between the Affymetrix and Illumina platforms is 18,037, representing approximately 75% of the current estimate for the number of genes in the human genome. Of the genes in this common set, 8,763 were concordant on both platforms and expressed in either normal or aneurysmal tissue. Several gene ontological categories were significantly different from that expected by chance such as "protein metabolism and modification" (overrepresented; $P = 1.87 \times 10^{-8}$), "cell communication" (underrepresented; $P = 3.04 \times 10^{-13}$), and "intracellular protein traffic" (overrepresented; $P = 9.05 \times 10^{-10}$).

Differential gene expression was also examined using a fold difference threshold set to four. It was necessary to use a fold difference measure due to limited samples on the Affymetrix platform. A total of 468 unique genes, out of the common gene set, met the criterion in both array platforms. Several of the genes in this list have been reported previously as being possibly important in AAA formation or growth such as MMP1,[5] MMP9,[6] and IL1B[7] to name a few. Analysis of the gene ontological categories of these differential genes showed that the Biological Process category "immunity and defense" was extremely overrepresented ($P = 2.04 \times 10^{-20}$) as was "cell communication" ($P = 2.74 \times 10^{-12}$) and "cell structure and motility" ($P = 9.77 \times 10^{-8}$).

In conclusion, these data provide global expression profiles for normal and aneurysmal abdominal aorta, and point to the importance of immune defense and tissue remodeling in the course of aneurysmal disease. Knowing which genes are actively transcribed in either normal or aneurysmal aorta is useful in identifying plausible positional candidate genes for diseases of the aorta. Thus, the insights provided by these data are valuable for future research and will aid in the discovery of therapeutic targets for the treatment of AAAs.

## ACKNOWLEDGMENTS

The study was supported in part by a grant from NHLBI (HL064310). Guy M. Lenk is a Pre-Doctoral Fellow of the American Heart Association.

## REFERENCES

1. ERNST, C.B. 1993. Abdominal aortic aneurysms. N. Engl. J. Med. **328:** 1167–1172.
2. LEDERLE, F.A., G.R. JOHNSON, S.E. WILSON, *et al.* 2000. The aneurysm detection and management study screening program: validation cohort and final results. Aneurysm Detection and Management Veterans Affairs Cooperative Study Investigators. Arch. Intern. Med. **160:** 1425–1430.
3. SHIBAMURA, H., J.M. OLSON, C. VAN VLIJMEN-VAN KEULEN, *et al.* 2004. Genome scan for familial abdominal aortic aneurysm using sex and family history as covariates suggests genetic heterogeneity and identifies linkage to chromosome 19q13. Circulation **109:** 2103–2108.
4. MI, H., B. LAZAREVA-ULITSKY, R. LOO, *et al.* 2005. The PANTHER database of protein families, subfamilies, functions and pathways. Nucleic Acids Res. **33:** D284–D288.
5. IRIZARRY, E., K.M. NEWMAN, R.H. GANDHI, *et al.* 1993. Demonstration of interstitial collagenase in abdominal aortic aneurysm disease. J. Surg. Res. **54:** 571–574.
6. NEWMAN, K.M., Y. OGATA, A.M. MALON, *et al.* 1994. Identification of matrix metalloproteinases 3 (stromelysin-1) and 9 (gelatinase B) in abdominal aortic aneurysm. Arterioscler. Thromb. Vasc. Biol. **14:** 1315–1320.
7. PEARCE, W.H., I. SWEIS, J.S. YAO, *et al.* 1992. Interleukin-1 beta and tumor necrosis factor-alpha release in normal and diseased human infrarenal aortas. J. Vasc. Surg. **16:** 784–789.

# Thoracic Aortic Compliance as a Determinant of Rupture of Abdominal Aortic Aneurysms

LUIGI RUSSO

*Senescence.Org, Cardiologia I livello, Ospedale San Camillo, Roma, Italy*

ABSTRACT: The relative importance of collagen and elastin in formation, expansion, and rupture of abdominal aortic aneurysms (AAAs) has been investigated extensively. Aortic compliance, which is a relevant component of cardiac afterload, is also determined by the relative amount of media proteins in large arteries as well as by pathological arterial processes. The objective of this study was to determine if thoracic aortic compliance was different in patients with ruptured AAAs compared to those undergoing elective AAA repair. The study was carried out in 43 patients with infrarenal AAAs in the postoperative period. The first group (A) included 17 patients undergoing emergency ruptured AAA repair. The second group (B) included 26 patients operated on for an AAA who underwent elective repair. Patients were studied by a noninvasive Doppler echocardiography. Pulse wave velocity (PWV) was determined in the descending thoracic aorta. Results show that patients with electively repaired AAAs had an accelerated pulse wave transmission, typical of an atherosclerotic aorta with a Gaussian distribution (PWV 9.26 m/sec $\pm$ 1.27). In contrast, patients with ruptured aneurysms presented in a distribution with three peaks. A striking increase in aortic compliance (41% of patients with PWV $<6$ m/sec in group A vs. 3% of group B) was observed in patients with ruptured AAAs.

KEYWORDS: abdominal aortic aneurysm; aortic compliance; aneurysm rupture; pulse wave velocity

## INTRODUCTION

Several recent papers have stressed that mortality for ruptured abdominal aortic aneurysms (AAAs) remains high despite advances in surgical technique and postoperative care. The high incidence of ruptured AAAs is an unsolved social, clinical, and scientific problem. Despite the diffusion of elective surgical repair, the number of patients with ruptured AAAs is not decreasing.

Address for correspondence: Dr. Luigi Russo, Senescence.org, Via Vigne Nuove 10, 00045 Genzano di Roma, Italy.
e-mail: aorta@senescence.org

Ann. N.Y. Acad. Sci. 1085: 363–366 (2006). © 2006 New York Academy of Sciences.
doi: 10.1196/annals.1383.026

The relative importance of collagen and elastin in the formation, expansion, and rupture of AAA has been investigated extensively.[1] Aortic compliance, which is a relevant component of cardiac afterload, is determined by the relative amount of media proteins in large arteries as well as by pathological arterial processes.[2]

## METHODS

Patients with AAAs were studied by a noninvasive Doppler echocardiography.[3] Pulse wave velocity (PWV) was determined in the descending thoracic aorta. Aortic velocities were recorded by pulse wave Doppler at two points: (1) at the isthmus, through the suprasternal window and (2) at the subdiaphragmatic aorta through a classical subcostal approach. PWV was calculated as: $PWV = (L/PWD)$ $(msec^{-1})$. (L was the sternal length and PWD was the isthmus-diaphragm pulse wave delay).

The study was performed on 43 patients with infrarenal AAAs in the postoperative period. The first group (A) included 17 patients operated on as emergencies for ruptured AAAs. The second group (B) included 26 patients operated on electively for AAA. Ages were comparable.

## RESULTS

Results show that patients with electively repaired AAAs have an accelerated pulse wave transmission, typical of atherosclerotic aorta, with a Gaussian distribution (PWV 9.26 m/sec $\pm$ 1.27). Patients with ruptured aneurysms presented in a distribution with three peaks. A striking increase in aortic compliance (41% of patients with PWV< 6 m/sec in group A vs. 3% of group B) was observed in patients with ruptured AAA (FIGS. 1 and 2). A statistical (nonparametric) analysis of data revealed a high significance of results ($P <$ 0.05).

Two cases are reported individually for their relevance:

Patient C.A. in group A. The patient was operated on for an AAA and a left iliac artery aneurysm, electively. At surgery, the iliac aneurysm had a contained rupture and was included in the group of ruptured aneurysms. PWV was 3.91 m/sec, the lowest value of the group.

Patient C.V. in group B. The patient presented with an AAA with a rapid expansion (1.5 cm/year). He had abdominal pain and was operated on with priority (electively). PWV was 5.86 m/sec and C.V. was the only patient in group A with a PWV < 6 m/sec.

Two out of 17 patients in group A presented with a highly rigid aorta (PWV > 15 m/sec). Rupture in these cases may be related to the high stress on the aneurysmal walls (mechanical rupture).

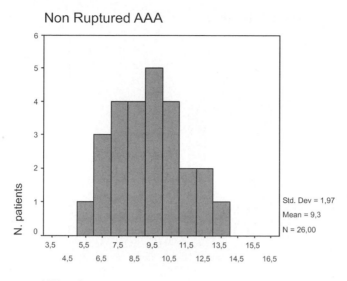

FIGURE 1. PWV in patients with electively operated AAA.

## DISCUSSION

AAA is a leading cause of death ranking 14th in the United States.[4] Most deaths are related to aneurysm rupture, which is associated with an estimated overall mortality (pre-, intra-, and postoperative) of approximately 80–90%, since many patients die before hospitalization. Clinical studies conducted on limited populations have demonstrated that the incidence of aneurysms presenting with rupture is not declining despite the increasing number of elective surgical procedures and diagnostic investigations.

Aortic compliance is due to the presence of elastin in aortic media and it is modified during one's lifetime by a series of factors: (1) an increase in connective tissue between endothelial cells in the intimae, (2) abnormalities in the elastic fibers, and (3) increases in collagen, ground substance, and calcium in the media. These factors are responsible for the high variation in values measured in this study. Therefore, patients with high thoracic aorta compliance may have a less severe deposition of calcium in the aorta as well as a variation in relative content or types (biochemical rupture) of elastin and collagen. Biochemical studies are necessary to identify the exact mechanism underlying this observation. Nevertheless, the effect of changes in compliance in a remote segment of aorta on AAA rupture may lead to the identification of a subtype of patients with congenital or acquired peculiarities of connective tissues.

From an epidemiologic standpoint, these data may help to explain the paradox of a nondecreasing incidence of ruptured AAAs even with an increased

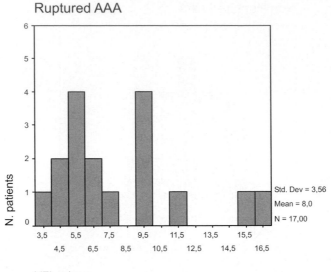

**FIGURE 2.** PWV in patients with ruptured AAA.

number of elective surgical procedures. It may be that patients with a high aortic compliance undergo a faster growth and an earlier rupture. This "fast track" in the evolution of such aneurysms probably precludes their early diagnosis and treatment.

In conclusion, the fundamental problem of AAAs is not only their recognition in asymptomatic patients, but also the definition of their risk of rupture. According to our observation, patients with ruptured AAA belong to a population separated (in most cases) from the "normal" AAA population. Thoracic aorta compliance may be relevant in determining which patients are at a high risk of rupture.

## REFERENCES

1. DOBRIN, P.B. 1989. Pathophysiology and pathogenesis of aortic aneurysms: current concepts. Surg. Clin. N. Am. **69:** 687–703.
2. DOBRIN, P.B. 1978. Mechanical properties of arteries. Physiol. Rev. **58:** 397–460.
3. DAHAN, M. *et al.* 1990. Doppler echocardiographic study of the consequences of aging and hypertension on the left ventricle and aorta. Eur. Heart J. (Suppl. G) **11:** 39–45.
4. REILLY, J.M. & M.D. TILSON. 1989. Incidence and etiology of abdominal aortic aneurysms. Surg. Clin. N. Am. **69:** 705–711.

# Female Gender Attenuates Cytokine and Chemokine Expression and Leukocyte Recruitment in Experimental Rodent Abdominal Aortic Aneurysms

INDRANIL SINHA, BRENDA S. CHO, KAREN J. ROELOFS,
JAMES C. STANLEY, PETER K. HENKE,
AND GILBERT R. UPCHURCH, JR.

*Department of Surgery, Jobst Vascular Research Laboratories, Section of Vascular Surgery, University of Michigan, Ann Arbor, MI 48109-0329*

ABSTRACT: Female gender appears to be protective in the development of abdominal aortic aneurysms (AAAs). This study sought to identify gender differences in cytokine and chemokine expression in an experimental rodent AAA model. Male and female rodent aortas were perfused with either saline (control) or elastase to induce AAA formation. Aortic diameter was determined and aortic tissue was harvested on postperfusion days 4 and 7. Cytokine and chemokine gene expression was examined using focused gene arrays. Immunohistochemistry was used to quantify aortic leukocyte infiltration. Data were analyzed by Student's $t$-tests and ANOVA. Elastase-perfused female rodents developed significantly smaller aneurysms compared to males by day 7 ($93 \pm 10\%$ vs. $201 \pm 25\%$, $P = 0.003$). Elastase-perfused female aortas exhibited a fivefold decrease in expression of the BMP family and ligands of the TNF superfamily compared to males. In addition, the expression of members of the TGF β and VEGF families were three to fourfold lower in female elastase-perfused aortas compared to males. Multiple members of the interleukin, CC chemokine receptor, and CC ligand families were detectable in only the male elastase-perfused aortas. Female elastase-perfused aortas demonstrated a corollary twofold lower neutrophil count (females: $17.5 \pm 1.1$ PMN/HPF; males: $41 \pm 5.2$ neutrophils/HPF, $P = 0.01$) and a 1.5-fold lower macrophage count (females: $12 \pm 1.1$ macrophages/HPF; males: $17.5 \pm 1.1$ macrophages/HPF, $P = 0.003$) compared to male elastase-perfused aortas. This study documents decreased expression of multiple cytokines and chemokines and diminished leukocyte trafficking in female rat aortas compared to male aortas following elastase perfusion.

Address for correspondence: Gilbert R. Upchurch, Jr., M.D., University of Michigan Hospital, 2210 THCC, 1500 East Medical Center Drive, Ann Arbor, MI 48109-0329. Voice: 734-936-5790; fax: 734-647-9867.
e-mail: riversu@umich.edu

Ann. N.Y. Acad. Sci. 1085: 367–379 (2006). © 2006 New York Academy of Sciences.
doi: 10.1196/annals.1383.027

These genes may contribute to the gender disparity seen in AAA formation.

KEYWORDS: AAAs; gender; cytokine; chemokine; gene array

# INTRODUCTION

Male gender is a well-established risk factor in the formation of abdominal aortic aneurysms (AAA). Clinically, men form AAAs at a 4:1 ratio compared to women.[1] However, AAA development becomes accelerated in women post-menopausal.[2] These observations support the tenet that circulating estrogens may play a protective role in limiting pathologic inflammation in the aortic wall associated with AAA formation.[3] In this regard, it is known that estrogen attenuates the inflammatory response and decreases leukocyte infiltration in many nonaneurysmal cardiovascular diseases.[4]

The mechanisms underlying the gender disparity in AAA formation are not well understood. Few studies have examined the role of gender in experimental AAA models. We reported the incidence and size of AAAs are significantly less in female rodents compared to males.[5] In this regard, female aortas also exhibit significantly decreased aortic wall macrophage secreting matrix metalloproteinase (MMP)-9, an enzyme critical for AAA formation.[5,6] In a separate study, tamoxifen, a selective estrogen receptor modulator, also attenuated experimental AAA formation and limited neutrophil infiltration.[7] The present study was undertaken to determine if gender disparities in cytokine and chemokine expression contribute to decreased leukocyte trafficking in experimental female AAAs.

# MATERIALS AND METHODS

All rats were obtained from Charles River Laboratories (Wilmington, MA, USA). All experiments were approved by the University of Michigan Universal Committee on the Use and Care of Animals (UCUCA No. 8566).

## *Aneurysm Induction*

Male and female Sprague-Dawley rats, weighing 190–210 g, underwent elastase perfusion as previously described.[8] Briefly, rats were anesthetized with 1–2% isoflurane inhalation and the infrarenal aorta was isolated. Temporary control of the aorta was obtained, lumbar branches were ligated, and an aortotomy was made near the bifurcation using a 30-gauge needle. The aorta was then perfused for 30 min with either 2 mL of normal saline or 12 units of porcine pancreatic elastase (Sigma, St. Louis, MO, USA) in 2 ml of normal saline.

Infrarenal aortic diameters were measured prior to perfusion, immediately postperfusion, and prior to harvest. This was accomplished using a Spot Insight Color Optical Camera (Diagnostic Instruments, Inc., Sterling Heights, MI, USA) attached to an operating microscope (Nikon, Melville, NY, USA) utilizing Image Pro Express software (Media Cybernetics, Inc., Silver Springs, MD, USA). Aortas harvested on 4 and 7 days postperfusion ($n = 5$ to 6 at each time point for both saline controls and elastase-perfused animals) were subjected to RNA (seems like total RNA was used) extraction and paraformaldehyde fixation.

## Gene Arrays

Total RNA was isolated by treatment of aortic segments harvested on postperfusion day 4 with TRIzol reagent (Life Technologies, Rockville, MD, USA). cDNA was produced by reverse transcription using oligo-(dT) primer and M-MLV reverse transcriptase (Life Technologies). Two micrograms of total RNA from each animal ($n = 4$ per gender, per array, for both saline controls and elastase-perfused aortas) were obtained for microarray experiments. RNA labeling was accomplished using the SuperArray Amplolabeling Linear Polymerase Reaction kit (SuperArray Bioscience Corp., Frederick, MD, USA) according to the manufacturer's specifications. Hybridization was performed using Oligo-GE Q-series Rat Gene Arrays, ORN-021 (Rat Cytokine) and ORN-022 (Rat Chemokines and Receptors) per provided protocol. Gene expression was standardized to all housekeeping genes included in the corresponding array. Gene arrays were visualized using the provided Superarray Chemiluminescent Detection Kit. Photographs were obtained using a CCD camera. All data analysis was done using online GEArray Expression Analysis Suite software (http://geasuite.superarray.com).

## Immunohistochemistry

Aortic tissue was fixed in 4% paraformaldehyde for 20 h, transferred to 70% ethanol, and subsequently embedded in paraffin for immunohistochemistry. Aortic tissue deparaffinization and rehydration were performed using xylene and graded alcohols. The sections were stained for macrophages and neutrophils using the following procedures. The aortic sections were deparaffinized in xylene and rehydrated in graded alcohols.

For neutrophil staining, blocking buffer was then applied to prevent nonspecific binding. Rabbit anti-rat neutrophil primary antibody (Accurate Chemical and Scientific Corporation, Westbury, NY, USA) was used for staining, followed by an antirabbit IgG biotinylated secondary antibody and avidin-biotin complex-AP reagent available in the Rabbit IgG Alkaline Phosphatase ABC Kit (Vector Laboratories, Burlingame, CA, USA). The sections were then visualized using the Vector Red Alkaline Phosphatase Substrate Kit I (Vector Laboratories) and counterstained with Hematoxylin QS (Vector Laboratories).

Macrophage staining entailed heat-induced epitope retrieval using 10 mM sodium citrate, pH 6.0, in a microwave. The sections were subsequently incubated with 3% hydrogen peroxide in methanol to block endogenous peroxidase activity, followed by a blocking buffer to prevent nonspecific binding. Mouse antirat CD68 primary antibody (Serotec, Raleigh, NC, USA) was used for staining, followed by an antimouse IgG biotinylated secondary antibody and an avidin-biotin-HRP complex, available in the Mouse IgG Elite Vectastain ABC Kit (Vector Laboratories). Sections were then visualized using a DAB Peroxidase Substrate Kit (Vector Laboratories) and counterstained with Hematoxylin QS (Vector Laboratories). All cell counts were done by a trained, blinded observer in 10 separate 100× high-powered fields (HPF) of both the adventitia and media. A mean value was then calculated for positively stained cells in each animal.

## Statistics

Data analysis was performed using nonpaired Student's *t*-tests and analysis of variance (ANOVA) with significance set as $P < 0.05$. All data are expressed as the mean ± standard error of the mean (SEM). Statistical analysis was performed using SigmaStat (Version 2.03, Copyright 1992–1997, SPSS Inc.).

## RESULTS

### Female Aortas Form Smaller Experimental AAAs

Saline-perfused aortas did not form aneurysms in either gender. Mean diameters of elastase-perfused male aortas increased 88 ± 2.7% and 201 ± 25.1% by postperfusion days 4 and 7, respectively. In contrast, the mean diameters of female elastase-perfused aortas increased 65 ± 4.4% ($P = 0.002$) and 93 ± 10% ($P = 0.003$) by postperfusion days 4 and 7, respectively (FIG. 1). Six of six elastase-perfused male aortas formed aneurysms as defined by a 100% increase in aortic diameter by postperfusion day 7 in contrast to one of six elastase-perfused female aortas.

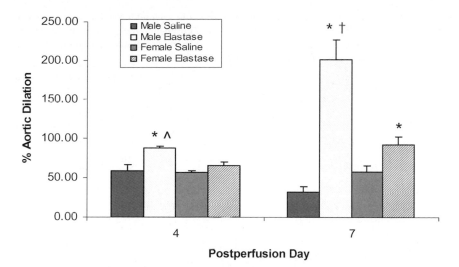

**FIGURE 1.** Attenuated experimental AAA formation in females. Elastase-perfused male aortas were significantly larger than elastase-perfused female aortas (N = 5 to 6 per group at each day of harvest) by postoperative day 7. Six of six elastase-perfused male aortas formed aneurysms by day 7 as defined by a 100% increase in aortic diameter. In contrast, only one of six female elastase-perfused aorta became aneurysmal by postperfusion day 7. No saline-perfused aortas became aneurysmal in either gender. *$P < 0.05$ for elastase-perfused aortas compared to same postperfusion day saline perfused control for that gender, †$P < 0.05$ for elastase-perfused male aortas compared to same postperfusion day elastase-perfused female aortas.

## Female Aortas Exhibited Decreased Expression of Multiple Cytokines and Chemokines by Gene Array on Postperfusion Day 4

No appreciable cytokine or chemokine expression was demonstrated in saline-perfused male or female control aortas on postperfusion day 4. Elastase-perfused female aortas compared to elastase-perfused male aortas exhibited a fivefold decrease in expression of multiple genes in the bone morphogenetic protein (BMP) family, including BMP1, BMP6, BMP7, and BMP15, and tumor necrosis factor superfamily ligands (TNFSF), specifically TNFSF4, TNFSF6, TNFSF9, and TNFSF14. The transforming growth factor beta (TGFβ) family, specifically TGFβ1, TGFβ2, and TGFβ3, as well as vascular endothelial growth factor VEGF1 and VEGF2, were three to fourfold lower in female elastase-perfused aortas compared to male elastase-perfused aortas. Multiple members of the interleukin (IL) family were detectable in only the male elastase-perfused aortas including IL8 receptor α and β, IL11, IL12, and IL13. Similarly, multiple genes of the CC chemokine receptor (CCR) family, specifically CCR2, CCR6, CCR7, and CCR9 as well as the CC ligand

**TABLE 1. Female gender and decreased cytokine and chemokine expression in experimental AAA formation. Note decreased cytokine and chemokine production in female elastase-perfused aortas on postperfusion day 4. ND (none detectable) denotes expression was present in males, but not detectable in female aortas**

| Cytokine/Chemokine | Fold decrease in females |
|---|---|
| Bone morphogenetic protein (BMP) family | |
| BMP1 | 6.1 |
| BMP6 | 6.3 |
| BMP7 | 5.6 |
| BMP15 | 6.3 |
| C-C Chemokine ligand family | |
| CCL24 | ND |
| CCL25 | ND |
| CCL28 | ND |
| C-C Chemokine receptor family | |
| CCR2 | ND |
| CCR7 | ND |
| CCR8 | ND |
| Interleukin (IL) family | |
| IL1 | 6.2 |
| IL2 | 6.1 |
| IL3 | 4.9 |
| IL5 | 4.9 |
| IL7 | 5.9 |
| IL8$\alpha$ | ND |
| IL8$\beta$ | ND |
| IL11 | 6 |
| IL12 | 6.3 |
| Transforming growth factor (TGF) family | |
| TGF$\beta$1 | 4.1 |
| TGF$\beta$2 | 4.2 |
| Tumor necrosis factor (TNF) family | |
| TNFSF4 | ND |
| TNFSF6 | ND |
| TNFSF9 | ND |
| TNFSF15 | ND |
| Vascular endothelial growth factor family | |
| VEGF1 | 3.6 |
| VEGF2 | 3.6 |

(CCL) family, specifically CCL3, CCL5, CCL24, CCL25, and CCL28, were detectable in male elastase-perfused aortas, but not in female elastase-perfused aortas (TABLE 1).

### Female Aortas Exhibit Decreased Neutrophil and Macrophage Infiltration

Minimal neutrophil and macrophage infiltration was detected in both male and female saline perfumed aortas. Male elastase-perfused aortas demonstrated $13.7 \pm 5.9$ positively staining cells/HPF in males compared to $5.0 \pm 0.5$

neutrophils/HPF ($P = 0.09$) in females on postperfusion day 4. By postperfusion day 7, male elastase-perfused aortas demonstrated a twofold greater neutrophil count ($40.75 \pm 5.2$ PMN/HPF) in comparison to female elastase-perfused aortas ($17.5 \pm 1.1$ PMN/HPF, $P = 0.01$) (FIGS. 2A and B). Male elastase-perfused aortas also demonstrated $12.2 \pm 5.1$ and $17.5 \pm 1.1$ CD68 positive cells (macrophages)/HPF on postperfusion days 4 and 7, respectively. Number of macrophages was significantly fewer in females ($4.7 \pm 1.1$ macrophages/HPF on postperfusion day 4, $P = 0.2$, and $11.8 \pm 1.1$ macrophages/HPF on postperfusion day 7, $P = 0.003$) (FIGS. 3A and B).

## DISCUSSION

This study confirms that female rodents develop significantly smaller experimental AAAs compared to males. Cytokine and chemokine gene arrays identified several cytokine and chemokine families, which were differentially expressed by gender including BMP, TNF, TGFβ, IL, CCR, and CCL gene families. Furthermore, female rat aortas exhibited significantly fewer infiltrating neutrophils and macrophages by postperfusion day 7.

It is possible that the known effect of estrogen in females on inflammatory processes in cardiovascular diseases may be associated with the observed decreased leukocyte cell infiltration in females and their apparent resistance to AAA formation.[9] Multiple studies have shown estrogen plays a protective role by attenuating inflammatory cell mediated damage by downregulating cytokine and chemokine expression. In two separate AAA models, female gender has been shown to limit experimental AAA formation, at least in part by limiting neutrophil and macrophage infiltrate.[4,10] In addition, Miller *et al.* observed that estrogen attenuation of the early inflammatory response following endoluminal vascular injury was associated with decreased expression of several cytokines and chemokines, especially the CXC chemokine family.[11] This was accompanied with decreased neutrophil and macrophage infiltration and vasoprotection through an apparent anti-inflammatory pathway.[11] Estrogen is also known to decrease myocardial inflammation and damage following ischemia-reperfusion injury by downregulating proinflammatory cytokines such as TNFα, IL1β, and IL6.[12]

Estrogen also attenuates inflammation-mediated damage in nonvascular tissue. Santizo *et al.* demonstrated that chronic estrogen depletion enhanced leukocyte adhesion in the rat cerebral circulation and suggested this was a mechanism underlying increased neural damage in ovariectomized females as compared to intact females.[13] In addition, estrogen has been observed to enhance wound healing through an anti-inflammatory effect by limiting neutrophil and macrophage infiltration and suppressing the production of numerous cytokines including TNFα and macrophage migration inhibitory factor (MIF).[14]

Estrogen is likely to decrease cytokine and chemokine expression through multiple mechanisms. First, estrogen decreases p38 mitogen activated protein kinase (MAPK), a crucial upstream proinflammatory regulator of numerous cytokines, including TNFα, IL1, IL4, IL6, and IL8.[15] Wang *et al.* demonstrated decreased p38 MAPK phosphorylation (activation) in control females compared to oophorectomized females and control males following ischemia/reperfusion injury.[12] Second, estrogen also decreases the activity of nuclear factor κB (NFκB), a key proinflammatory transcription factor.[16] Finally, estrogen decreases oxidant stress, a stimuli for the production of multiple inflammatory cytokines in ischemia/reperfusion injury.[15]

**(A)**

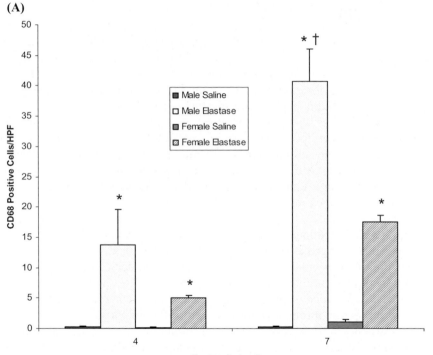

**FIGURE 2.** Female gender and decreased aortic wall neutrophil infiltration. (**A**) Immunohistochemistry (100×) by postoperative day 7 revealed significantly increased neutrophil infiltration in the adventitia of male aortas compared to female aortas. Few positively stained cells were identified in saline-perfused controls of either gender. *$P < 0.05$ for elastase-perfused aortas compared to same postperfusion day saline-perfused control for that gender, †$P < 0.05$ for elastase-perfused male aortas compared to same postperfusion day elastase-perfused females, N = 4 per group at each day of harvest. (**B,C**) Representative images of positively staining cells (arrows) in the adventitia of elastase-perfused male (**B**) and fewer positively staining cells in the female aortas (**C**) (100×). [Saline-perfused aortas not shown.]

**(B)**

**(C)**

**FIGURE 2.** Continued.

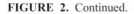

The present intervention demonstrates multiple cytokine families that were differentially regulated by gender, although their role in AAA pathogenesis has not been thoroughly investigated. Others have provided some insight into this subject. Dai *et al.* have previously shown that adenoviral delivery mediated exogenous overexpression of TGF-β1 stabilized preformed experimental AAAs.[17] However, no studies to date have examined gender differences in TGFβ regulation in experimental AAAs. Similarly, the TNF superfamily is known to have a role in AAA pathogenesis, but no studies have assessed gender difference in AAA formation.[6] Kobayashi *et al.* demonstrated VEGF to be upregulated in AAAs, but a role in AAA pathogenesis remains unclear.[18] Certain ILs are known to be critical to AAA formation, but no evidence exists for the roles of IL11, IL12, or IL13.[6]

A limited number of investigators have examined the role of chemokines in AAA formation. Zhao *et al.* demonstrated that macrophage inhibitory protein (MIP)1α (also known as CCL3), which was differentially expressed by gender in the present study, and MIP2 (CXCL2) were important in experimental AAA formation.[19] Similarly, Yamagishi *et al.* observed an elevenfold increase in CXCR2 production in human AAAs compared to control healthy aortas.[20] However, no studies to date have elucidated gender differences in the patterns of chemokine expression.

**(A)**

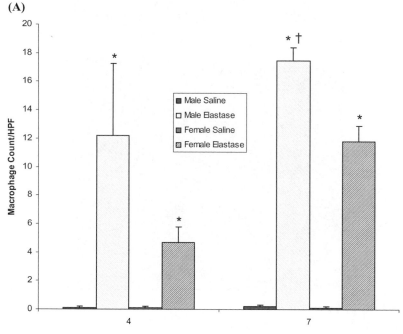

**FIGURE 3.** Female gender and decreased aortic wall macrophage infiltration. **(A)** Immunohistochemistry (100×) by postoperative day 7 revealed significantly increased macrophage infiltration in the adventitia of male aortas compared to female aortas. Minimally positively stained cells were identified in saline-perfused controls of either gender. *$P < 0.05$ for elastase-perfused aortas compared to same postperfusion day saline-perfused control for that gender, †$P < 0.05$ for elastase-perfused male aortas compared to same postperfusion day elastase-perfused females, N = 4 per group at each day of harvest. **(B,C)** Representative images of positively CD68 staining cells (arrows) in the adventitia of elastase-perfused male **(B)** and minimal positively staining cells in the female aortas **(C)** (100×). (Saline-perfused aortas not shown.)

**(B)**

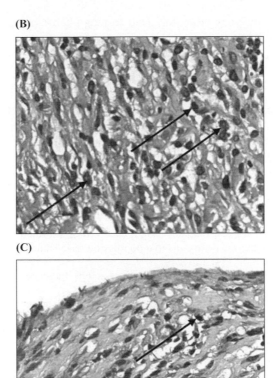

**(C)**

**FIGURE 3.** Continued.

The present investigation supports the speculation that a number of cytokines and chemokines may be differentially regulated by gender and may contribute to vessel wall injury. More reliable polymerase chain reaction or northern blotting data will be required to confirm these observations. This study also only examined postperfusion day 4 and therefore does not take into account genes that may be upregulated either earlier or later in experimental AAA formation. Additionally, it will be necessary to determine if gender differences in cytokine and chemokine differences are intrinsic to the wall or secondary to diminished leukocyte trafficking into female aortas. Nevertheless, this study has identified multiple gene families that deserve further consideration for a potential role in gender differences during AAA formation. Furthermore, continuing research is needed to more fully elucidate the mechanism by which estrogen acts to decrease cytokine and chemokine expression. A better understanding of gender disparities may ultimately lead to new pharmacological targets for the treatment of AAAs.

## ACKNOWLEDGMENTS

This work was supported by NIH KO8 (HL67885-02) (GRU), Von Liebig Award-Lifeline Foundation (GRU), the Lifeline Medical Student Research Award (IS), the Griswold and Margery H. Ruth Alpha Omega Alpha Medical Student Research Fellowship (IS), and the Jobst Foundation.

## REFERENCES

1. SINGH, K., K.H. BONAA, B.K. JOCOBSEN, et al. 2001. Prevalence and risk factors for abdominal aortic aneurysms in a population based study: the Tromso study. Am. J. Epidemiol. **154:** 236–244.
2. BENGTSSON, H., B. SONESSON & D. BERGVIST. 1996. Incidence and prevalence of AAA. N. Y. Acad. Sci. **800:** 1–24.
3. LAVECCHIA, C., A. DECARLI, S. FRANCESCHI, et al. 1987. Menstrual and reproductive factors and the risk of myocardial infarction in women under fifty-years of age. Am. J. Obstet. Gynecol. **157:** 1108–1112.
4. BAKER, L., K.K. MELDRUM, M. WANG, et al. 2003. The role of estrogen in cardiovascular disease. J. Surg. Res. **115:** 325–344.
5. AILAWADI, G., J.L. ELIASON, K.J. ROELOFS, et al. 2004. Gender differences in experimental aneurysm formation. Arterioscler Thromb. Vasc. Biol. **24:** 2116–2122.
6. AILAWADI, G., J.L. ELIASON & G.R. UPCHURCH. 2003. Current concepts in the pathogenesis of abdominal aortic aneurysms. J. Vasc. Surg. **38:** 584–588.
7. GRIGORYANTS, V., K.K. HANNAWA, C.G. PEARCE, et al. 2005. Tamoxifen up-regulates catalase production, inhibits vessel wall neutrophil recruitment, and attenuates development of experimental abdominal aortic aneurysms. J. Vasc. Surg. **41:** 108–114.
8. ANIDJAR, S., J.L. SALZMANN, D. GENTRIC, et al. 1990. Elastase induced experimental aneurysms in rats. Circulation **82:** 973–981.
9. LEINWAND, L.A. 2003. Sex is a potent modifier of the cardiovascular system. J. Clin. Invest. **112:** 302–307.
10. MARTIN-MCNULTY, B., D.M. THAM, C. DA, et al. 2003. 17 β-estradiol attenuates development of angiotensin II-induced aortic abdominal aneurysm in apolipoprotein E-deficient mice. Arterioscler Thromb. Vasc. Biol. **23:** 1627–1632.
11. MILLER, A.P., W. FENG, D. XING, et al. 2004. Estrogen modulated inflammatory mediator expression and neutrophil chemotaxis in injured arteries. Circulation **110:** 1664–1669.
12. WANG, M., B.M. TSAI, K.M. REIGER, et al. 2006. 17-β-estradiol decreases p38 MAPK-mediated myocardial inflammation and dysfunction following acute ischemia. J. Mol. Cell. Cardiol. **40:** 205–212.
13. SANTIZO, R. & D.A. PELLIGRINO. 1999. Estrogen reduces leukocyte adhesion in the cerebral circulation of female rats. J. Cereb Blood Flow Metab. **19:** 1061–1065.

14. ASHCROFT, G.S., S.J. MILLS, K. LEI, *et al.* 2003. Estrogen modulated cutaneous wound healing by downregulating macrophage migration inhibitory factor. J. Clin. Invest. **111:** 1309–1318.
15. KHER, A., M. WANG, B.M. TSAI, *et al.* 2005. Sex differences in the myocardial inflammatory response to acute injury. Shock **23:** 1–10.
16. DESHPANDE, R., H. KHALILI, R.G. PERGOLIZZI, *et al.* 1997. Estradiol down-regulates LPS-induced cytokine production and NFκB activation in murine macrophages. Am. J. Reprod. Immunol. **38:** 46–54.
17. DAI, J., F. LOSY, A.M. GUINAULT, *et al.* 2005. Overexpression of transforming growth factor-beta1 stabilizes already formed aortic aneurysms: a first approach to induction of functional healing by endovascular gene therapy. Circulation **112:** 1008–1015.
18. KOBAYASHI, M., J. MATSUBARA, M. MATSHUSHITA, *et al.* 2002. Expression of angiogenesis and angiogenic factors in human aortic vascular disease. J. Surg. Res. **106:** 239–245.
19. ZHAO, L., M.P. MOOS, R. GRABNER, *et al.* 2004. The 5-lipoxygenase pathway promotes pathogenesis of hyperlipidemia-dependent aortic aneurysm. Nat. Med. **10:** 966–973.
20. YAMAGISHI, M., T. HIGASHIKATA, H. ISHIBASHI-UEDA, *et al.* 2005. Sustained upregulation of inflammatory chemokine and its receptor in aneurysmal and occlusive atherosclerotic disease: results from tissue analysis with cDNA macroarray and real-time reverse transcriptional polymerase chain reaction methods. Circ. J. **69:** 1490–1495.

# Features and Genomic Origins of Matrix Cell Adhesion Molecules-1 and -2 Expressed by Fibroblasts of Human Aortic Adventitial Origin

M.D. TILSON III

*Columbia University and the St. Luke's-Roosevelt Hospital Center, New York, New York, USA*

ABSTRACT: Precursor mRNAs for proteins that we have called matrix cell adhesion molecules-1 and -2 (Mat-CAM-1 and Mat-CAM-2) were cloned from fibroblasts cultured from a specimen of human abdominal aorta. Both protein sequences have the unusual feature that there is an immunoglobulin kappa (Igκ)-like domain at the N terminus and they are glycine/proline rich in the C-terminal domain. Antibodies were raised in rabbit against peptides synthesized for a specific unique sequence of Mat-CAM-1 and Mat-CAM-2, respectively (not detected in any other proteins referenced in GenBank). Both antibodies were immunoreactive with adventitial microfibrils of the aorta and some additional arteries. Mat-CAM-1 was detected in the common/internal iliac arteries, but it was not detected in the external iliac artery. Conversely, Mat-CAM-2 was conspicuous in the external iliac artery, but not the common/internal iliac arteries. Thus, these proteins show features of site-specific expression within the arterial tree. Computerized searches show that the genomic origins of Mat-CAM-1 and -2 are in the so-called nasopharnygocarcinoma (NPC) gene on chromosome 2, which is a putative oncogene. Expression of the two different gene products from the same genomic sequence requires shifts of reading frame. Further studies will be required to determine whether these proteins are prototypes for a larger family of tissue-specific matrix proteins arising from alternative transcriptions of the same genomic sequence.

KEYWORDS: Mat-CAM-1; fibroblasts; aortic adventitia; Nasophyarngo-carcinoma gene (NPC); aneurysm; alternate splicing

Address for correspondence: M. David Tilson III, M.D., Department of Surgery, St. Luke's-Roosevelt Hospital Center, 1000 Tenth Avenue, New York, NY 10019. Voice: 212-523-7780; fax: 212-523-6495. e-mail: mdt1@columbia.edu

Ann. N.Y. Acad. Sci. 1085: 380–386 (2006). © 2006 New York Academy of Sciences. doi: 10.1196/annals.1383.017

# BACKGROUND

The cDNAs for molecules we named matrix cell adhesion molecules-1 and -2 (Mat-CAM-1 and Mat-CAM-2) were cloned from an expression library developed from a surgical specimen of abdominal aortic aneurysm (AAA). They were originally referenced as recombinant clones-1 and -5 (r-CL-1 and r-Clone-5),[1] We have also referred to them as "kappafibs" because (1) both proteins have N-terminal domains that resemble Ig-κ light chains and (2) they are detected in fibroblasts and microfibrils of connective tissue matrix.[2] A revision of the sequence of the precursor mRNA was reported to GenBank (Accession No. AF186176) in 2001.[3]

We additionally referenced Mat-CAM-1 (and also the aneurysm-associated-antigenic-protein-40kDa, AAAP-40) as "aorta-specific-antigenic proteins" (ASAPs). However, we found that this definition was too "specific," because the proteins were detected in other arterial vessels.[4] The acronym ASAP is still acceptable for "artery-specific antigenic proteins" because immunoreactivity is only minimally detectable in tissues other than arteries. Here we report additional studies on the tissue and cellular localization of Mat-CAM-1 and Mat-CAM-2, and we confirm previously reported differences based on the study of arterial specimens from a single autopsy cadaver with all specimens harvested at one time and processed in the same batch of immunohistological preparations.

In another publication, we traced similarities of the putative protein sequences for Mat-CAMs-1 and -2 to a collagen-associated fibrinogen-like protein of the dermis of the sea cucumber.[5] Here we report a computer-based search for the origin of the Mat-CAM-1 gene itself in the human genome.

# METHODS

The following methods were adopted:

(1) Antibodies were raised in rabbit by a commercial vendor for synthetic peptides based on unique sequences in the predicted proteins (e.g., not detected elsewhere in the human protein database [GenBank NR]) as previously described.[2,5] Serial sections were cut from specimens of multiple arterial segments harvested at a single human autopsy and they were used for comparative immunohistochemistry (IHC). All slides were processed as a single batch and laid out on a desktop scanner for imaging as a single high-resolution visual display. These steps were taken to avoid any possible sources of artifact in the selection of sections of interest for photomicroscopy and comparison.

(2) Similar preparations were performed on sections from an autopsy of a C57-BL6 mouse as dissected by my student, D. Syn (1999), and photographed in FIGURE 1.

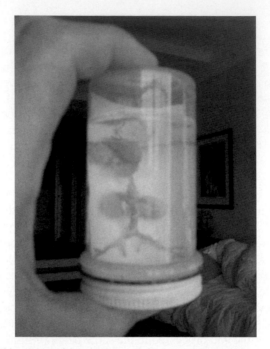

**FIGURE 1.** Dissection of the arterial tree of a C57-BL6 laboratory mouse for immuno-histochemical studies of the regional distribution of Mat-CAMs-1 and -2 in the murine arterial tree.

(3) Immunohistochemistry was performed on fibroblast cell cultures from normal human aorta and skin by my students, J. Gefen and D.R. Ewing (2000) and A. Bhatti and T. Jordan (2001).

(4) A search for the genomic origin of Mat-CAM-1was carried out with BLASTn available at the web site of the NCBI and referenced to the USC BLAT Human Genome Assembly.

(5) Alternate splicing was detected by inspection of the aligned DNA and protein sequences with assistance of word processor software (WP5.1 under DOS).

## RESULTS

The results can be summarized as:

(1) Immunoreactivity (IHR) of human arterial specimens for Mat-CAM-1 antibody was conspicuous in the microfibrils of the adventitia of the aorto-common internal iliac system, but IHR was not detected in the external iliac artery. Conversely, antibody against Mat-CAM-2 showed maximal IHR in the external iliac artery. These findings are illustrated in FIGURE 2.

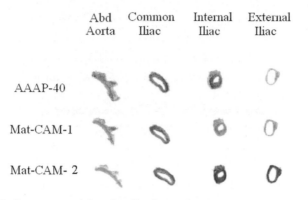

|  | Abd Aorta | Common Iliac | Internal Iliac | External Iliac |
|---|---|---|---|---|
| AAAP-40 | | | | |
| Mat-CAM-1 | | | | |
| Mat-CAM- 2 | | | | |

**FIGURE 2.** Immunoreactivity of antibodies against Mat-CAM-1 and Mat-CAM-2 for aorta, common, internal, and external iliac arteries based on serial sections of paraffin blocks of tissue harvested at a single human autopsy. Original slides were scanned together on a flatbed office machine so that all comparisons would be comparable. There was no initial magnification in the flatbed scan.

(2) IHR in mouse for Mat-CAM-1 and -2 was similar in distribution to the pattern observed in human (not shown).

(3) IHR for Mat-CAM-1 was strongly positive in cultured aortic fibroblasts as shown in FIGURE 3, but IHR in cultured dermal fibroblasts was not detectable. As in the studies of arteries obtained at a single human autopsy, the converse results were obtained with antibody against Mat-CAM-2.

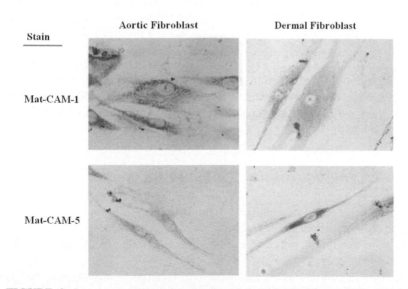

| Stain | Aortic Fibroblast | Dermal Fibroblast |
|---|---|---|
| Mat-CAM-1 | | |
| Mat-CAM-5 | | |

**FIGURE 3.** Immunoreactivity of antibodies against Mat-CAM-1 and Mat-CAM-2 in cell cultures of human aortic fibroblasts and human dermal fibroblasts.

Search for genomic origin of Mat-CAM-1

(908 letters)

Distribution of 41 Blast Hits on the Query Sequence

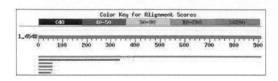

Leads to chromosome 2 reference genomic sequence

## NT_015805

**which is the
so-called**

# Nasopharyngocarcinoma

# Gene

**FIGURE 4.** A BLASTn search for the genomic origin of Mat-CAM-1 localizes to the NPC gene on chromosome 2.

(4) The origin of both the N-terminal and C-terminal domains of Mat-CAM-1 are in the nasopharyngealcarcinoma gene (NPC) on chromosome 2p11.2. Our initial search gave e @ ~ (-176). Another search shown in FIGURE 4 gave $e = 0.0$

(5) The observed cDNA sequence of Mat-CAM-1 can be explained by frameshifts in the transcription of a portion of the NPC gene as illustrated by the boxes of clusters of amino acid sequences in the hypothetical protein in FIGURE 5. A similar situation was observed in the translation of Mat-CAM-2 (data not shown).

## DISCUSSION AND SPECULATIONS

In consideration of these observations, Mat-CAM-2 can no longer be considered to be an ASAP as it was abundantly detected in skin.

We also found immunoreactivity for Mat-CAM-2 in other tissues including peritoneal surfaces.

Mat-CAMs 1 and 2 may be representative of a larger family of genes based on alternative splicing of a single genomic sequence. Tissue-specific communications from matrix molecules to resident or transient cellular elements should

Coding sequence of the NPC gene:

```
CCGCCAUCUGAUGAGCAGUUGAAAUCUGGAACUGCCUCUGUUGUGUGCCUGCU
UUCUAUCCCAGAGAGGCCAAAGUACAGUGGAAGGUGGAUAACGCCCUCCAAUCC
UCCCAGGAGAGUGUCACAGAGCAGGACAGCAAGGACAGCACCUACAGCCUCAGC
```

Translations of coding sequence in three frames. Red boxes highlight the shifts in reading frame that are inferred from the experimentally determined sequence of Mat-CAM-1:

```
P P S D E Q L K S G T A S V V C L L N N
R H L M S S * N L E L P L L C A C *I T
A I * * A V E I W N C L C C V P A E * L
```

```
F Y F R E A K V Q W K V D N A L Q S G N
S I P E R P K Y S G R W I T P S N R V T
L S Q R G Q S T V E G G * R P P I G * L
```

```
S Q E S V T E Q D S K D S T Y S L S S T
P R R V S Q S R T A R T A P T A S A A P
P G E C H R A G Q Q G Q H L Q P Q Q H P
```

**FIGURE 5.** Shifts in reading frame in expression of a region of the NPC gene are required to explain the mRNA sequence and hypothetical amino acid sequence of Mat-CAM-1. The boxes in the figure illustrate the hypothetical shifts in the reading frame.

be approachable by future studies. The great diversity of these phenomena may be too complex to permit explanation on the basis of our parsimonious repertoire of only ~30,000 genes unless some genes serve multiple tissue-specific functions. The author has previously speculated that the sudden evolutionary appearance of the diversity of the soluble Ig family might be explained by millions of previous years of diversification of molecules based on alternative splicing of Ig-like molecules with matrix functions that are more primitive than soluble immunity.[5] At that particular juncture in evolutionary history, a few mutational events may have enabled matrix cells to circulate as B cell precursors and release soluble Igs. This hypothesis is highly speculative, but there has never been a satisfying explanation for the sudden Big Bang in the development of soluble immunity.

## CONCLUSION

Mat-CAM-1 has a regional distribution in the arterial tree that resembles the specificity of aneurysm-prone vessels (e.g., common and internal iliac, but not external iliac arteries). Mat-CAM-1 is expressed by fibroblasts of aorta, but not fibroblasts from skin. The converse tissue distribution is observed for Mat-CAM-2. The genomic sequences for these mRNAs are in the NPC gene and their expression requires the hypothesis of tissue-specific alternative splicing.

## REFERENCES

1. OZSVATH, K.J., S. XIA, H. HIROSE & M.D. TILSON. 1996. Two hypothetical proteins of human aortic adventitia, with Ig kappa, collagenous, and aromatic-rich motifs. Biochem. Biophys. Res. Commun. **225:** 500–504.
2. OZSVATH, K.J., H. HIROSE, S. XIA, *et al*. 1997. Expression of two novel recombinant proteins from aortic adventitia (kappafibs) sharing amino acid sequences with cytomegalovirus. J. Surg. Res. **69:** 277–282.
3. TILSON, M.D., *et al*. 2001 (Aug. 22). NCBI Gen Bank. Accession #AF186176.
4. CHEW, D.K., J. KNOETGEN, III, S. XIA, *et al*. 1999. Regional distribution in human of a novel aortic collagen-associated microfibrillar protein. Exp. Mol. Pathol. **66:** 59–65.
5. TILSON, M.D. & A. RZHETSKY. 2000. A novel hypothesis regarding the evolutionary origins of the immunoglobulin fold. Curr. Med. Res. Opin. **16:** 88–93.

# Arterial Aneurysms in HIV Patients

## Molecular Mimicry versus Direct Infection?

M.D. TILSON III AND L. WITHERS

*Columbia University and the St. Luke's-Roosevelt Hospital Center, New York, New York, USA*

ABSTRACT: There is growing literature on the subject of aneurysmal degeneration of arteries in patients who are infected with HIV. A patient recently seen at our medical center with an aneurysm of the carotid artery stimulated our interest in reviewing the mechanisms by which HIV may initiate or predispose to these pathologies. There are at least three major possibilities: (1) immunodeficiency allows bacteria that are known to cause mycotic aneurysms to proliferate without immune restraint; (2) one or more of the HIV envelope proteins sufficiently resemble one or more artery-specific-antigenic proteins (ASAPs) that may trigger an autoimmune response (molecular mimicry); and (3) the HIV virus itself infects arterial-resident cells that maintain the integrity of the load-bearing matrix. The computational searches reported here suggest that the ASAP, matrix cell adhesion molecule-1 (Mat-CAM-1), has a high degree of similarity to known ligands for HIV envelope proteins gp41 and gp120. No similarities of Mat-CAM-1 to the HIV envelope glycoproteins were detected. Accordingly, among the possibilities for explaining the HIV/aneurysm connection, direct infection of aortic fibroblasts by the HIV virus is more likely to be the pathogenetic mechanism than the process of molecular mimicry.

KEYWORDS: carotid; aneurysm; molecular mimicry; infection; HIV; Mat-CAM-1; autoimmunity; epitopes

## INTRODUCTION

The first cases of "cerebral arteriopathy" were reported in pediatric AIDS patients in 1987.[1] In 1989 Sinzobahamvya et al.[2] reported four cases of aneurysms of the carotid artery. The authors attributed three of the cases to infection by microorganisms known to cause mycotic aneurysms, but they suggested that the fourth case might be due to primary infection by the HIV virus. The recent presentation of a 49-year-old male patient at our institution

Address for correspondence: M. David Tilson III, M.D., Department of Surgery, St. Luke's-Roosevelt Hospital Center, 1000 Tenth Avenue, New York, NY 10019. Voice: 212-523-7780; fax: 212-523-6495. e-mail: mdt1@columbia.edu

Ann. N.Y. Acad. Sci. 1085: 387–391 (2006). © 2006 New York Academy of Sciences. doi: 10.1196/annals.1383.018

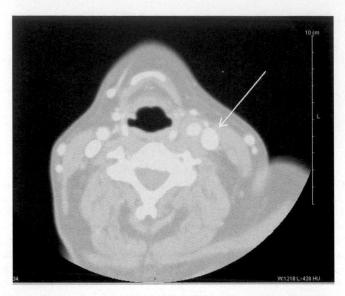

**FIGURE 1.** CT scan of the patient with HIV infection and AAA. There is a zone of low attenuation surrounding the central enhancing lumen and deep to the vessel wall at the level of the left carotid bulb. There is a mild degree of luminal narrowing and irregularity. There are inflammatory changes of the surrounding fat. These findings suggest an inflammatory aneurysm of the left carotid artery.

with an aneurysm of the left common and internal carotid artery prompted our interest in reviewing this subject. The CT scan of this patient is illustrated in FIGURE 1.

Arterial aneurysms in HIV are not limited to the cerebral circulation. In 1995, 16 cases of aneurysms affecting a variety of arteries were described during a 4-year period at a single hospital.[3] By 1999, arterial aneurysms in HIV patients were described as a "distinct clinicopathological entity."[4] However, the association of vasculopathy and HIV has been described as "enigmatic."[5,6] Here we report the results of GenBank searches relevant to the molecular mechanisms of the disease process.

## BACKGROUND FOR DATABASE SEARCHES

Ten years ago we reported the cDNA sequences of two clones from an expression library derived from abdominal aortic adventitia,[7] which encoded unique hypothetical proteins with an N-terminal immunoglobulin-kappa (Igκ)-like domain. The C-terminals had domains with glycine/proline-rich and aromatic amino acid-rich motifs suggestive of proteins of extracellular matrix. The deduced amino acid sequence for "clone 1" in that report has been renamed matrix cell adhesion molecule–1 (Mat-CAM-1) by customary usage in our

```
 1     M D M R V P A Q L L G L L L L W L P G A        20

21     R C D I Q L T Q S P S L L S A S V G D R        40

41     V M I T C R A S Q A I S S F L A W Y Q Q        60

61     K P G K A P K L L I H A A S S L Q T G V        80

81     P S R F S G S G S G T                          91
```

**FIGURE 2.** Amino acid sequence deduced from the Mat-CAM-1 cDNA sequence.

laboratory. A revised edition of the experimentally determined cDNA was posted to GenBank in 2001.[8]

The cDNA sequence translates without any ambiguities over a span of 273 base pairs and specifies the amino acid residues shown in FIGURE 2.

In theory, if the envelope proteins of HIV1 (gp41 or gp120) share epitopes with an ASAP such as Mat-CAM-1, infection with HIV may trigger an autoimmune response against the arterial matrix. This situation has been described as "molecular mimicry." However, if Mat-CAM-1 has a high degree of homology with Igs that are HIV-ligands, the virus may be infecting arterial fibroblasts directly when Mat-CAM-1 is expressed on the surfaces of the cells and provides a site for attachment of the virus.

## RESULTS OF SEARCHES

No candidate epitopes were detected in Mat-CAM-1 by NCBI BLAST-p to support the hypothesis of "molecular mimicry." However, there were significant similarities of the variable domain of Mat-CAM-1 with antibodies against gp41 and gp120 as shown in FIGURES 3 and 4.

```
>gi|732746|emb|CAA84391.1| antibody, light chain variable region to HIV1 gp41
[Homo sapiens]
Length=115

 Score = 135 bits (340),  Expect = 3e-32
 Identities = 66/73 (90%), Positives = 70/73 (95%), Gaps = 0/73 (0%)

Query  18   PGARCDIQLTQSPSLLSASVGDRVMITCRASQAISSFLAWYQQKPGKAPKLLIHAASSLQ  77
            PGARCDIQLTQSPS LSASVGDRV ITCRASQ ISS+LAWYQQKPGKAPKLLI+AAS+LQ
Sbjct  1    PGARCDIQLTQSPSFLSASVGDRVTITCRASQGISSYLAWYQQKPGKAPKLLIYAASTLQ  60

Query  78   TGVPSRFSGSGSG  90
            +GVPSRFSGSGSG
Sbjct  61   SGVPSRFSGSGSG  73
```

**FIGURE 3.** Results of a BLAST search with the Mat-CAM-1 cDNA sequences showing similarity to an antibody against the HIV1 gp41 sequence.

```
>gi|732738|emb|CAA84388.1| antibody light chain variable region to HIV1 gp120
[Homo sapiens]
Length=111

 Score =  125 bits (314),  Expect = 3e-29
 Identities = 61/73 (83%), Positives = 68/73 (93%), Gaps = 0/73 (0%)

Query  19   GARCDIQLTQSPSLLSASVGDRVMITCRASQAISSFLAWYQQKPGKAPKLLIHAASSLQT   78
            GARCDIQ+TQSPS LSASVGDRV ITC+ASQ IS++L WYQQKPGKAPKLLI+ AS+L+T
Sbjct  2    GARCDIQMTQSPSSLSASVGDRVTITCQASQDISNYLNWYQQKPGKAPKLLIYDASNLET   61

Query  79   GVPSRFSGSGSGT   91
            GVPSRFSGSGSGT
Sbjct  62   GVPSRFSGSGSGT   74
```

**FIGURE 4.** Results of a BLAST search with the Mat-CAM-1 cDNA sequences showing similarity to an antibody against the HIV1 gp120 sequence.

## CONCLUSION

An HIV-associated carotid aneurysm was diagnosed at our medical center with clinical similarities to previously reported cases. The molecular similarity of Mat-CAM-1 to HIV-ligands may be a coincidence. However, our initial interpretation of this information is that direct infection of arterial matrix fibroblasts is more likely to be the pathobiologic mechanism for arterial degeneration than the phenomenon of molecular mimicry. We hypothesize that the presentation of a ligand for HIV1 on the surface of the aortic adventitial fibrobast may provide an attachment site for the virus, initiating a pathway for HIV1 infection that may be similar to the process for the infection of susceptible T cells. This hypothesis could be approached by direct experimental methods. Because no substantial similarities of Mat-CAM-1 to potential epitopes in the HIV gp41 and gp120 proteins themselves were detected, the case for HIV1 triggering an autoimmune response against the aortic fibroblast is not compelling.

## REFERENCES

1. JOSHI, V.V., B. PAWEL, E. CONNOR, *et al.* 1987. Arteriopathy in children with acquired immune deficiency syndrome. Pediatr. Pathol. **7:** 261–275.
2. SINZOBAHAMVYA, N., K. KALANGU & W. HAMEL-KALINOWSKI. 1989. Arterial aneurysms associated with human immunodeficiency virus (HIV) infection. Acta Chir. Belg. **89:** 185–188.
3. MARKS, C. & S. KUSKOV. 1995. Pattern of arterial aneurysms in acquired immunodeficiency disease. World J. Surg. **19:** 127–132.
4. NAIR, R., A. ABDOOL-CARRIM, R. CHETTY & J. ROBBS. 1999. Arterial aneurysms in patients infected with human immunodeficiency virus: a distinct clinicopathology entity. J. Vasc. Surg. **29:** 600–607.
5. CHETTY, R., S. BATITANG & R. NAIR. 2000. Large artery vasculopathy in HIV-positive patients: another vasculitic enigma. Hum. Pathol. **31:** 374–379.

6. CHETTY, R. 2001. Vasculitides associated with HIV infection. J. Clin. Pathol. **54:** 275–278.
7. OZSVATH, K.J., S. XIA., H. HIROSE & M.D. TILSON. 1996. Two hypothetical proteins of human aortic adventitia, with Ig kappa, collagenous, and aromatic-rich motifs. Biochem. Biophys. Res. Commun. **225:** 500–504.
8. TILSON, M.D., *et al*. 2001 (Aug. 22). NCBI Gen Bank. Accession #AF186176.

# HLA–DQA Is Associated with Abdominal Aortic Aneurysms in the Belgian Population

GERARD TROMP,[a] TORU OGATA,[a] LUCIE GREGOIRE,[b]
KATRINA A.B. GODDARD,[c] MAGDALENA SKUNCA,[a]
WAYNE D. LANCASTER,[a,d] ANTONIO R. PARRADO,[c] QING LU,[c]
HIDENORI SHIBAMURA,[a] NATZI SAKALIHASAN,[e] RAYMOND LIMET,[e]
GERALD L. MACKEAN,[f] CLAUDETTE ARTHUR,[f] TAIJIRO SUEDA,[g]
AND HELENA KUIVANIEMI,[a,h]

[a]Center for Molecular Medicine and Genetics, Wayne State University School of Medicine, Detroit, MI, USA

[b]Department of Immunology and Microbiology, Wayne State University School of Medicine, Detroit, MI, USA

[c]Department of Epidemiology and Biostatistics, Case Western Reserve University, Cleveland, OH, USA

[d]Department of Obstetrics and Gynecology, Wayne State University School of Medicine, Detroit, MI, USA

[e]Department of Cardiovascular Surgery, University of Liège, Liège, Belgium

[f]Department of Surgery, Dalhousie University, Halifax, Canada

[g]Department of Surgery, Graduate School of Biomedical Science, Hiroshima University, Hiroshima, Japan

[h]Department of Surgery, Wayne State University School of Medicine, Detroit, MI, USA

ABSTRACT: Chronic inflammation and autoimmunity likely contribute to the pathogenesis of abdominal aortic aneurysms (AAAs). The aim of this study was to investigate the role of autoimmunity in the etiology of AAAs using a genetic association study approach with human leukocyte antigen (HLA) polymorphisms (HLA–DQA1, –DQB1, –DRB1 and –DRB3–5 alleles) in 387 AAA cases and 426 controls. We observed an association with the HLA–DQA1 locus among Belgian males, and found a significant difference in the HLA–DQA1*0102 allele frequencies between AAA cases and controls. In conclusion, this study showed potential evidence that the HLA–DQA1 locus harbors a genetic risk factor for AAAs suggesting that autoimmunity plays a role in the pathogenesis of AAAs.

Address for correspondence: Helena Kuivaniemi, M.D., Ph.D., Center for Molecular Medicine and Genetics, Wayne State University School of Medicine, 3317 Gordon H. Scott Hall of Basic Medical Sciences, 540 E. Canfield Ave., Detroit, MI 48201, USA. Voice: 313-577-8733; fax: 313-577-5218.
e-mail: kuivan@sanger.med.wayne.edu

Ann. N.Y. Acad. Sci. 1085: 392–395 (2006). © 2006 New York Academy of Sciences.
doi: 10.1196/annals.1383.045

KEYWORDS: autoimmunity; Chromosome; 6p21.31; genetic association study; riskallele

An aneurysm is a dilatation of a blood vessel and most are characterized by chronic expansion that ultimately results in rupture. The expansion process is accompanied by increased turnover and remodeling of the extracellular matrix. The processes characteristic of the pathological changes observed in abdominal aortic aneurysms (AAAs) are chronic inflammation, loss of vascular smooth muscle cells, and destructive remodeling of the extracellular matrix.[1] It has previously been suggested that immunity, specifically local immune responses and autoimmunity, is an important factor in the pathogenesis of AAA.[2,3] Observations of infiltrating monocytes, macrophages, plasma cells, and T lymphocytes including both CD4 and CD8 positive T cells, in the AAA walls, support this suggestion.[4]

The genes that define histocompatibility are important determinants of immune function. The major histocompatibility complex (MHC) is divided into three classes: HLA class I, class II, and class III. The locus is on chromosome 6p21.31 and is the most gene-dense and polymorphic region of the human genome identified so far.[5] Class I antigens are present on the surface of most types of cells in the human body, whereas class II antigens are expressed by a few types of antigen-presenting cells, namely B lymphocytes, macrophages, dendritic cells, thymic epithelial cells, and activated T lymphocytes;[6,7] consequently, class II locus polymorphisms have been associated with a number of immune and autoimmune disorders.[5,7]

There are five isotypes of the HLA class II molecules, all of which function as protein heterodimers with $\alpha$ and $\beta$ chains.[7] HLA–DQ and –DR proteins present foreign peptide antigens from bacteria, viruses, or autoimmune antigens to CD4$^+$ T cells. These antigens stimulate CD4$^+$ T-cell responses that activate B cells and macrophages. The structure of the peptide binding groove of the HLA–DQ or –DR dimers differs substantially depending on which DQA1, DQB1, and DRB1 alleles form the dimers.[8] The different alleles thereby increase or decrease the ability of HLA–DQ or –DR molecules to bind and properly present foreign antigens to the CD4$^+$ T cell.[7,9] The genetic variants may therefore have an important effect on the intensity of any specific immune response and can predispose individuals to particular types of autoimmune diseases.

At present, the events or factors that initiate the chronic inflammatory response leading to AAA have not been identified. Nevertheless, HLA loci, particularly the HLA–DQ and HLA–DR antigens, because of their role in the cellular inflammatory response and in autoimmunity, are functional candidate genes.

The aim of this study was to investigate the role of autoimmunity in the etiology of AAAs using a genetic association study approach with HLA polymorphisms. HLA–DQA1, –DQB1, –DRB1, and –DRB3–5 alleles were determined in 387 AAA cases (180 Belgian and 207 Canadian) and 426 controls (269 Belgian and 157 Canadian) by a polymerase chain reaction (PCR) and single-stranded oligonucleotide probe hybridization assay. Relevant regions of the HLA locus were amplified, immobilized on nylon membranes, and radiolabeled allele-specific oligonucleotides were hybridized to the immobilized DNA under standardized conditions. The membranes were washed and X-ray film was exposed to the radiolabel. The films were developed and scored. The genotype data were analyzed with the CLUMP[10] and Haplostats[11] programs. Empirical $P$ values were generated to ensure that the large numbers of alleles at the loci did not inflate significance due to low cell counts.

We observed an association with the HLA–DQA1 locus among Belgian males (empirical $P = 0.027$, asymptotic $P = 0.071$). Specifically, there was a significant difference in the HLA–DQA1*0102 allele frequencies between AAA cases (67/322 alleles, 20.8%) and controls (44/356 alleles, 12.4%) in Belgian males (empirical $P = 0.019$, asymptotic $P = 0.003$). In haplotype analyses, marginally significant association was found between AAA and haplotype HLA–DQA1–DRB1 ($P = 0.049$ with global score statistics and $P = 0.002$ with haplotype-specific score statistics). This study showed potential evidence that the HLA–DQA1 locus harbors a genetic risk factor for AAAs providing genetic support for the suggestion that autoimmunity plays a role in the pathogenesis of AAAs.

## ACKNOWLEDGMENTS

This work was supported in part by grants from the National Heart, Lung, and Blood Institute (HL064310 to H.K.), the National Human Genome Research Institute (HG01577 to K.G.), and the National Center for Research Resources (RR03655).

## REFERENCES

1. STEINMETZ, E.F., C. BUCKLEY & R.W. THOMPSON. 2003. Prospects for the medical management of abdominal aortic aneurysms. Vasc. Endovasc. Surg. **37:** 151–163.
2. HIROSE, H. & M.D. TILSON. 2001. Abdominal aortic aneurysm as an autoimmune disease. Ann. N.Y. Acad. Sci. **947:** 416–418.
3. BROPHY, C.M., J.M. REILLY, G.J. SMITH & M.D. TILSON. 1991. The role of inflammation in nonspecific abdominal aortic aneurysm disease. Ann. Vasc. Surg. **5:** 229–233.
4. KOCH, A.E., G.K. HAINES, R.J. RIZZO, et al. 1990. Human abdominal aortic aneurysms. Immunophenotypic analysis suggesting an immune-mediated response. Am. J. Pathol. **137:** 1199–1213.

5. PRICE, P., C. WITT, R. ALLCOCK, *et al.* 1999. The genetic basis for the association of the 8.1 ancestral haplotype (A1, B8, DR3) with multiple immunopathological diseases. Immunol. Rev. **167:** 257–274.
6. SIMMONDS, M.J., J.M. HOWSON, J.M. HEWARD, *et al.* 2005. Regression mapping of association between the human leukocyte antigen region and Graves disease. Am. J. Hum. Genet. **76:** 157–163.
7. MARSH, S.G.E., P. PARHAM & L.D. BARBER. 2000. *In* The HLA Facts Book. Academic Press, San Diego.
8. TROWSDALE, J. & S.H. POWIS. 1992. The MHC: relationship between linkage and function. Curr. Opin. Genet. Dev. **2:** 492–497.
9. ALTMANN, D.M. 1992. HLA–DQ associations with autoimmune disease. Autoimmunity **14:** 79–83.
10. SHAM, P.C. & D. CURTIS. 1995. Monte Carlo tests for associations between disease and alleles at highly polymorphic loci. Ann. Hum. Genet. **59**(Pt 1): 97–105.
11. SCHAID, D.J., C.M. ROWLAND, D.E. TINES, *et al.* 2002. Score tests for association between traits and haplotypes when linkage phase is ambiguous. Am. J. Hum. Genet. **70:** 425–434.

# Toward a Model for Local Drug Delivery in Abdominal Aortic Aneurysms

JONATHAN P. VANDE GEEST,[a,b,c] BRUCE R. SIMON,[a,c]
AND ARIANE MORTAZAVI[a]

[a]Department of Aerospace and Mechanical Engineering, The University of
Arizona, Tucson, Arizona, USA

[b]Bio5 Institute for Collaborative Research, The University of Arizona, Tucson,
Arizona, USA

[c]Biomedical Engineering Graduate Interdisciplinary Program, The University
of Arizona, Tucson, Arizona, USA

ABSTRACT: The formation of an abdominal aortic aneurysm (AAA) may
eventually result in rupture, an event associated with a 50% mortality
rate. This work represents a first step toward improving current stress
estimation techniques and local transport simulations in AAA. Toward
this aim, a computational parametric study was performed on an axisymmetric cylindrical FEM of a 5 cm AAA with a 1.5 cm thick intraluminal
thrombus (ILT). Both the AAA wall and ILT were modeled as porohyperelastic PHE materials using estimated values of AAA wall and ILT
permeability. While no values for AAA wall permeability could be found
in the literature, the value of ILT permeability was taken from a previous investigation by Adolph et al.[7] Peak stresses, fluid velocities, and
local pore pressure values within the ILT and wall were recorded and
analyzed as a function of the cardiac cycle. While peak wall stress values for the PHE models did not largely differ from corresponding solid
finite element simulations (186.2 N/cm$^2$ vs. 186.5 N/cm$^2$), the stress in
the abluminal region of the ILT increased by 17.4% (7.7 N/cm$^2$ vs. 6.5
N/cm$^2$). Pore pressure values were relatively constant through the ILT
while there were significant pore pressure gradients present in the AAA
wall. The magnitude of fluid velocities varied in magnitude and direction
throughout the cardiac cycle with large fluctuations occurring on the luminal surface. The combination of the patient-specific PHE AAA FEMs
with mass transport simulations will result in spatially and time-varying
concentration distributions within AAA, which may benefit future pharmaceutical treatments of AAA.

KEYWORDS: aneurysm; stress; porohyperelasticity; local drug delivery

Address for correspondence: Jonathan P. Vande Geest, Ph.D., Department of Aerospace and
Mechanical Engineering, The University of Arizona, 1130 N Mountain Ave, P.O. Box 210119, Tucson,
Arizona, 85721. Voice: 520-621-2514; fax: 520-621-8191.
e-mail: vandegeestjp@ame.arizona.edu

Ann. N.Y. Acad. Sci. 1085: 396–399 (2006). © 2006 New York Academy of Sciences.
doi: 10.1196/annals.1383.047

# INTRODUCTION

The formation of an abdominal aortic aneurysm (AAA) may eventually result in rupture, an event associated with a 50% mortality rate. Knowledge of the mechanical environment within the AAA may help to better diagnose AAAs that require immediate operative treatment.[1] While recent reports have suggested that pharmacological treatments may inhibit aneurysm growth,[2,3] it remains unclear whether the mass transport of drugs locally to the aneurysm wall in humans is possible. This work represents a first step toward improving current stress estimation techniques and local transport simulations in AAA.

Current methods for assessing the stresses within the AAA and the intraluminal thrombus (ILT) use finite element models that assume the ILT and AAA to be a solid continuum. Porohyperelastic (PHE) finite element modeling allows the simulation of multiphasic (solid and fluid) materials in the computational modeling of soft tissues.[4–6] Application of this type of modeling to the AAA wall and ILT allows several primary advantages: (1) more realistic representation of the biomechanical environment within the ILT and AAA wall, (2) investigation of local fluid velocities in the ILT and AAA wall, and (3) the coupling of PHE modeling with mass transport simulations to emulate the local drug delivery of pharmacological agents in the ILT and AAA.

The purpose of this work was to investigate the use of PHE FEMs in determining local stress, pore pressure, and fluid velocity within the AAA wall and ILT. Such results are required to quantify the local delivery (concentrations) of drugs within AAA tissues.

# MATERIALS AND METHODS

Toward this aim, a computational parametric study was performed on an axisymmetric cylindrical FEM of a 5 cm AAA with a 1.5 cm thick ILT. Both the AAA wall and ILT were modeled as PHE materials using estimated values of AAA wall and ILT permeability. While no values for AAA wall permeability could be found in the literature, the value of ILT permeability was taken from a previous investigation by Adolph *et al.*[7] Peak stresses, fluid velocities, and local pore pressure values within the ILT and wall were recorded and analyzed as a function of the cardiac cycle.

# RESULTS

Typical results displaying the pore pressure and fluid velocities within the AAA wall and ILT are shown in FIGURE 1. While peak wall stress values for the PHE models did not largely differ from corresponding solid finite element simulations (186.2 N/cm$^2$ vs. 186.5 N/cm$^2$), the stress in the abluminal region of the ILT increased by 17.4% (7.7 N/cm$^2$ vs. 6.5 N/cm$^2$). Pore pressure values

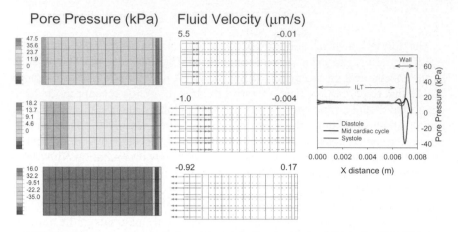

**FIGURE 1.** Pore pressure (*left, right*) and fluid velocity (*middle*) in the PHE FEM.

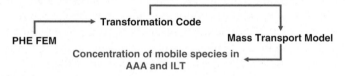

**FIGURE 2.** Strategy for coupling current PHE FEM data with mass transport for modeling local distributions of mobile species.

were relatively constant through the ILT, while there were significant pore pressure gradients present in the AAA wall (Fig. 1). The magnitude of fluid velocities varied in magnitude and direction throughout the cardiac cycle with large fluctuations occurring on the luminal surface.

## DISCUSSION

Ongoing research within our laboratory will include PHE simulations with more realistic AAA geometries, the experimental determination of PHE and mass transport properties for AAA and ILT, and the coupling of mass transport with PHE (Fig. 2). The combination of the patient-specific PHE AAA FEMs with mass transport simulations will result in spatially and time-varying concentration distributions within AAA, which may benefit future pharmaceutical treatments of AAA.

## REFERENCES

1. VORP, D.A. & J.P. VANDE GEEST. 2005. Biomechanical determinants of abdominal aortic aneurysm rupture. Arterioscler Thromb. Vasc. Biol. **25:** 1558–1566.

2. BARTOLI, M.A. *et al.* 2006. Localized administration of doxycycline suppresses aortic dilatation in an experimental mouse model of abdominal aortic aneurysm. Ann. Vasc. Surg. **20(2):** 228–236.
3. BAXTER, B.T. 2001. Regarding use of doxycycline to decrease the growth rate of abdominal aortic aneurysms: a randomized, double-blind, placebo-controlled pilot study. J. Vasc. Surg. **34:** 757–758.
4. SIMON, B.R. *et al.* 1998. Porohyperelastic finite element analysis of large arteries using ABAQUS. J. Biomech. Eng. **120:** 296–298.
5. SIMON, B.R. *et al.* 1998. Identification and determination of material properties for porohyperelastic analysis of large arteries. J. Biomech. Eng. **120:** 188–194.
6. SIMON, B.R. *et al.* 1996. A poroelastic finite element formulation including transport and swelling in soft tissue structures. J. Biomech. Eng. **118:** 1–9.
7. ADOLPH, R. *et al.* 1997. Cellular content and permeability of intraluminal thrombus in abdominal aortic aneurysm. J. Vasc. Surg. **25:** 916–926.

# Gender-Related Differences in the Tensile Strength of Abdominal Aortic Aneurysm

JONATHAN P. VANDE GEEST,[a,b] ELLEN D. DILLAVOU,[e]
ELENA S. DI MARTINO,[d] MATT OBERDIER,[e,f] AJAY BOHRA,[e]
MICHEL S. MAKAROUN,[e] AND DAVID A. VORP[e,f]

[a]Department of Aerospace and Mechanical Engineering, The University of Arizona, Tucson, Arizona, USA

[b]Bio5 Institute for Collaborative Research, The University of Arizona, Tucson, Arizona, USA

[c]Biomedical Engineering Graduate Interdisciplinary Program, The University of Arizona, Tucson, Arizona, USA

[d]Institute for Complex Engineered Systems, Carnegie Melon University, Pittsburgh, Pennslyvania, USA

[e]Division of Vascular Surgery, Department of Surgery, University of Pittsburgh Medical Center, Pittsburgh, Pennsylvania, USA

[f]Department of Bioengineering, University of Pittsburgh, Pittsburgh, Pennsylvania, USA

ABSTRACT: A recent study investigated the association of gender with the growth rate of AAAs and found a significant increase in the growth rate of AAAs in women than in men. On the basis of these observations, we hypothesize that there are gender-associated differences in AAA wall integrity and mechanical strength. The purpose of this study was to explore this hypothesis by comparing the tensile strength of freshly resected AAA tissue specimens between women and men. Seventy-six rectangular specimens (20 mm long × 5 mm wide) from 34 patients (24 male, 10 female) were excised from the anterior wall of patients undergoing open repair of their abdominal aortic aneurysm and tested in a uniaxial tensile tester. Ultimate tensile strength (UTS) was taken as the peak stress obtained before specimen failure. While there were no statistical differences in strength between specimens taken from male and female patients, there was a trend toward a decrease in strength in females as compared to males ($87.6 \pm 6.7$ N/cm$^2$ vs. $67.6 \pm 8.1$ N/cm$^2$, p = 0.09). To the authors knowledge this work represents the first report of differences in biomechanical properties as a function of gender. The nearly

Address for correspondence: Jonathan P. Vande Geest, Ph.D., Department of Aerospace and Mechanical Engineering, The University of Arizona, 1130 N Mountain Ave, PO Box 210119, Tucson, AZ 85721. Voice: 520-621-2514; fax: 520-621-8191.
e-mail: vandegeestjp@ame.arizona.edu

Ann. N.Y. Acad. Sci. 1085: 400–402 (2006). © 2006 New York Academy of Sciences.
doi: 10.1196/annals.1383.048

**significant decrease in UTS in women versus men reported here may be important in assessing the risk of rupture in AAA. Further testing is warranted to confirm the current trends.**

KEYWORDS: **aneurysm; stress; strength, rupture potential**

## INTRODUCTION

Although the frequency of abdominal aortic aneurysm (AAA) among men is 2–4 times higher than among women in the same age group, epidemiologic studies have shown a higher risk of rupture of AAA in women.[1,2] A recent study investigated the association of gender with the growth rate of AAAs and found a significant increase in the growth rate of AAAs in women compared to men.[3] These differences may be a result of biological differences, for example, the estrogen-mediated reduction in macrophage matrix metalloproteinases (MMP)-9 production found in women.[4] On the basis of these observations, we hypothesize that there are gender-associated differences in AAA wall integrity and mechanical strength. The purpose of this study was to explore this hypothesis by comparing the tensile strength of freshly resected AAA tissue specimens between women and men.

## METHODS

Seventy-six rectangular specimens (~20 mm long × 5 mm wide) from 34 patients (24 male, 10 female) were excised from the anterior wall of patients undergoing surgical repair of their abdominal aortic aneurysm. The specimens were placed in a previously validated uniaxial tensile testing system and continuously wetted with saline solution at $37°C$[5–7] (FIG. 1). The force and deformation applied to each specimen were measured continuously as the specimen was stretched to failure. These data were converted to stress versus strain as described in FIGURE 1 and elsewhere.[5] The ultimate tensile strength (UTS) was taken as the peak stress obtained before specimen failure (FIG. 2). Differences in the average strength per patient between groups were investigated using a Student's *t*-test with $P < 0.05$ determining significance.

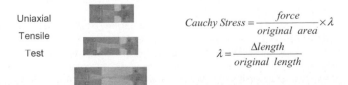

Uniaxial Tensile Test

$$Cauchy\ Stress = \frac{force}{original\ area} \times \lambda$$

$$\lambda = \frac{\Delta length}{original\ length}$$

**FIGURE 1.** Uniaxial tensile test (*left*) and corresponding calculation of Cauchy stress (*right*).

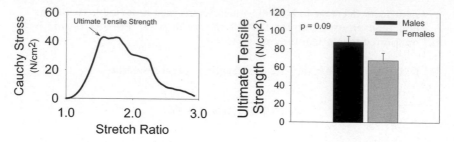

**FIGURE 2.** Representative stress-strain curve (*left*) and differences in UTS with gender (*right*).

## RESULTS

While there were no statistical differences in strength between specimens taken from male and female patients, there was a trend toward a decrease in strength in females as compared to males ($87.6 \pm 6.7$ N/cm$^2$ vs. $67.6 \pm 8.1$ N/cm$^2$, $P = 0.09$) (FIG. 2).

## DISCUSSION

To the authors' knowledge this work represents the first report of differences in biomechanical properties as a function of gender. While the differences in strength between males and females reported here were not significant at the $P = 0.05$ level, the trend of lower strength values for females suggests gender may be important in the assessment of the risk of rupture of an AAA. The decrease in wall strength in females reported here should be confirmed with additional *ex vivo* uniaxial tensile tests.

## REFERENCES

1. BENGTSSON, H., B. SONESSON & D. BERGQVIST. 1996. Ann. N.Y. Acad. Sci. **800:** 1–24.
2. LILLIENFELD, D.E., P.D. GUNDERSON, J.M. SPRAFKA & C. VARGAS. 1987. Ateriosclerosis **7:** 637–643.
3. SOLBERG, S., K. SINGH, T. WILSGAARD & B.K. JACOBSEN. 2005. The Tromso Study. Eur. J. Vasc. Endovasc. Surg. **29:** 145–149.
4. AILAWADI, G., J.L. ELIASON, K.J. ROELOFS, *et al*. 2004. Arterioscler. Thromb. Vasc. Biol. **24:** 2116–2122.
5. RAGHAVAN, M.L., M.W. WEBSTER & D.A. VORP. 1996. Ann. Biomed. Eng. **24:** 573–582.
6. WANG, D.H., M. MAKAROUN, M.W. WEBSTER & D.A. VORP. 2001. J. Biomech. Eng. **123:** 536–539.
7. RAGHAVAN, M.L. & D.A. VORP. 2000. J. Biomech. **33:** 475–482.

# Identification of c-Jun N-Terminal Kinase as a Therapeutic Target for Abdominal Aortic Aneurysm

KOICHI YOSHIMURA,[a] HIROKI AOKI,[a] YASUHIRO IKEDA,[a]
AKIRA FURUTANI,[b] KIMIKAZU HAMANO,[b]
AND MASUNORI MATSUZAKI[a,c]

[a]Department of Molecular Cardiovascular Biology

[b]Department of Surgery and Clinical Science

[c]Department of Cardiovascular Medicine, Yamaguchi University School
of Medicine, 1-1-1 Minami Kogushi, Ube, Yamaguchi 755-8505, Japan

ABSTRACT: Despite the advances in molecular cell biology, identification
of a therapeutic target in a given disease still poses a significant challenge.
Here we report a strategy for identification of the therapeutic target
in abdominal aortic aneurysm (AAA). We screened for various signaling molecules in human AAA samples and identified c-Jun N-terminal
kinase (JNK) as a prominently activated molecule. The JNK pathway-
oriented transcriptome analyses revealed that activation of JNK leads to
enhancement of the activity of matrix metalloproteinases and, concurrently, suppression of the extracellular matrix biosynthesis, suggesting
that JNK may represent a novel therapeutic target in AAA.

KEYWORDS: abdominal aortic aneurysm; AAA; c-Jun N-terminal kinase; JNK; matrix metalloproteinase; MMP; extracellular matrix; ECM

## INTRODUCTION

Abdominal aortic aneurysm (AAA) is a highly prevalent disease that is
characterized by chronic inflammation and degradation of extracellular matrix
(ECM) by matrix metalloproteinases (MMPs).[1] Recently, we identified c-Jun
N-terminal kinase (JNK, also known as stress-activated protein kinase) as a
proximal signaling molecule in the pathogenesis of AAA.[2]

Address for correspondence: Koichi Yoshimura, M.D., Ph.D., Department of Molecular Cardiovascular Biology, Yamaguchi University School of Medicine, 1-1-1 Minami Kogushi, Ube, Yamaguchi
755-8505, Japan. Voice: +81-836-22-2361; fax: +81-836-22-2362.
e-mail: yoshimko@yamaguchi-u.ac.jp

Ann. N.Y. Acad. Sci. 1085: 403–406 (2006). © 2006 New York Academy of Sciences.
doi: 10.1196/annals.1383.049

## ACTIVATION OF JNK IN HUMAN AAA WALLS

We analyzed various signaling proteins for their phosphorylated forms to identify signaling pathway that is involved in the pathogenesis of AAA. We observed a significant increase in JNK phosphorylation in human AAA walls compared with the level in the nonaneurysmal aorta (FIG. 1 A). Other mitogen-activated protein kinases did not show such an obvious activation in AAA. In addition, no significant change was found in the phosphorylation level of IκB-α, Akt, p70S6K, or p90RSK, although there was an elevation in the phosphorylation level of STAT3 in AAA walls (unpublished observation by KY). Active JNK levels showed a highly positive correlation with levels of MMP-9 expression in human AAA walls (FIG. 1 B). Most of the active JNK was localized in macrophages, which secrete proinflammatory cytokines and MMPs, but some active JNK was also present in vascular smooth muscle cells (VSMCs), which synthesize ECM and secrete MMPs. These results prompted us to further investigate the link between JNK activation and ECM degradation in AAA.

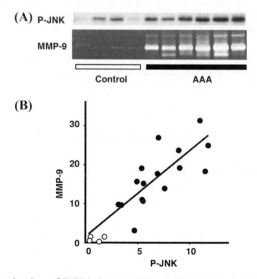

**FIGURE 1.** Activation of JNK in human AAA walls. **(A)** Protein expression of phosphorylated JNK (P-JNK) and MMP-9 in human control aorta and AAA, determined by Western blotting and gelatin zymography, respectively. **(B)** A linear correlation ($r = 0.76$) between the levels of P-JNK and MMP-9 is shown. Open and closed circles indicate control and AAA samples, respectively. (Modified from Yoshimura *et al.*[2])

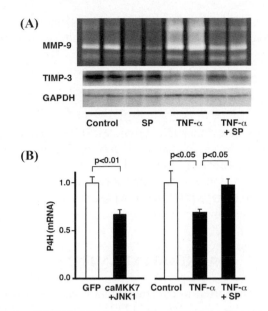

**FIGURE 2.** Role of JNK in ECM metabolism. **(A)** The effect of a specific JNK inhibitor, SP600125 (SP), on MMP-9 was examined in human AAA *ex vivo* culture with or without stimulation by TNF-α. The level of secretion of MMP-9 was determined by gelatin zymography and the protein level of TIMP-3 was determined by Western blotting. Glyceraldehyde-3-phosphate dehydrogenase (GAPDH) was used as an internal control. **(B)** mRNA expression of P4H in rat VSMCs was determined by Northern blotting. JNK was either activated by overexpression of constitutively active Mitogen-activated protein kinase kinase 7 (MKK7) and JNK1, or inhibited by SP600125. Green fluorescent protein (GFP) was used as a negative control. (Modified from Yoshimura *et al.*[2]).

## ROLE OF JNK IN ECM METABOLISM

To obtain insight into the role of JNK in AAA, we screened for JNK-dependent genes in VSMCs. We adopted the gain-of-function and the loss-of-function strategy for the JNK pathway in the transcriptional profiling in rat VSMCs to identify genes that are regulated by JNK. Interestingly, a number of JNK-induced genes were those for positive regulators of MMP-9. In fact, SP600125, a specific JNK inhibitor,[3] significantly suppressed the secretion of MMP-9 and MMP-2 and prevented collagen degradation in human AAA walls in *ex vivo* culture (FIG. 2 A). In addition, SP600125 restored the level of expression of the tissue inhibitor of metalloproteinase (TIMP)-3, which had been strongly suppressed by TNF-α (FIG. 2 A).

Furthermore, microarray data showed that JNK downregulates the gene expression of crucial ECM biosynthetic enzymes including lysyl hydroxylase (procollagen-lysine, 2-oxoglutarate 5-dioxygenase; PLOD; essential for the stability of collagen fibers), lysyl oxidase (LOX; responsible for the cross-linking and deposition of collagen and elastin fibers), and prolyl 4-hydroxylase (P4H; the rate-limiting enzyme for collagen biosynthesis), which was confirmed by the gene-specific analysis (FIG. 2 B).

## CONCLUSION

These findings suggest that JNK promotes ECM degradation and concurrently suppresses ECM biosynthesis. In fact, we demonstrated that selective JNK inhibition *in vivo* not only prevented the development of aortic aneurysm but also caused regression of established aortic aneurysm in two mouse models.[2,4] JNK-targeted therapy may thus provide a nonsurgical therapeutic option for AAA.

## ACKNOWLEDGMENTS

This work was supported in part by Grants-in-aid for Scientific Research (KAKENHI 12770651, 14657284, and 17591337 to KY; 12670673, 12204081, 14370229, and 16390365 to HA; and 16209026 to MM) from MEXT Japan and a Grant from the Sankyo Company to the Department of Molecular Cardiovascular Biology, Yamaguchi University School of Medicine.

## REFERENCES

1. THOMPSON, R.W., P.J. GERAGHTY & J.K. LEE. 2002. Abdominal aortic aneurysms: basic mechanisms and clinical implications. Curr. Probl. Surg. **39:** 110–230.
2. YOSHIMURA, K. *et al*. 2005. Regression of abdominal aortic aneurysm by inhibition of c-Jun N-terminal kinase. Nat. Med. **11:** 1330–1338.
3. BENNETT, B.L. *et al*. 2001. SP600125, an anthrapyrazolone inhibitor of Jun N-terminal kinase. Proc. Natl. Acad. Sci. USA **98:** 13681–13686.
4. YOSHIMURA, K. *et al*. Regression of abdominal aortic aneurysm by inhibition of c-Jun N-terminal kinase in mice. Ann. N. Y. Acad. Sci. This volume.

# Concluding Remarks

HELENA KUIVANIEMI[a,b] AND GILBERT R. UPCHURCH, JR.[c]

[a] Center for Molecular Medicine and Genetics, [b] Department of Surgery, Wayne State University School of Medicine, Detroit, Michigan, USA

[c] Department of Surgery, University of Michigan, Ann Arbor, Michigan, USA

We have spent an exciting two and a half days enjoying presentations and posters, and were filled with excitement from the new discoveries about the genetics, pathophysiology, and molecular biology of abdominal aortic aneurysms (AAAs). Ten years had passed since the previous AAA meeting organized by M. David Tilson, and the consensus of the participants of the current meeting is that we cannot wait another 10 years but should organize another AAA meeting within 2 to 3 years.

The progress made during the past 10 years has been phenomenal! Multidisciplinary approaches are now being used to address important research questions. This type of approach has paid off. For example, the evidence linking genetic risk factors with AAA development has become increasingly strong with two genetic loci identified. Also, family history for AAA is considered an important risk factor and plays a role even when estimating AAA rupture risks using biomechanical approaches with three-dimensional computer modeling. A large number of studies also shed light on the importance of the inflammatory component of AAA as well as the key role that extracellular matrix-degrading enzymes play in AAA pathogenesis. A great deal of enthusiasm about potential treatment modalities for small AAAs was expressed, and it is expected that clinical trials will occur in the not-too-distant future.

For the field to keep progressing and to foster the many promising leads and advances, significant resources are needed. The National Heart, Lung, and Blood Institute of the National Institutes of Health will continue to support AAA research and seek new initiatives to encourage multidisciplinary approaches. We are grateful for the leadership of Momtaz Wassef in this regard.

Addresses for correspondence: Helena Kuivaniemi, Wayne State University School of Medicine, 3317 Gordon H. Scott Hall of Basic Medical Sciences, 540 East Canfield Avenue, Detroit, MI 48201. Voice: 313-577-8733; fax: 313-577-5218.
  e-mail: kuivan@sanger.med.wayne.edu

Gilbert R. Upchurch, Jr., Department of Surgery, University of Michigan, 1500 East Medical Center Drive, Taubman Center 2210N, Ann Arbor, MI 48109-0329. Voice: 734-936-5790; fax: 734-647-9867
  e-mail: riversu@umich.edu

Ann. N.Y. Acad. Sci. 1085: 407–408 (2006). © 2006 New York Academy of Sciences.
doi: 10.1196/annals.1383.051

The meeting would not have been possible without the dedicated work of M. David Tilson. He has been a passionate advocate for AAA research for many decades. Many of us consider him a true pioneer responsible for bringing AAA research to the level it is today. His group made many of the initial discoveries on which current AAA research is now based. He was, for example, the first to report on a large collection of multiplex families with AAA. His laboratory also suggested that extracellular matrix-degrading enzymes play an important role in AAA. He worked tirelessly to get the meeting program together in a truly interdisciplinary fashion while covering a comprehensive list of topics and inviting many experts in the field. We feel truly honored for having had the opportunity to work closely with him on the details of the meeting. Dr. Tilson is also an excellent musician, and the participants got a taste of his musical skill during one of the poster sessions when he sat down to play the keyboard wearing his cowboy hat and boots.

"The important thing is not to stop questioning. Curiosity has its own reason for existing," said Albert Einstein, the most famous AAA patient. We have many important unanswered questions about the genetics, pathophysiology, and molecular biology of AAA. Addressing these questions will require more than just knowledge. It will require innovative approaches and greater investment of resources to solve the mysteries of AAA, the silent killer.

# Index of Contributors